Abattoir Practices, By-products and Wool Technology

AF640514

nipa books for everyone PAPERBACKS

NIPA® GENX ELECTRONIC RESOURCES & SOLUTIONS P. LTD.

New Delhi-110 034

About the Authors

Dr. V.P. Singh has been a meritorious student throughout his studentship. He did his graduation in veterinary science and animal husbandry from G.B. Pant University of Agriculture and Technology, Pantnagar and Master's degree in Livestock Products Technology from Indian Veterinary Research Institute, Izatnagar. He obtained his Doctoral Degree in Livestock Products Technology from U.P. Pt. Deen Dayal Upadhyay Pashu Chikitsa Vigyan Vishwa Vidyalaya Evam Go Anusandhan Sansthan, Mathura, U.P. He is currently working in the capacity of Assistant Professor in Department of Livestock Products Technology at U.P. Pt. Deen Dayal Upadhyay Pashu Chikitsa Vigyan Vishwa Vidyalaya Evam Go Anusandhan Sansthan, Mathura, U.P. He is engaged in teaching of U.G. classes of veterinary science and animal husbandry as well as P.G. and Ph. D of Livestock Products Technology. He started his career as Veterinary officer in State Veterinary Services of U.P. Government and served for about ten years. He is having more than fifty research and fifty five technical/ review articles to his credit in different reputed National and International Journals. He is also an author of two books titled "Principles of Meat Technology" and "Dairy Technology" and compiled five teaching manuals of Livestock Products Technology. He is an examiner and paper setter of different institutions of India. He is also the member of Editorial Board of the Journal "International Journal of Agro Veterinary and Medical Sciences" and "Meat Science International". He is also serving as member in scientific committee of International Journal of Livestock Research and reviewer of the several National and International Journals.

Dr. Neelam Sachan has had colourful academic record. She did her graduation in veterinary science and animal husbandry from G.B. Pant University of Agriculture and Technology, Pantnagar and Master's degree in Veterinary Public Health from Indian Veterinary Research Institute, Izatnagar. She has doctorate degree from M.J.P. Rohilkhand University, Bareilly. She has more than twelve years experience as Veterinary Officer in U.P. Government and about five years as Assistant Professor in the Department of Veterinary Public Health at U.P. Pt. Deen Dayal Upadhyay Pashu Chikitsa Vigyan Vishwa Vidyalaya Evam Go Anusandhan Sansthan, Mathura, U.P. As Veterinary officer she served for State Veterinary Services of U.P. government and held different posts including divisional laboratory. She is recipient of Junior Research fellowship in her Master's Degree programme. She is having more than fifty research and technical articles to her credit in different reputed National and International Journals.

Abattoir Practices, By-products and Wool Technology

Authors

V.P. Singh (M.V.Sc, Ph.D)

Assistant Professor
Department of Livestock Products Technology
U.P. Pt. Deen Dayal Upadhyay Veterinary University Evam
Go Anusandhan Sansthan, Mathura
Uttar Pradesh- 281001

Neelam Sachan (M.V.Sc, Ph.D)

Veterinary Officer
Department of Animal Husbandry
U.P. Government

nipa books for everyone
PAPERBACKS

NIPA® GENX ELECTRONIC RESOURCES & SOLUTIONS P. LTD.

New Delhi-110 034

nipa books for everyone
PAPERBACKS

NIPA® GENX ELECTRONIC RESOURCES & SOLUTIONS P. LTD.

101,103, Vikas Surya Plaza, CU Block
L.S.C. Market, Pitam Pura, New Delhi-110 034
Ph : +91 11 27341616, 27341717, 27341718
E-mail: newindiapublishingagency@gmail.com
www: www.nipabooks.com

For customer assistance, please contact
Phone: + 91-11-27 34 17 17
Fax: + 91-11- 27 34 16 16
E-Mail: feedbacks@nipabooks.com

ISBN 978-81-96053-64-2

Composed & Designed by NIPA

Preface

Livestock is an important source of income for farmers and rural poor people. This sector thus contributes to poverty alleviation. The livestock sector of India is expanding as well as adapting to emerging socio-economic, environmental and technological forces. India is possessing vast livestock population including 200 million cattle, 106 million buffaloes, 71.5 million sheep, 140.5 million goats, 11.3 million pigs. As per the report of Central Statistical Organization, the Indian livestock sector is contributing approximately 4.07 percent GDP and over 27 percent to the agricultural GDP. Therefore, the importance of livestock in Indian economy is enormous and cannot be underestimated. The global demand of livestock products is expanding very fast and it is an opportunity for India to cater the demand of world food and earn foreign revenues. Indian wool sector is also contributing great to livestock sector but very few trend persons are available in India.

India is earning nearly two billion dollars through the export of meat and provides lucrative outlet for rural livestock producers. Industry is also providing employment to over fifty thousand people in India. Thus major concern in India is in meat production for export purposes and domestic meat production units are facing great crises. The by-products and waste generated in this sector is highly neglected which is posing the environmental threads to human health. Though some organized sector is taking lead to produce quality meat, utilizes most of the by-products generated in abattoirs. The shearing, wool processing and testing is an expert operation but trained persons in the sector are not sufficient to handle the great challenges of natural fibre with great inherent variability.

In view of requirement of technical expertise in abattoir, by-products utilization and wool technology authors tried to compile the relevant information on these aspects. The fundamentals of abattoir establishments, slaughter procedures for quality meat production, scientific evaluation of food animals and carcasses are thus discussed in most effective manners. The sustainability of meat industry and meat food sector is basically dependant on abattoir by-products utilization. So different types of by-products generated in abattoir i.e. blood, hide and skin, intestines, bones, glandular by-products etc. are taken up in more understandable way. The waste generated and sanitary requirement of abattoir is also discussed in more realistic approach. All aspects of wool technology starting from shearing, sampling, wool structure, physico-chemical properties, processing and testing are elaborated in best possible efforts.

Authors are very confident that the book titled 'Abattoir Practices, By-products and Wool Technology' will be of great value to serve the source of knowledge and information on these aspects for the persons engaged in meat and wool profession, business, planning and research. The critical comments and suggestions are always welcome.

V.P. Singh
Neelam Sachan

Contents

Chapter 1

Layout and Management of Abattoirs

Animal protein has a great importance in human health by providing essential amino acids. It is supplied by the milk, meat, fish, eggs etc. Specifically meat has a prime position in the human's diet particularly for those who are non- vegetarians. As per Indian Council of Medical Research (ICMR) recommendations a normal human being requires 60 gram protein in a day with the net protein utilization (NPU) of 65. In ideal cases 30 to 50 percent of daily protein intake should be from animal sources to get optimal range of amino acids. In present scenario human beings all over the globe are getting 29 gram of protein while developing countries have 15 g per day availability and developed nations are getting 60 grams protein per day per head. However, in India availability of protein is only 10 grams/day/head.

India is having vast livestock resources and variety of food animals. However, livestock is not specifically meant for meat purpose and most of the meat is produced from the spent animals (who passed their productive life in primary field). The production of meat is traditionally based on the ritual methods and modern plants that came up in the country are mainly producing 'Halal' meat. It might be due to engagement of person of a particular religion in slaughter business and export to the gulf countries.

Table 1. Status of meat production in India

Livestock type	Number of live stock (million)	Global share (%)	World rank	Meat production (million tones)	Extraction rate (%)	Meat share in Indian total meat (%)	Growth rate (%)
Cattle	210	12.5	IInd	1.09	7.9	17.34	1.83
Buffalo	111	56.7	Ist	1.46	10.0	23.33	1.84
Goat	154	17	IInd	0.59	37.9	9.36	3.10
Sheep	74	7	IIIrd	0.29	47.9	4.61	3.87
Pigs	11.13	1.5	-	0.33	88.9	5.31	-4.74
Poultry	649	3.1	Vth	2.29	-	36.68	7.33
Others	-	1.4	-	0.21	-	3.37	-

Abattoir or slaughter house is a place specified by the authority to convert the food animals into edible products and useful by-products by slaughtering the animals in various manners. In abattoir, carcasses are handled and processed in most hygienic and efficient manner. The most commonly slaughtered animals in a slaughter house include cattle, buffalo, sheep, goat, pigs and poultry. Now a day deer, rabbit and other small animals are also utilized for meat production. The steps involves in planning of an abattoir includes daily kill of animals, species of animals to be slaughtered, disposal of slaughterhouse waste and processing of edible and inedible by-products etc.

Prime considerations for abattoir

1. Religious considerations must be kept in mind during planning an abattoir.
2. There should be separate slaughter house for pigs and horses. The slaughter house of pigs should be separate from cattle/buffalo and sheep/goat. Sheep and goat slaughter house may be together but clear cut separation is required.
3. Depending on capital and land availability there should be separate floors for clean and dirty operations.
4. There should also be the facility of handling of edible and inedible by-products separately.
5. In site selection for abattoir, rural or nominated industrial site is generally preferred and urban site is always avoided.

6. The actual site of slaughter house must be connected with the road and rail transport.
7. The site must be in vicinity of the animal market to ensure the continuous supply of animals.
8. There should be three phase electric supply and sufficient availability of potable water in minimal charges.
9. Selected land for abattoir must be good for foundation and drainage.
10. Site for abattoir must be away from other industries producing smoke, odour, dust, ash, pollutants etc.
11. The site of abattoir must be dispute free, in particular religious disputes.
12. The abattoir must be away from human dwellings and airport.
13. The land should be sufficient enough for various slaughter operations, drainage, waste treatment and also for future expansion.
14. The site for abattoir must be authorized by the authority specified in slaughter acts.
15. Abattoir must have all the basic facilities required for slaughter operations.
16. The facilities for handling the animals as per livestock unit must be there. One livestock unit is equal to one adult bovine or two pigs or three calves or five sheep.
17. There should be ample availability of skilled labourers in the vicinity of the slaughter house.
18. There should be the sewage line near the abattoir.
19. For domestic consumption slaughter house should be near by the meat market because in India consumers like to eat the fresh meat.
20. The entrance of animals should be separate from the final meat produced.

Classification of abattoir

- Abattoir
  - On the basis of unit killings
    - Small abattoir — Unit killing <100; Area in acres 1-2
    - Medium abattoir — 100-200; 2-4
    - Large abattoir — >200; 4-6
  - On the basis of managemental practices
    - Service abattoirs
      - Booth system abattoir
      - Line system abattoir
    - Commercial abattoirs
      - Modern abattoirs
      - Semi modern abattoirs

Abattoir may be classified on the basis of the utility of slaughter house and management practices carried out in the slaughter house to produce the meat for domestic as well as export purposes. For domestic consumption meat is mainly produced by the *booth system* abattoirs in which animal are slaughtered on the floor provided by the municipal authorities. The municipal officers are charging fees from butchers for slaughter house maintenance and waste material is also sold to the market by these authorities. The ante-mortem and post mortem of the animals and carcasses are carried out by the government veterinarians. It has very limited facilities like knife; axe etc. and carcasses is hoist for lifting the carcasses. Skinning cradles for flaying are used with cattle, and they help to keep the carcasses away from floor contact. It is older system but adopted till date due to traditional practices. This is common system for cattle/ buffaloes and sheep/goat in traditional ways of slaughter. For pigs due to essentials of scalding some different management is required.

For commercial production of quality meat, an ideal abattoir operation uses the line-slaughter system. "*Line slaughter*" entails hoisting up the carcass at an early stage, preferably beginning with the bleeding. All subsequent slaughtering and dressing procedures are carried out with the carcass suspended on and moving along an overhead rail (or line). Line slaughter is suitable for bovines, small ruminants and pigs. Line slaughter procedures are adopted in the modern and semi modern slaughter house owned by the traders or taken up on lease from the municipal authorities. The ante-mortem and post mortem is carried out by the expert veterinarians appointed either by the traders or municipal corporations. It facilitates the quality meat production and easy as well as faster rate of killings of animals. However, high initial cost is the prime drawback of this system.

The third type of abattoir may be called as *semi modern or workable slaughter house*, generally used to slaughter the small ruminants like sheep/ goat and other animals. In this system of slaughter animals are killed on the floor and dressing is done in hanging position. The chances of contamination are more though washing of carcasses is carried out in hanging position. The initial cost involvement is comparatively low than commercial abattoirs.

Requirements for an abattoir

1. *Building construction*: the building should be compact with clear cut demarcation of clean and unclean areas are preferred. Double story building with top floor for clean operations and ground floor for unclean operations with impervious floor, tiled walls and adequate ventilation is suitable for abattoir. Building must be constructed in such a manner which can facilitate the easy cleaning and sanitation.

Floor and walls should be easy in cleaning and made up of non-toxic and non-absorbent material like concrete, ceramic, steel or polymer tiles. Floor of abattoir should be non-slippery and 50 mm slope is required for every 3 meter area. Floor of slaughter halls, lairage, work and chill rooms should be covered at all junctions and rounded at corners. Walls should be faced with a smooth, hard, impervious material upto a height of not less than 3m from the floor preferably reaching the ceiling.

Doors should be wide enough to allow passage of product without contact with doorway. A width of 4.5ft is usually adequate. Doors must be constructed of rust-resistant material and automatic closure is required.

2. *Equipments and instruments*: all the equipments and instruments used in an abattoir should be made up of non-toxic, non-corrosive material. Most preferably they should be made up of stainless steel or plastic and should be free from rust. The other equipments like overhead rails, working platforms, knocking pen etc. which are not coming in direct contact of meat should be galvanized steel. Commonly used equipments and instruments in abattoir are stunning gun, electric head tongs and mechanical stunners, sticking knives (15 cm sharpened on both side), skinning knives (15 cm curved), sharpening steel, oil and water sharpening stone, scabbard and belt for holding knives, meat saw, block and tackle or chain hoist,

dressing cradles (pritch, clocks or skinning rack), a strong beam, tripod or track (2.4 to 3.4 meter away from the floor), spreader (gambrel or metal pipe), buckets, working platform, scalding barrel or tank, system of boiling, bell scrapers, solid scraping table or platform, thermometer, balance, hog or hay hook, torch or flame for singeing etc. Some additional equipments are also required for specialized operations like knocking pen, bleeding hooks, blood catching trough, wash trough for sanitation of hands and tools, hand wash basin, sterilizers etc.

3. *Water requirement*: for continuous and abundant supply of water to various slaughter operations there should be main water supply with a pressure of at least 20 psi at all points. There should be separate supply lines for hot and cold water. Water supply in the slaughter houses must be of potable type. Alongwith the continuous water supply there must be the facility of water storage for at least one day's consumption. Recommended water requirement for different animals slaughter operations are as follows:

   For pigs - 454 litres/day/pig plus 25% extra water for cleaning

   For bovine - 272 litres/day/bovine plus 25% extra water for cleaning

   For sheep - 45 litres/day/sheep plus 25% extra water for cleaning

4. *Electricity requirement*: for smooth running of slaughter operations in abattoir electricity must be continuous, uninterrupted with three phases industrial power supply. There must be the facility of generators for emergency.

5. *Light requirement*: in each and every corner of abattoir there should be ample natural light. However, facility of artificial light is also essential throughout the meat plant. Artificial light provided to the abattoir must not distort colours. Recommended overall intensity of light at different places of abattoir is as follows:

   At all inspection points - not less than 540 lux(50 foot -candles)

   In work rooms - not less than 220 lux(20 foot -candles)

   In other places - not less than 110 lux(10 foot -candles)

6. *Ventilation*: proper ventilation in abattoir is also essential to prevent excessive heat, steam, condensation, accumulation of odour, dust etc. Opening ventilators and windows should be screened to prevent the entrance of insects, flies and other vermins.

7. *Drainage*: Drainage is an essential requirement in abattoirs. In wet areas drainage should be with ½ inch/foot (6.35cm/3.05m)gradient

and special care is required at the site of blood, intestine and stomach collection. The provision of floor drains fitting with sub drains and main drains is also necessary. One drain for each 400 sq. ft (37.2 sq.m) of floor area is required. Care must be taken that all the drains must be meshed and must be free from vermins and insects breeding point. So the maintenance and sanitation of drains is an essential step in proper sanitary maintenance in the plant.

8. *Insect and pest control facilities*: the entry and movement of birds, rats, mice and insects like flies and cockroaches must be totally prohibited. It is also necessary to prevent the entry of food-poisoning, spoilage organisms and to prevent the spread of zoonotic diseases through meat. So for pests and insects control, proper cleaning, sanitization, disinfection and use of ultraviolet light, electrocutors, mesh screens etc. are some of the preventive measures must be adopted in abattoir. The spray of insecticidal drugs must be restricted to the non-meat sectors of the abattoir.
9. *Hygienic requirement*: all the parts of the abattoir must be cleaned and washed at the end of each day operations. The immediate removal of dirty material is also enhances the sanitary status of abattoir. To maintain the good hygienic conditions in abattoir, all the walls, floors, platforms, gullies etc. should be cleaned for all materials and debris followed by washing with strong cleaning solution and disinfectants. Equipment used in slaughter house must also be cleaned first with soap and detergents followed by complete sanitizing with hot water maintained at 82^{0}C and then rinsing with approved chlorine or iodine solution. Finally equipments other than stainless steel should be coated with light mineral oil to prevent the rust.

Personnel hygiene is utmost important to produce the quality meat. It includes good clothing, use of coat and gowns, aprons, hairnet, gloves, gumboots etc. All the workers of abattoir must be sound in health and disease free. Sanitary condition of the workers is also important and bad habits like spouting, coughing, sneezing; scratching of body parts, placing fingers in and around the nose and mouth should be prohibited. Chewing of tobaccos, smoking and drinking of alcohols in abattoir should also be banned. Fingernails should be short and there should be proper washing of hands after daily routine works.

10. *Refrigeration facility*: the areas like meat cutting, handling of carcasses and processing other than slaughter unit should be maintained at 10-12^{0}C. The rooms holding carcasses should be maintained at 7^{0}C and offals at 3^{0}C. The storage room of meat till dispatch should have the temperature near -18 to -22^{0}C.

Abattoir components

To complete all the slaughter operations smoothly and for quality meat production there should be some separate provisions in the abattoir. They must have the basic requirements and facilities to carry out the work designated in these areas. These components must be in good maintenance and working conditions. The basic components require for slaughter of large and small animals may be summarized as:

1. *Entry and exit points*: entry and exit points in the abattoir should always be separate to maintain the hygienic status and facilitate the raw and finish product quality. Gates must be sufficiently wide so that truck or other vehicles get entry into abattoir easily. The check post is another requirement at this point. Gateman must be acquainted with the communication system and should be in proper uniform. There should also be booth for security arrangements and routine checkup. It must be well organized and good looking condition because it is a main point to provide the aesthetic image of the slaughter house.

2. *Unloading ramp*: loading and unloading procedures of slaughter operations are considered as most stressful events for both animals and handlers. So to facilitate easy and safe unloading of animals from vehicles like truck or railway wagons in slaughter premises, an elevated non-slippery concrete structure with the height of about 1.2 m with gentle slope known as unloading dock or ramp is required. Unloading ramp also facilitate the examination of animals by veterinarians for soundness and other abnormalities like fatigue, transit tetany etc.

3. *Lairage*: lairage is a lifeline of slaughter house because it provides the input to the slaughter operations. Lairage is a specified covered area to provide the rest to the animals before slaughter. The other parts in lairage include a covered space for ante-mortem examination and an isolation pan for suspect and sick animals. Lairage floor should be hard, impervious, non-slippery, having gradient slope towards drainage. Lairage roofs should preferably be made up of galvanized iron sheets, light roofing materials, aluminium sheets or hatch. The lairage construction should be in such a way that provides proper air and ventilation to the animals. Lairage space should be sufficient for 3 days supply of cattle/buffaloes and 2 day supply of sheep or pigs. There should be sufficient space in lairage to provide the rest to the animals. It should not be less than 2.8 sq.mt. per large animal and 1.6 sq.mt. per small animal. A pan of 7.6 x 6 m area

may be sufficient for 20-25 cattle/ buffalo and sheep/ goat pan should be 0.9 x0.9 m and height of the pan should also be of 0.9 m. However, pig pan is preferably constructed with stouter rails but care should be taken that the space in between two rails should be 15 cm to prevent the pig head putting between the rails. As a thumb rule 2.8, 0.6 and 0.5 m^2 space may be sufficient for cattle/buffalo, pigs and sheep/goat respectively. There should be sufficient daily maintenance labour for proper cleaning and sanitation of lairage.

The rest provided in the lairage is dependent on the condition of animals. Depending the condition of animal minimum 8 hrs and maximum 36 hrs is a time for providing rest to the animals. The most preferred rest time for normal animal is 12-24 hrs. For poultry it may be 6-12 hrs. If the rest beyond 36 hrs is provided then it may not be profitable due to high shrinkage and chances of cross contamination by several organisms (most common is salmonella infection). In lairage animals are generally withdrawn from feed atleast 12 hrs prior to slaughter but ample amount of water should be provided to the animals till slaughter. It is essential to facilitate the flushing of intestines and easy dressing of animals. It also reduces the cross contamination of carcasses through intestinal contents and makes the evisceration and flaying easier. This step also enhances the bleeding rate.

The *ante-mortem room* in lairage must have the basic facilities for thorough examination of animals prior to slaughter. It is performed on the day of animals enters in the lairage and if time span in lairage reaches beyond 24 hrs then again ante-mortem examination is required. If animals found in suspect or sick conditions then they may be shifted to *isolation pan* and can be slaughtered at the end of the day or can be kept under supervision of the veterinarian and can be slaughtered under his/her supervision. It may be attached with the detained meat room for proper disposal of the condemned parts.

4. *V-race area*: it is a tapering narrow race (V-shaped area) in between lairage and slaughter hall. The space length for V-race area should be at least 10 meters. The length of V-race area may be upto 36 meter depending on the overall throughput of the meat plant. It is an important area of abattoir to ensure even flow of animals to the slaughter. Identification and checking of slaughter sequence numbers is carried out at this place.

5. *Slaughter hall*: It is a main component of the abattoir and known as the heart of abattoir. It is so because all the slaughter operations like stunning, bleeding, dressing, washing and inspection are carried out at this section of the abattoir.

a. *Stunning area*: stunning area must have the facilities of stunning (mechanical, electrical or gaseous) of animals as per the species requirement. Stunning area may have the noiseless, durable and easy to operate stunning box/knocking pen. It facilitates the easy restraining of animals during stunning and revolving door or automatic slide door provides easy ejection of animals after stunning.

b. *Dry land area*: the area in front of the stunning pen should be at least 3 m width to opposing the wall or bleeding trough and be fitted with upright bars 5 cm in diameter and 1.2 m high, spaced 50 cm intervals for safety purposes. When improperly stunned animals regain their feets the handler may safe himself at this place. The floor of this area should be properly drained, posses' high impact and non-slip property.

c. *Bleeding area*: after stunning animals reach to the bleeding section where they are subjected for bleeding as per the procedures given in below mentioned table. The bleeding area should preferably be 5 x3.5 m size. The blood can be collected at this point in containers or stainless steel bleeding trough at least 1.5 m wide. In modern abattoirs bleeding is carried out on rails known as bleeding rails. The height of bleeding rails for cattle/ buffaloes should be 2.7 m and width around 1.1 to 1.2 m while height of bleeding rails for sheep/goat and pigs should be around 1.5 to 2.0 meters. It may also be collected with the help of hollow knife for edible and pharmaceutical purposes. The disposal of blood is an essential step in animal slaughter because it may choke the sewage system if not properly managed. It is also important because blood has highest biological oxygen demand (BOD) than other products obtained in animal slaughter which is an indicator of pollution.

Species of animal	Method of sticking	Bleeding time(min.)	Superior bleeding posture
Cattle	Bilateral severance of the carotid arteries and jugular veins by an incision across the throat region caudal to the larynx. Incision in jugular furrow at the base of the neck, the knife being directed towards the entrance of the chest to severe the branchiocephalic trunks and anterior venacava.	6-7	Vertical
Sheep & Goat	By an incision in the jugular furrows close to the head, severing both carotid arteries and jugular veins and in some cases the trachea ,oesophagus and spinal cord at the occipitoatlantal junction. However thoracic inlet bleeding is superior.	5-6	Horizontal
Pigs	The knife is inserted in the midline of the neck at the depression in front of the sternum and is then pushed forward to sever the anterior venacava brachiocephalic trunk at the entrance of the chest; sometimes the carotid artery is also pierced.	6-7	Horizontal

d. *Dressing area*: dressing area is a specified part of the slaughter hall in which dressing is carried out. Traditionally a block or booth is used where carcasses are hoisted on chain and dressed for meat production. In modern meat plant or abattoirs, on line dressing or rail dressing is generally practiced and most of the dressing is completed on rails by a single operator or many operators. It makes the dressing easier and high number of animals dressing can be completed in shorter period of time. Other benefits of on-the rail dressing system includes: more hygienic, heavy carcasses can handled easily, enhances throughput, high quality meat and offals can be obtained, safer for handlers etc. Generally four types of on-the rail dressing systems are in use like:

On-the rail system	Operational system	Capacity	Comments
i. Gravity rail system	Carcasses are suspended in spreader and single wheel trolley or runners which move from one point to another with gravity, manually stop at each point and move forward for next operation.	10-40 animals/hr	System is economical, compact and simple in design. Optimum pitch of the rail is required.
ii. Intermittent powered system	In this system mechanical moving of carcass suspended on a gambrel takes place which stops at certain points with pre-set timing depending on slaughter rate.	10-75 animals/hr	-
iii. Continuous powered system	In this system dressing line remain in continuous motion with electric supply and carcass moves in full 360^0on the rail which allows the operators to work on all sides from one position.	40-120 animals/hr	Suitable for higher throughput and mechanical hide puller, moving top inspection table like sophisticated equipments are used.
iv. Canpak system	It is a continuous conveyorized method in which carcasses are suspended in a heavy trolleys or runners from the overhead rails instead of gambrels.	50-150 animals/hr	This system was patented by Canada packers limited Toronto and is common system adopted by modern meat plants.

The height of dressing rail for various animals should be 3.3 m, 2.7 m and 3.4 m for cattle/buffaloes, sheep/ goat and pigs respectively. The operations which are carried out on the rail system depend on the animal slaughtered. However, some routine practices which are taken place on rail includes: forelegs removal, hind leg removal, skin/hide removal started from hind leg to belly, chest, neck, foreleg etc. head removal, dropping of tongue, trachea and brisket removal' tieing of weasand, caul removal and abdomen evisceration, thorex removal' reed removal, pluck removal (pluck includes larynx, trachea, lungs, heart and liver in calf/cattle/buffaloes while spleen also in sheep and in pigs spleen as well as oesophagus is also included in pigs), carcass splitting, neck shaping, tail and channel fat removal, trimmings, weighing and packaging.

e. *Cutting room*: to make the cuts of choice a room with adequate facilities like equipments, supply of hot and cold water and waste disposal system is essential to meet the hygienic requirements. Cutting room should be maintained at or below 10^{0}C along with sufficient refrigeration facilities to maintain the internal temperature of meat not more than 7^{0}C and offals 3^{0}C.

6. *Chilling or freezing room*: chilling or freezing room is also a essential component of the modern abattoir depending on the choice of meat utility and storage need of particular type of meat. This room should be made up of impervious material and must have good insulation and drainage facility. Walls of chilling/freezing room should be made up of durable, high impact materials such as stainless steel, aluminium or reinforced plastics. Carcasses or meat are immediately shifted to this room for cooling. So it must have the facility of chilling at 7^{0}C and freezing at -18^{0}C. In general, the minimum space between the carcasses on the rails should be 0.3 to 0.4 m. Whereas, space requirement between rails for various meat species should be as follows:

   Beef and buffalo meat - 0.9 m^2

   Pork - 0.7 m^2

   Mutton and chevon - 0.5 m^2

7. *Dispatch area*: dispatch area for fresh meat should be a separate outlet inside the abattoir. It should be roofed, free from pest and paved with tiles and only vehicle entrance is permitted in this area. It must be opened a side and floor of this area must be equal to the height of the vehicle floor. This area should be away from all unclean areas and used to dispatch the carcasses or cuts in loading vehicles. The temperature inside the dispatch area should be refrigeration temperature (7^{0}C) or freezing temperature (-18^{0}C).

8. *Emergency slaughter hall*: emergency slaughter hall should be attached with the detained meat room and lairage. It must have all the facilities as required in miniature slaughter hall meant for diseased or suspected as unfit animals are slaughtered. Emergency slaughter hall is used to slaughter the animals that are in acute pain and delay in slaughter should be contrary to the animal welfare. The conditions like acute fractures, injuries, uterine prolapsed etc may lead to animals under the emergency slaughter.

9. *Detained meat room*: detained meat room is generally used to hold the meat having some doubt and needs laboratory results and confirmatory diagnosis to pass as a food for consumption. This section of abattoir should be well connected with the main slaughter line, miniature slaughter and emergency slaughter hall. It should also be well connected with the chill room, condemned meat room and meat plant laboratory in which meat has to go after final decision. This room should have light intensity at least 540 lux to examine the detained meat properly. It should also have good drainage and cleaning facility. There should also have the facility of adequate sterilization of equipments and record keeping facility.

10. *Condemned meat*: meat and other parts of the carcass which are unfit for human consumption should be stored in this lockable room. It should be directly connected to one side from main slaughter hall and on other side from rendering unit or incineration for further disposal.

11. *By-product processing unit*: to sustain the meat industry and to earn profit from the abattoir it is utmost important to utilize the slaughter house by-products in most proper way. So for proper utilization of by-products they should be collected in different slaughter operations through stainless steel chutes in the separate sections.

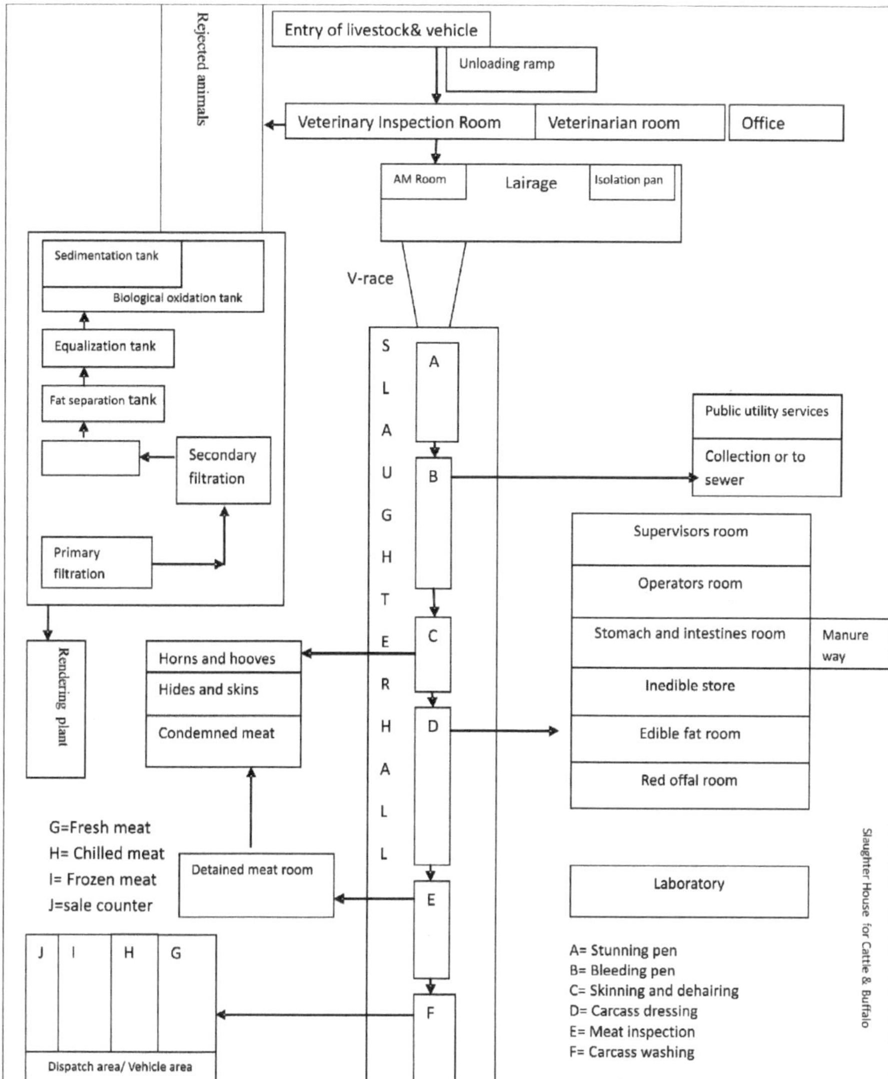

By-products processing section must have following essential compartments:

a. *Hide and skin store*: hide or skin section should be attached with the flaying section of slaughter hall. In this section primary treatment of hides and skin such as washing, removal of flesh and fat, salting and bundling is carried out. This store can also be used to receive the feet of animals for further disposal.

b. *Gut and tripe store*: gut and tripe section should be attached with the evisceration part of the slaughter hall. In this section separation and emptying of stomach and intestines is normally carried out. This section should be associated with moving top tables and arrangement for discharging intestinal and stomach contents for composting or feed manufacturing unit. It should also have the approach to the manure way if requires for manure preparation.

c. *Edible fat store*: edible fat store room should be near the gut room to receive the raw material easily. It must have the temperature near refrigeration to prevent the oxidation of fat. It should not have the direct exposure of light.

d. *Edible offal store:* edible offal store is generally used for collection, washing and storage of edible offals such as liver, lungs, heart, spleen, oesophagus and kidneys. It should be maintained at 3^0C and can also be used for collection of brains for consumptions.

e. *Inedible store:* All materials unfit for human consumption except hides and skins is stored in this section. The material collected in this section can be utilized to produce the slaughter meal or can be disposed of by incineration if not utilized.

12. *Facilities for veterinary services*: to receive the healthy livestock for slaughter and to provide the wholesome meat to the consumers veterinary services are utmost important. The prime duty of veterinarian in slaughter house is to conduct the ante-mortem and post mortem examination to ensure the healthy stock and wholesome meat.

a. *Veterinarian room*: there should be a lockable room for veterinary officer or meat inspector with the facilities of all necessary equipments, washing and changing room. All the essentials for inspection can be held in this room alongwith the seating arrangements for veterinarians.

b. *Veterinary laboratory*: There should be a well equipped laboratory for disease diagnosis as well as to maintain hygienic standards in the meat plant. It must be acquainted with basic facilities like microscope, microbiological examination facility, trichnoscope, biochemical testing facility etc.

13. *Rendering plant*: abattoir must have the facility of dry and wet rendering through digesters to produce different valuable by-products such as meat meal, bone meal, carcase meal, poultry feed, fertilizer etc. from condemned meat, offals, seized meat and other inedible by-products. Fat can also be rendered and can be used in soap, paint and cosmetics industry. This unit should be attached with an incinerator for proper disposal of infectious material.

14. *Effluent treatment plant*: slaughter house also have facility of primary treatment i.e. screening, fat removal etc and secondary treatment in a form of aerobic and anaerobic treatments of the effluent. It is also necessary to have the chlorination facility of waste before discharge of the abattoir waste into domestic sewage. This unit can also be used as an alternative source for production of heat, light and gas.

15. *Vehicle area*: There should be a provision of separate route for vehicles carrying livestock and meat. It is also necessary to have the facility of vehicle cleaning, washing and sanitation. The proper maintenance of the vehicle is the prime need for meat industry.

16. *Manure way*: there should be a covered area to hold the waste material from the slaughter house and gut/ intestinal parts of the animal. The contents of stomach can also be stored in this section. It may be converted into manure and composts. It is essential to reduce or minimize the pollution in the abattoir.

17. *Public utility services:* public utility service room must be in one corner of the slaughter house and should have well sanitized area. As per the specification, on 25 workers one latrine, two urinals, one wash basin and one bathroom is essential. If workers exceeds 25 to 50 than requirement doubles and if exceeds 50 to 100 these requirements triples and if exceeds above 100 these facilities' requires five times as compared to the requirements of 25 workers in abattoir. All sanitary measures must be adopted in this room.

Additional requirements to slaughter the specific animals including poultry

Pig slaughter house: pig slaughter is generally constructed in a separate building and normally away from the cattle/buffalo slaughter house and even separately from sheep and goat slaughter house. Pig slaughter should also be a separate entity due to religious believes in India. Along with all facilities for slaughtering the cattle/buffaloes pig requires a separate platform of 5 m with the partition of 3 m high to perform the scalding, depilation, scrapping, singeing etc. As the most common stunning procedure for pigs is gaseous anesthesia so all the facilities for Co_2 anesthesia should be maintained in stunning section. A separate scalder with the facility of hot water and a dehairing machine is also required to perform these operations in proper way. Now a day to minimize the contamination of carcasses during scalding a double walled tunnel is designed and steam passes over the carcasses in this tunnel for scalding.

The temperature (62-64^{0}C) in scalding tunnel is normally maintained with thermostat.

Sheep/goat slaughter house: sheep/goat slaughter house may be constructed with the cattle/buffalo slaughter house but a clear cut separation must be done in between both slaughter houses. Though, some sections of cattle/ buffalo slaughter can be utilized for rest and slaughter of the sheep/goat in emergency or with special conditions. For sheep/goat quality meat production automatic pelt remover can be utilized. In sheep and goat slaughter bleeding is normally carried out in horizontal position in twin conveyors by suspending the carcasses with forelegs. Floor chutes may also be utilized in sheep/goat slaughter house for several operations.

Poultry slaughter house: in addition to the routine facilities, poultry slaughter must have some additional things to perform the poultry slaughter. Poultry lairage should have the facility of cages to provide the rest to the birds. Stunning is normally or generally not practices in broilers but it is a part of chicken slaughter. Stunning is generally performed with the help of electric shocker or by dipping the head or leg for a fraction of seconds in water bath through which electric current passes. The electric current generally used for poultry is 50 volts AC for 1 min but it may vary depending on the poultry species slaughtered. Poultry slaughter is generally performed by decapitation of head and dressing is on hanging platform or rails. For scalding, poultry requires scalders to loosen the feathers. It may be performed either by dipping the poultry after bleeding in hot water maintained at 50-80^{0}C depending on the choice of poultry slaughtered. Automatic feather plucker is also required for fast feather removal. There should also be the facility of wax pickers and singeing to remove the pinfeathers and filoplumes. Removal of filoplumes (hair like appendeges over the poultry carcass) is performed over the blue flames and process is called singeing. Washing of carcass requires steam and rubber scrubbers to clean the carcasses. Giblet makes the edible portion of the carcass and normally kept inside the body cavity. Poultry giblet generally includes heart without pericardium, liver without gallbladder and gizzard after removal of outer layer. For chilling of poultry carcasses internal temperature of carcass should be 4^{0}C.

Abattoir planning and management is a key to provide the wholesome meat to the consumers. The facilities and components of an abattoir is solemnly dependant on the species of animals to be slaughter, daily throughput, capital available, purpose of meat production and religious requirements etc. However, quality meat is a reality of today and implementation of standards and techniques make it in realistic way.

The hygienic quality of abattoir, animals and workers are other important factors to be taken in account during production of meat.

References

1. BIS (2005). Indian standards basic requirements for an abattoir (first revision). Indian Standards Institution, New Delhi. pp 4-24.
2. Gracey, J.F. and Collins, D.S. (1994). Meat plant construction, equipments and operations. *In:* Reprint of 9th edition, Meat Hygiene, ELBS, The Bath Press, Avon. pp 87-108.
3. Mountney, G.J. (1970). Processing poultry. *In:* 2nd edition, Poultry Products Technology, The AVI Publishing Company Inc, Westport Connecticut, London. pp 123-136.
4. Mountney, G.J. and Parnell, E.D. (1958). Proper slaughtering for good carcass quality. Poultry Processing and Marketing, 64(11): 14-15.
5. Sharma, B.D. (1999). Pre-slaughter handling, transport and dressing of poultry. *In:* 1st edition, Meat and Meat Products Technology including Poultry Products Technology, Jaypee Brothers Medical Publishers (P) Ltd, New Delhi. Pp 99-103.
6. Sharma, B.D. (2003). Organization, layout and management of slaughter houses. In:1st edition, Modern Abattoir Practices and Animal Byproducts Technology, Jaypee Brothers Medical Publishers (P) Ltd, New Delhi. pp 11-25.
7. Singh, V.P.Singh and Pathak, V. (2011). Laboratory manual Abattoir practices and animal products technology, DUVASU, Mathura. pp 13-23.
8. Waskar, V.S. (2008). Management of an abattoir. In: Universal Meat Hygiene in Public Health care, International Book Distributing Co. Lucknow. pp 161-175.

Chapter 2

BIS Standards on Organization and Layout of Abattoirs

To streamline the slaughter activities throughout country and to produce the quality meat for domestic as well export market, Bureau of Indian Standards (BIS) formulated certain standards related to abattoir and other food items. It also harmonizes the standards as per the requirement of importing country. So that traders can easily meet out the demand of importing country. Under the standard provisions of BIS, each and every aspect of abattoir as well as its processing aspect is very well described in these standards. These standards are written and documented and easily available to know how about their implementations.

Bureau of Indian Standards (BIS)

National standardization activity started in India in 1947 with the establishment of Indian Standards Institution (ISI) as a society under the Societies Registration Act 1860, to prepare and promote the adoption of national standards. In 1952, the Institution was given the responsibility of operating a certification marking scheme under an Act of Parliament. In 1986 the national authorities made a review of the structure and status of ISI and assessed the impact made by it on the national economic development and the technological growth of various sectors of Indian industry. The Government of India felt that a new thrust had to be given to standardization and quality control activities and that a national strategy had to be evolved for giving appropriate recognition and importance to standards and for integrating them with the growth and development of production and exports in different sectors. The Government of India therefore decided to create a statutory organization as the national standards body which was named as the Bureau of Indian Standards (BIS) with adequate autonomy as well as flexibility in its operations to achieve harmonious development of the activities of standardization, certification, marking and connected matters. The Bureau of Indian Standards Act was passed by the Parliament in 1986 and BIS came into action on 1 April 1987. It has its headquarter at Manak Bhawan, New Delhi with a network of regional offices at Mumbai, Calcutta, Chandigarh and Chennai and branch offices at Ahmedabad, Bangalore, Bhopal, Bhubneshwar, Guwahati, Hyderabad, Jaipur, Kanpur, Patna and Trivandrum.

Structure of BIS: BIS is a corporate body consisting of members from Central and State Governments, Industry, Scientific and Research Institutions. Minister of Civil Supplies, Consumer Affairs and Public Distribution is the president of BIS and has administrative control over it. It is assisted by Executive Committee in which Secretary to the Ministry and Director General BIS are the ex-officio members. Its functioning bodies are Executive Committee and Advisory Committees which are engaged in dealing with finance, certification, standards, formulations, laboratories and planning.

For the formulation of standards on meat and meat products ISI constituted meat and meat products sectional committee under the Agricultural and Food Products Division Council (AFDC 18) in 1958 to prepare Indian Standards for meat industry. In this committee research scientists, technologists, manufacturers, Government agencies and consumers are the member participants. BIS committee provides familiar monogram 'ISI' after thorough examination of the products.

Functions of BIS

i. Formulation and publication of Indian standards on products, commodities, materials and processes.

ii. Promotion for adoption and implementation of these standards throughout the country.

iii. Certification of various articles and processes.

iv. Establishment, maintenance and recognition of laboratories for standardization and quality control.

v. Conduction of research for standards formulations.

vi. To provide information, documentation and other relevant services to consumers.

vii. Conduction of conferences, seminars and symposia to make aware of the consumers regarding standards and quality control measures.

viii. Provides guidance and consultancy services on standards and quality control measures.

ix. Harmonize standards and quality control activities in the country.

x. Provides guidance and recognition of quality assurance system in manufacturing and processing units.

xi. Publications of handbooks, guides and other special publications on Indian Standards.

BIS Standards for Indian Meat Industry

Standards for abattoir and sale of meat

IS: 4393-1979	Basic requirement for an abattoir (Ist revision)
IS: 7053-1973	Basic requirements of stall for sale of meat of small animals
IS: 8700-1977	Basic requirements of stall for sale of meat of large animals

Standards for ante-mortem and post-mortem examinations of meat animals

IS: 1982-1971	Code of practice for ante-mortem and post mortem inspection of meat animals
IS: 6559-1972	Code of practice for ante-mortem and post mortem inspection of poultry

Standards for meat plant hygiene

IS: 8182-1976	Code of hygienic conditions for processed meat products
IS: 8182-1976	Code of hygienic conditions for processing plant

Specifications for meat processing equipments

IS: 3545-1982	Specifications for meat choppers
IS: 6628-1972	Specifications for slide rails used in abattoir
IS: 7891-1975	Specifications for inedible offals trolleys
IS: 6782-1972	Specifications for hog gambrels
IS: 7909-1975	Specifications for electrical stunning tongs for pigs
IS: 994-1964	Specifications for butchers knives and fish knives
IS: 6696-1972	Specifications for egg washing machine

Specifications for slaughter house by-products

IS: 8895-1978	Guidelines for handling, storage and transport of slaughterhouse by-products
IS: 1981-1978	Specifications for animal casings
IS: 4054-1966	Specifications for neats foot oil

The standards of BIS on basic requirements are mainly deals with the Schedule-VI and the standards must confirm the IS: 4393-1979 and as amended from time to time.

Terminology related to BIS standards as mentioned in IS: 1982-1971

Animal: Cattle means a bull, cow, ox, heifer, calf, stear, bullock and includes buffalo. Sheep term is used for sheep, lamb, ewe, wether and ram wheres goat term applied for wether, goat, she goat, buck and kid. However, term pig is applied for pig, barrow, boar, hog, stag, pigling, gilt, rig and sow.

Butcher: The person producing or dealing with meat intended for human consumption.

Carcass: The dead body or any part thereof including the viscera of any animal which has been slaughtered.

Condemned: Carcasses, parts or organs so marked unfit for human consumption meant to be destroyed or rendered unfit for food purposes.

Flayer: The person who skins the animals and dresses the carcass.

Local Authority: A local area which is a municipality, the municipal board or municipal corporation; cantonment, the cantonment authority: a notified area, the notified area committee or any other local area, such as may be prescribed by the central or state governments.

Meat: Flesh and other edible parts of a carcass.

Meat Inspector: Qualified veterinarian. In his absence, the Medical Officer of Health or any other qualified officer appointed by a local authority and vested with the power to inspect and examine animals and meat intended for human consumption.

Veterinarian: Any duly qualified veterinarian appointed or employed by a local authority or a local government to act in that capacity.

Nuisance: Includes any act, omission, place or thing which causes or is likely to cause injury, danger, annoyance or offence to the sense of sight, smell or hearing, or which is or may be dangerous to life or injurious to health or property.

Public Street: All street over which the public have a right of way or here to fore levelled, paved, metalled, channelled, sewered, or repaired out of municipal or other public funds.

Slaughter hall: The actual place where the animals are slaughtered for food purposes.

Abattoir: Any building/ premises, or place licensed as an abattoir by the local authority for slaughter of animals intended for human consumption.

Slaughter man: The person who slaughters the animal.

Layout of abattoirs as mentioned in IS: 4393-1979

For the purpose of assuring the quality of meat, it shall be ensured that the abattoir where the animals are slaughtered shall meet with the following requirements as specified by the BIS in IS: 4393-1979 as a "Basis requirement for an Abattoir".

Detail	Requirements	Special arrangements
Locations	Abattoir should be outside or on the periphery of a city or city and shall be away from airport.	Main services like potable water, electricity and proper hygienic sewage disposal is a prerequisite.
Layout plan	Abattoir must have the facilities like animal resting, ante-mortem inspection, human slaughter, flaying, dressing and washing of carcasses. Other facilities include carcasses and offal hanging, by-products handling, meat inspection, condemned meat disposal, laboratories, detained meat, water supply. Workers and staff supply is also a essential component.	In addition rendering and incineration facilities are also essential. Clear cut separation between clean and unclean points is mandatory.
Abattoir units	1. *Reception area*: It is having an adequate size place where animals are primarily	If animals are transported other than hoof then a ramp is required which directly opens to the veterinary

inspected by veterinarians for 24 hrs rest in lairage.	inspection room attached with the office. The examination and watering facilities must be in reception area.
2. *Isolation pan*: used to hold the animals suspected for contagious and infectious disease. Fractious animals are also kept in this section.	It should have the facilities of watering and feeding.
3. *Lairage*: space should not be less than 2.8 m^2 per large animal and 1.6 m^2 per small animal with adequate facility of watering and ante-mortem examination.	It must have the facilities for protection of animals from adverse weather. If lairage is meant for Jhatka, Halal and Jewish slaughter than clear cut separation among each other is essential and separate entry is mandatory.
4. *Slaughter hall*: separate space for stunning, bleeding and carcasses is essential. Knocking section and dry land area is also recommended.	There should be the facility of separate sheep/goat Halal, Jhatka and Jewish, pig and large animals. *Curbing* of 150mm x 100 mm with top slope of atleats 45^0 is essential. *Bleeding* should be in containers and must be cleaned immediately. There should be the facility of immediate disposal of *hides/skin, legs, horns, hooves* etc. *Viscera inspection room* must have the facility of inspection, hand washing, tool sterilization and condemned parts disposal. Jet facility for carcass washing and 33 mm per meter floor drains is required.
5. *Ancillary accommodation*: there should be stomach and intestine room, pluck, viscera, edible and inedible room, laboratory, condemned meat room, labour welfare facilities, hide/skin room, rendering plant, refrigeration room and a freezer room.	Slaughter floor except one or two connecting doorways should be solid, self closing and completely covered. There should be a toilet, bathroom, drinking water and washing facilities. A canteen and first aid facility should also be there. Hanging halls in refrigeration room must be maintained at temperature < 10^{0}C. In case of higher incidences of *Cysticercus bovis* freezing at -9.5^{0}C for 10 days is practiced.

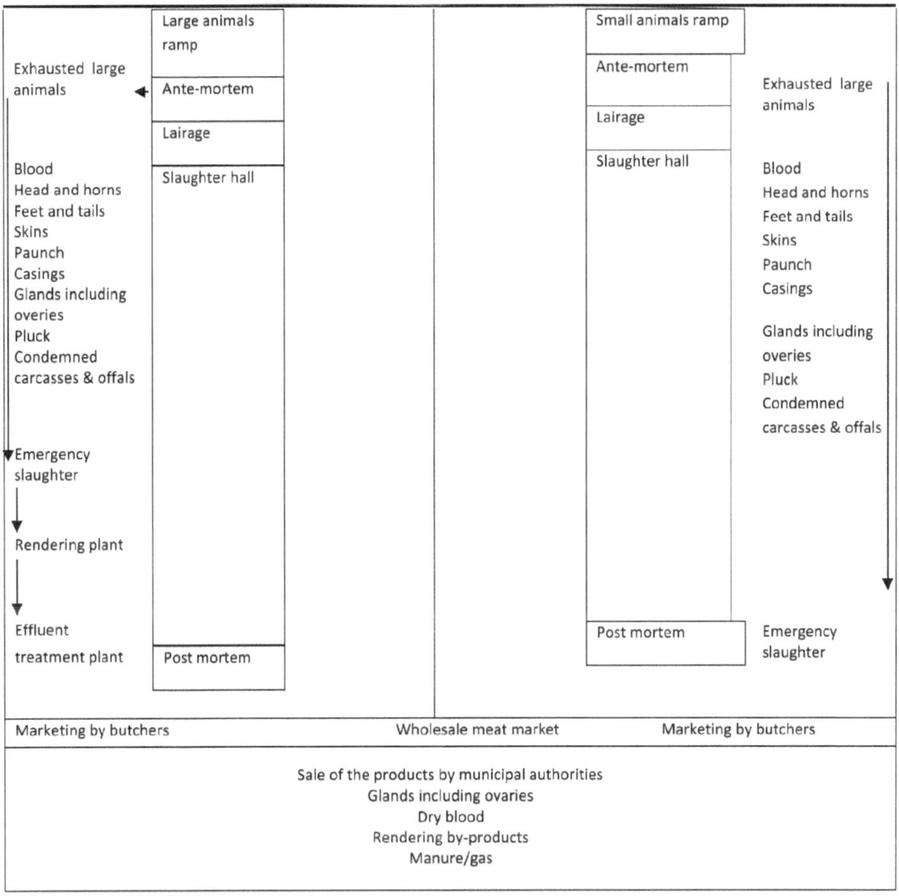

Fig 2.1 Abattoir for large and small animals

Provisions under BIS for slaughter house

1. Abattoir must have the facilities for resting, adequate facilities for ante-mortem inspection, flaying, dressing and washing, post-mortem inspection, disposal of meat unfit for human consumption , adequate water supply etc.

2. All the inspection areas and pan must be made up of impervious material such as concrete, bricks, pitched hearing, bone type and non-slippery which should be suitable for stand wear and tear. There should also be the adequate drainage facility and pen should always be covered.

3. Building material for abattoir or slaughter house should be impervious, easy in cleaning and resistant to wear and corrosions. Floor should be non slippery, non absorbent with suitable drain. There should be >100 mm coves, interior of walls should be washable upto the height of 2 meter and should be made up of smooth and impervious material. Ceiling should be atleast 5 meter high and may be painted with water resistant paint. Window should be atleast 1200 mm above the floor lebel and window ledges should have the slope of 45^0. Doors should be made up of rust resistant metal, tight soft wood with the doorways width of 1500 mm and 3000 mm height. There should be proper mesh, screens facility, fly repellent and rodent proofing facility. Stairs should be of impervious material and atleats 300 mm high.
4. All the vehicle areas should be paved with concrete with well drainage. It should be extended at least 6 meters from building, leading decks or livestock platforms shall be provided at places where vehicles are loaded or unloaded. The facilities like pressure washing jets and disinfection for trucks carrying animals should also be there. The refrigerated or freezing vehicles are now a day used to carry the carcasses and foods of animal origin.
5. All the points of abattoir where wet operations are carried out must have proper drainage facility. The slop of about 20 mm per meter is generally preferred in these areas except freezing and dry storage areas.
6. As thumb rule one drainage inlet should be provided for each 37 m^2 of floor space. Deep seal trap of P^-, U^- or S-shape is constructed on drainage lines. The provision of sanitary drainage lines should be there and drainage lines from toilet, urinals should not connected with the other drainage lines of the plant. All the floor drain lines should be U-shaped. Special drainage facility is required for some of the sections like floor drainage valley under the dressing rails for hogs, calves and sheep. These valleys should be integrated and 600 mm wide with 10 mm per meter slope.
7. There should be sufficient natural as well as artificial light except in refrigeration section. Colourless and high transmissibility of light glass may be used in skylights and windows. The overall 200 Lux intensity of light is required throughout the slaughter hall including the workable areas whereas; inspection areas must have the light intensity atleast 500 Lux. Proper ventilation is mandatory.
8. Water supply in abattoir should be potable, constant and sufficient with adequate pressure. Clean hot (82^0C) water supply shall be

available in the slaughter hall and work rooms during working hours. The water supply for washing hands and other uses for persons working in the abattoir should be in separate line. There should be sufficient water pressure in the supply. In general, floor cleaning area requires 200 to 330 kPa pressure and pressure in the carcass washing area should be atleast 1000 to 1700 kPa.

9. All the equipments in abattoir should be of rust resistant metal like stainless steel or galvanized metal.
10. Working platforms should be at the height of 800 mm to 860 mm for efficient and convenient working.
11. There should be the facility of sample collection and testing for doubtful carcasses and carcass parts.
12. Rail hooks must be rust proof made up of metal or mild steel. The BIS requirements for bleeding and dressing rails as well as carcass rails is given below:

Animal/ carcass type		Bleeding rails		Dressing rails		Carcass hanging rails		
		Height (mm)	Length (mm)	Height (mm)	Length (mm)	Space rails (mm)	Distance between rails (mm)	Height of rails (mm)
Sheep and goat		2200-3000	450	2000-2200	900	300-400	300-400	2000-2200
Pigs	Average	2200-3000	450	2000-2200	900	-	-	-
	Pigs >70 kg	-	-	-	-	450-600	450-600	2000-2200
	Pigs <70 kg	-	-	-	-	300-400	300-400	2000-2200
Large animals		4500-5000	600	3200	1800 for legging and dehiding and 2400 for evisceration	450-600	800-1000	3200 for halves and 2000-2200 for quarters

Provisions for ante-mortem and post-mortem inspection

All the required facilities for ante-mortem and post-mortem inspection should be there in the abattoir premises. For post mortem examination fresh carcasses or halves or quarters shall be stacked on clean racks at least 30 cm from the ceiling, 10 cm from the walls and 20 cm from the floor. Whereas, frozen and packed carcass or meat or mince shall be stacked on clean racks at least 30 cm from the ceiling, 20 cm from the floor and 20 cm from the walls and cartons shall be stacked one over the other. After thorough examination of carcasses and animals a certificate from qualified veterinarian is mandatory.

Provisions for Sanitary and phytosanitary requirements in meat processing plant

1. There should be a clear cut separation in between the clean and unclean areas.
2. There should be easy accessibility for cleaning and inspection in product zone areas.
3. The proper protective measures must be adopted to avoid the entry of dogs, cats, rodents, insects, flies, fires, crows, bats, cobwebs, spiders and vultures in meat processing plants. However, provision of poisons of any kind to protect from these animals shall always be prohibited.
4. Meat processing abattoir should be a separate entity and if the facility of processing of marine or other food products is in same premise it should be maintained in high sanitary condition and atleast seven days gap is essential in between various operations.
5. The meat processing operations are always performed on the specified platforms or structures where all the hygienic measures must be adopted. The contact of carcasses or meat with walls, floor and other surfaces shall always be restricted.
6. The proper cleaning, disinfection and deodorizing operations must be performed well in time to maintain the high quality hygiene in the premises. Lime washing, colour washing or painting as the case may be, shall be done at least once a year.

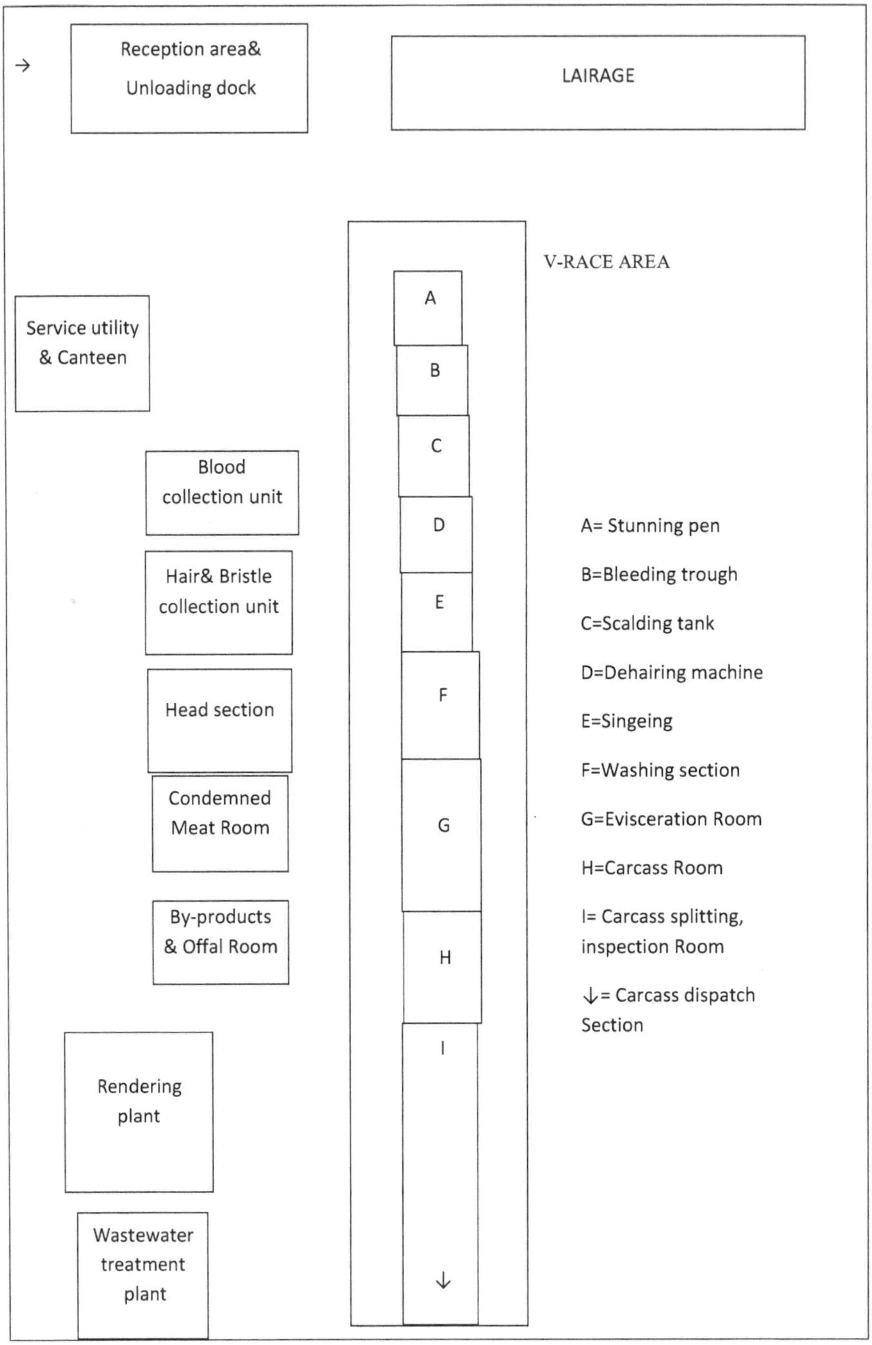

Fig. 2.2: Pig abattoir

7. Some materials like copper and its alloy in equipment used for edible products, cadmium in any form in equipment handling edible products, equipment with painted surface in product zone, enamel containers or equipment and lead in any form is not desirable in the abattoir.
8. All the equipments should be installed atleast 300 mm distance of walls to facilitate the easy cleaning and disinfection. However, wall mounted equipments should be atleast 25 mm from wall.
9. There should be a sound system for plant waste disposal, waste management, waste treatment, alongwith with the arrangement of catch basin, manure removal and disposal.
10. There should be the facility of hot and cold water in washing areas. Ample amount of detergents and harmless antiseptic solutions are also required in wash areas and wash basins.
11. Personnel hygiene is another aspect must be taken care. Persons having infections or contagious diseases must not work in the abattoir or meat processing plant. Regular health check up of workers must be adopted. Spitting, chewing, smoking, hair combing and blowing or cleaning of nose shall be prohibited in the processing areas. Other personnel practices like trimming of finger nails, hairs, bearing of aprons, headwears, hand gloves and footwear with good cleaning and disinfection conditions must be adopted. There must be facilities of changing of cloths etc.
12. There should be the restricted entrance in the premises. Facility of foot bath at entrance and exit of the slaughter house, hall and processing areas is another pre-requisite.
13. There should be sufficient latrines and wash basins for employees. Employees above 25 requires 2 urinals, 1 each of latrine, wash basin and bathroom while employees in-between 25-50 needs double of the number of assets mentioned previously. Similarly employees in between 50-100 require 6 urinals and 3 each of latrines, wash basins and bathrooms. If employs are above 100 then there should be 10 urinals and 5 each of latrines, wash basins and bathrooms. The requirement of both male and females must be kept in mind depending on the number of employees of a particular sex. These assets must be hygienically well maintained and properly sanitized.
14. There should be proper disposal of waste and by-products facility. The waste storage area shall be cleaned and disinfected at least once a day.

15. There should be a proper sanitization and cleaning schedule for premises as well as for each and every compartment or section of the abattoir and meat processing plant.

16. There should be proper refrigeration and freezing facilities to avoid the spoilage and development of pathogens in the carcasses and other food items.

The above norms and regulations are the integral part of BIS. However, many more norms and regulations are also in force for foods of animal origin. The basic motto of all the norms and regulations is to ensure the safe and quality food to the consumers. In general, strict hygienic and sanitary measures are the key of the quality meat production. Above all the maintenance of premises, environment and personnel hygiene are the key issues to be discussed before the meat plant or abattoir construction.

References

1. IS: 4393-1979. Indian Standards: Basic requirements for an abattoir (first revision). UDC637-513. Indian Standards Institution, New Delhi.

2. Sahoo, J., Sahmoon, A.H., and Yadav,K.N. (1993). Standards formulation and quality control aspects of Indian meat industry- a perspective review. The Journal of Remount and Veterinary Corps. 211-225.

Chapter 3

Pre-slaughter Care, Handling and Transport of Meat Animals Including Poultry

The aim of pre-slaughter care of animals is to arrange physiologically normal animals for slaughtering without loss of weight and to minimize stress to the animals. Pre-slaughter care of meat animals includes proper handling of animals during loading, unloading, transportation, lairage care and handling of animals just prior to slaughter. Thus due care must be adopted in this stage not only for welfare point of view but also for production of good quality meat. Proper care and handling is also essential to reduce the chances of bruises, cuts, tears and deformities on the animals/birds body.

Precautions to be taken in pre-slaughter care of meat animals

1. Good condition cows in temperate countries should not be held for long period during winter because of the possibility of development of hypomagnesaemic tetany.
2. Spring lambs require relatively shorter period of rest than adult sheep and tend to lose weight with prolonged holding.
3. Facilities should be checked to ensure that there should not be any defect which could cause bruising or even death.
4. Always avoid projections and sharp corners in the lairage and if rails are being used for pen partitions it is essential that there is no possibility of animals getting their heads between rails and being strangled; rail gaps must be of the proper width.
5. Aggressive animals and females in estrus as well as horned from polled stock must be isolated. Mixing of animals from different origins leads to fighting and injury.

6. The use of fine sprays of water on pigs awaiting slaughter in lair ages has been shown to have a beneficial effect in the prevention of fighting.

7. The aim should be to arrange physiologically normal animals for slaughter without any loss of body weight.

8. In lairage rest is main criteria to minimize stress to the animals. The factors determining the resting period are species of animals, age and sex of animals, condition of animals, length of journey, mode of transportation etc. Minimum resting period should be 6 hrs in case of normal large animals and 2-3 hrs for pigs. However, 12- 24 hrs rest is recommended in case of tired and agitated animals. But maximum holding period should not exceed 36 hrs otherwise there may be the development of hypomagnesaemic tetany and Salmonellosis etc.

9. Animals should be provided ample amount of drinking water during rest period. It is essential to minimize the bacterial load in intestines and facilitates removal of the hide or pelt during dressing of the carcass.

10. Animals should be withdrawn feed atleats 12 hrs before slaughter. Among butchers throughout the world the practice of withholding food from animals prior to slaughter has long been observed, it is being contended in support of this practice that fasted animals bleed better, that the carcass is easier to dress and that it has a brighter appearance. Scientific evidence for such assertions is lacking and the hungry animal does not settle as well as an animal which has been fed. It is also a known physiological fact that although cattle and sheep are better able to withstand cold than are the other farm animals, resistance to the shock of a severe fall in atmospheric temperature is greater in the fed animal than in one which has been starved.

    In poultry, feed withdrawal practice not only help in early evisceration but risk of contamination of meat by the intestinal contents is also minimized. By this practice we can reduce the spread of pathogens such as *Salmonella* and *Compylobacter*. Pigs lose weight faster after withhold of the feed. And after, Pigs rested for 24 hours after a journey do not regain normality unless they are fed. Indeed, the fatigue and restlessness engendered by hunger in pigs, in which definite excitement pyrexia appears to occur in those animals not used to handling may render the flesh unsuitable for preserved meat products. It has also been shown that the feeding of sugar rapidly restores the energy-yielding carbohydrate reserve (glycogen) of the muscles and liver, allowing the development of normal acidity in the former and preventing loss of weight in the latter. The feeding of up to 1.3 kg of sugar for three or more days before slaughter of cattle or pigs increased daily weight gains, killing-out percentages and liver weights.

11. Animals and birds should be handled humanly during handling for transportations.

Handling of animals and poultry birds

To avoid stress to the animals and poultry birds they must be handled with due care. It is not necessary only for quality meat production but also necessary for animal welfare point of view. For that purpose following cares must be adopted.

1. The minimal force of any type should be applied during handling of animals.
2. The attendant should be expert in their operations and calm in their attitude. Otherwise he/she may excite, confuse and antagonize the animals which will make the handling of animals more difficult.
3. Animals should be provided a flight zones around them.
4. The movement of sheep may be facilitated by the use of 'decoy'or 'Judas' sheep. This procedure utilizes the innate tendency of sheep to follow one another by 'training' one particular sheep.
5. Always avoid excessive noise during handling of animals otherwise it will create stress to the animals particularly in pigs.
6. Catching and crating of poultry birds is a most difficult, labour intensive and unpleasant task. All feeders, waterers and other accessory equipments should be arranged in corner of the house before catching the birds. The appropriate time of catching broilers is at night under very dim light. Whereas, culled and spent hens are caught in the cooler hours of the day preferevely in afternoon. The birds are caught manually by the shank in a human manner.

Transportation of livestock and poultry

Most countries have detailed regulations for humane transport of animals. In Great Britain a series of orders dating back to 1919 had been promulgated, viz. *Conveyance of live poultry order 1919, Transit of Animals orders 1927, as amended 1931; Animals (Sea Transport) order 1930, The Transit of Horses order 1951, The Houses (Sea Transport) order 1952, 1958; Transit of calves 1966, The Transit of Animals. (General) order 1973, The transit of Animals (Road and Rail) order 1975, 1979.* According to the above orders,

1. Exposure to inclement weather, transport of injured birds, use of unsuitable receptacles, mixed consignments and unnecessary long confinement in crates is prohibited.
2. Animals must be protected from injury and unnecessary suffering while being loaded, unloaded and during transport.
3. These orders outline the general provisions for road and rail vehicles and receptacles, deals with the separation of animals during transport, concerns cleansing and disinfections.
4. The transport of unfit animals and those likely to give birth during the journey is prohibited. Road vehicles must be provided with fittings for attachment of partitions. Floors and ramps must be fitted with suitable battens to prevent animals from slipping. All vehicles, which have more than one floor, must be provided with a suitable ramp or mechanical lifting gear to move animals from one floor to another. Ventilation must be adequate. Road vehicles are to be provided with suitable rigid sides and protective overhead coverings.
5. Different classes of livestock such as horned cattle, polled cattle, calves, ewes with unweaned lambs, rams over 6 months of age, weaned piglets etc are separately traveled. In India, horses and swine shall not be carried together in same vehicle, divided or undivided. Horned and polled cattle may be carried together provided all are secured by the head or neck.
6. Cleaning and disinfection of vehicles must be carried as soon as practicable after unloading and before loading of livestock.
7. Overcrowding of animals, which would result in injury and unnecessary suffering, is forbidden.
8. Adequate and suitable food and water must be offered to the animals at least every 12 h during the journey, except where a journey is completed within 15 h.
9. Unfit animals and those likely to give birth during the journey are not permitted to travel.
10. Carcasses must not be carried in vehicle in which a live animal is being carried.
11. According to American regulations, the minimum floor space required during transport is 335 cm^2 for pigs, 213 cm^2 for sheep and 271 cm^2 for calves.

As per Indian transportation rules

1. Transportation of animals must be meant to avoid injury, stress, loss of weight and disease conditions.
2. Only healthy animals certified by veterinarian to be free from infectious diseases and ectoparasites and fit for journey are allowed to transport.
3. Transportation of pregnant animals is avoided.
4. Animals from endemic areas of diseases shall be vaccinated, quarantined and then transported.
5. Vehicle should be checked for their safety, cleanliness and sanitation before loading.
6. Proper bedding, feeding, watering, ventilation shall be provided to the animals during transport.
7. Attendant with first aid equipment shall accompany the animals.
8. Males and females shall not be mixed.
9. All consignment shall bear proper labels with pertinent information on the kind of animals, address of consigner and consignee and instructions regarding feeding and watering.
10. Secured and unsecured animals may not be carried in the same undivided vehicle except unweaned and young with their mother. Horses and swine shall not be carried together in same vehicle, divided or undivided. Horned and polled cattle may be carried together provided all are secured by the head or neck.
11. Adequate and suitable food and water must be offered to the animals at least every 12 h during the journey, except where a journey is completed within 15 h.
12. Carcasses must not be carried in vehicle in which a live animal is being carried.

Livestock transport code

It is utmost important to keep the livestock healthy, in good condition and as clean as possible right from production to slaughter point. To achieve these goals, it is important to slaughter the animals as close as possible to the point of production. Loading and unloading of animals during vehicle transportation is considered most stressful both for animals and handlers. To minimize the stress during this stage ramp with the slope of 20^0 with the width of 1.5 meter is recommended.

Cattle/Buffalo: If animals are transported by truck or railway wagon then average 2m^2 space per animal should be provided. If transported by goods train than not more than 10 adult cattle or 15 calves on a broad gauge and not more than 6 adult cattle or 6 calves on narrow gauge are to be permitted.

When transported by truck not more than 6 cattle per lorry are permissible and the animals should preferable face the engine. Speed of the truck shall not exceed 40 km per hour. Unloading ramp of 1.5 meter width inclination not exceeding 30^0 should be used.

Sheep/Goats: Space requirement depends upon the weight of sheep and goat.

Weight of sheep and goat (kg)	Space requirement (m^2)
Upto 20	0.19
21-25	0.20
26-30	0.23
>30	0.28

Maximum number of animals which can be transported in different railway wagons are-

1. Broad gauge wagon -70-100
2. Meter gauge wagon-50-60
3. Narrow gauge wagon-25

Animals when transported with trucks then partition must be provided to prevent overcrowding and trapping. The speed of truck shall not exceed 40 km/hr. Unloading ramp should be atleast 0.75 meter width with 0.75 meter high walls and cleats on the floor.

Pigs:

Type of animal	Floor Space requirement (m^2)
Weaner	0.30
Young pig	0.45
Adult	0.60
Sow & litter	1.20

Maximum capacity of animals loading in different wagons of railways:

Type of animal	Broad gauge	Meter gauge	Narrow gauge
Weaner	70-100	50-60	40
Young pig	50-60	25-40	25
Adult	35-50	20-35	20
Sow & litter	18-20	10-14	10

Truck speed shall not exceed 40 km/hr and unloading ramp same as sheep and goats.

Poultry:

Category of birds	Minimum floor space requirement (cm^2)	Dimensions of container (cm)			Maximum number of birds in a container
		Length	Width	Height	
One month old chicken	75	60	30	15	24
Three months old chicken	230	55	50	35	12
Adult stock (excluding geese & turkey)	480	115	20	45	12
Geese & Turkey	900	120	75	75	10 young
	1300	75	35	75	2 growers
	1900	55	35	75	1 grower

The transportation of poultry birds are generally done in a van loaded with crates, coops or cages. In transportation process care must be taken to avoid overcrowding and suffocation to the poultry birds. Catching of birds for transportation is a tedious job which must be done judiciously to avoid stress and injuries to the poultry birds. Catching of birds must be done in cooler parts of the day for culled/spent poultry and broilers during night time with very dim light. All the equipments and accessories must be kept a side before start to catch the birds. In humane manner, birds should be caught manually by holding the shank. Another method of crating the birds is Novel Mechanical method which consists of a herding system where the birds are herded on to a conveyor and fully automatic harvesting system is used. It contains a catching unit, a truck unit and a crate-loading unit. In this system birds are directed by a long rubber fingers towards the crating area. The loading of birds is carried out in dim light either early morning or late evening to avoid excitement. The transportation should be done in cool period without much exposure to sun to prevent excessive shrinkage.

Poultry birds are generally transported in loose or fixed type plastic crates. Now a day's steel frame modules containing 4-16 crates or compartment are generally preferred instead of plastic trays. These frames may be taken in house by a fork lift truck to facilitate handling. Another system of crating birds is novel mechanical system in which birds are herded in conveyor attached with automatic harvesting system. It contains catching unit, trunk unit, crate loading unit and birds directing long rubber fingers.

Mode of transportation

1. **Driving on foot:** Movement of animals especially of cattle by foot with adequate grazing, watering and rest is still an excellent procedure. Animals are transported on foot in the cooler part of the day or night with proper treatment enroute for short distance under favourable conditions. These animals will not show signs of physical stress. Animals should not be beaten on the way or treated inhumanly.

2. **By Road:** Road transport is a second preferable mode of transport the animals but certain precautions are to be taken during the road transport.

   i. There should be provision of sufficient floor space and cubic space for the animals.

   ii. Hygienic requirements must be fulfilled.

   iii. There should not be overcrowding.

   iv. Loading and unloading should be done on unloading ramp.

   v. Stoppage should be minimum to minimize chances of bruises.

   vi. There should be a provision of protection against adverse climate but proper ventilation should be there.

   vii. Partition in the vehicles used for separating animals must be atleast 1.27 m high for cattle and horses and 76 cm for other species.

   viii. Adequate food and water must be offered to the animals as per the norms.

ix. The pregnant animals and those likely to give birth are not permitted for transport.

3. **Rail transport:** Similar to road transport except that the animals have long stoppage during journey and may require special attention. It is time taking transport and give more shrinkage. Cow shrinks more as compared to bulls and calf under normal condition. Shrinkage during first 24 hrs of transport is relatively greater than the next 24hrs. For example cattle shrinkage is about 5-6% of the live weight with in 70 hrs whereas 3-4% in 36 hrs.
4. **Sea transport:** Sea transport of food animals is not generally favored since it is too slow and greater weight loss. Animals may suffer from travelling sickness, shipping fever, muscular hemorrhages etc.
5. **By air**: It is costly and animals intended for slaughter are generally not transported. This method is used for transporting show animals.

Directives for transportation of animals by air

i. Only those animals which are in perfect health and are well fed may be accepted for transportation.

ii. The animals which are shortly going to give birth to young ones must not be accepted for transportation unless the owner signs a statement to the effect that he will bear all the risk.

iii. The animals must be delivered for shipment in suitably constructed and hygienically maintained cages and crates etc.

iv. During high altitude flights the animals must be kept in pressurized flight cabins.

v. At each air port where there is a comparatively long stop, the animal must be placed in well ventilated building.

vi. There should be an attendant to take care of animals during transport and instructions regarding feeding, watering etc. should be given to the attendant.

vii. There should be a provision of veterinary services in advance in cases of emergency on the next landing airport.

Conditions induced by transport

1. **Shrinkage:** Shrinkage is a loss of weight during transport. It is mainly loss of water by sweating and respiration and waste materials in the urine and faeces. The extent of shrinkage depends upon body condition of animals, season and journey time etc.

Loss of weight in various species is mentioned below

Species	Loss of weight	
	Live wt. (kg)	Carcass wt. (kg)
Pigs, 24 h transport	2.2 to 5.4	-
Sheep, 24 h in lairage	0.9 to 1.8	-
Sheep, 24 h transport	3.6	-
Calf of 149.6 kg. live wt. in Ist day travel	4.0	-
IInd day"	1.8	-
Bullock of 609.6 kg. live wt. in Ist day travel	30.0-40.0	-
IInd day	5.0-7.0	-
Bacon pig, per day journey	-	0.9
Pigs, over exertion, excitement during transit	-	6-7 % wt. of liver
Cattle, 161 KM journey	-	1.48
402 – 482 KM "	-	2.10
Poultry	3-4%	-

Loss in live weight and carcass weight due to journey is being compensated to great extent in cattle due to regain of tissue moisture during pre-slaughter rest. Adult merino sheep after a 3 days rail transport, when given 24 hr rest with feed and water showed beneficial effect on carcass yield. The amount of weight loss increased with an increase in temperature and decrease in relative humidity in case of pigs. When large white pigs are sprayed with cold water in an uncovered lorry during 80 Km travel, the weight loss can be reduced by 50%. Temperature and relative humidity appeared to be involved in the development of DFD meat in cattle.

2. **Stress -** During the process of loading, unloading, detention in lairage and subsequent handling up to the point of slaughter, the animal is subjected to many stressors, which may have adverse effects with subsequent deleterious changes in the carcass. In addition to physical trauma, other stresses in the form of sound, light, humidity, cold, wind and fear cause abnormal bodily changes at slaughter. There are two reactions of the animals exposed to stresses.

   i) Alarm or emergency reaction

   ii) General adaptation syndrome (fight-or-flight syndrome)

The alarm reaction is the result of sudden adverse stimuli and takes place immediately. There is an increased activity of the sympathetic nervous system which supplies the involuntary muscles, secreting glands and the heart. The result is an outpouring of catecholamines, nor adrenaline and adrenaline by the medulla of the adrenal (suprarenal gland, leading to increased heart rate and force of contraction, constriction of peripheral blood vessels, elevated blood pressure, dilatation of bronchi, cessation of digestion and mobilization of liver glycogen with increase in blood sugar. Glucagons, secreted from α-cells of the islet of langerhans in the pancreas, are more powerful than adrenaline in the production of blood glucose from liver glycogen.

The general adaptation syndrome is the essential stress reaction and is longer-lasting. Adrenocorticotrophic hormone (ACTH) is released by the anterior pituitary gland brings about the production of corticosteroids such as cortisal (hydrocortisone) and cortisone from cortex of adrenal, which regulate the general metabolism of carbohydrates, proteins and fats. There is a decrease in carbohydrate metabolism and increase in protein metabolism, the amino acid being converted into glycogen in liver. Fat is mobilized from fat depot and is metabolized in the liver producing ketone bodies. The overall result is high blood glucose level and ketosis. There is adrenal hypertrophy, eosinopenia, lymphopenia, polynucleosis and increased susceptibility to disease.

Changes in the meat quality are associated with a decreased glycogen level with the formation of less lactic acid after slaughter, a higher pH and poor keeping quality of meat. In case of accelerated glycolysis with rapid postmortem pH decline, while the temperature of carcass is still high, there is muscle protein denaturation with production of pale, soft, exudative (PSE) meat. Similarly dark, firm, dry (DFD) condition is associated with stressful situation prior to slaughter. PSE meat is more common in pig and DFD meat in cattle.

3. **Bruising -** The causes of bruising in meat animals and birds are many. These are rough handling, vehicle design and defects, presence of horns, temperature of the animal, stunning box design, mixing of animals, transport condition, breed of animal etc. Bruising causes downgrading of carcass and quantitative loss. This depends upon time and extent of bruising. A bruise may be dated approx. by appearances:

Red and hemorrhagic	0-10 h old
Dark coloured	24 h old
Watery consistency	24-38 h
Rusty orange colour and soapy to the touch	3+days

The time of bruising can be estimated by Bilirubin test. It is based upon the formation of bilirubin from hemoglobin in the area of the bruise. A sample of bruised meat is soaked in Fouche's reagent (trichloroacetic acid and ferric chloride); bruises up to 50 h old give no reaction, those 60-72 h old turn the solution light blue; those 4-5 days old give a dark green reaction. The age of a bruise can also be estimated by measuring the electrical conductivity of the tissue, which increases up to a maximum at 40 h.

4. **Transport mortality** - Deaths in classes of livestock occur during transportation. Sheep and pigs are frequently found dead as a result of suffocation during transport. In most of the countries the incidence is less than 1%. Death of pigs during transport has become an increasingly serious problem in many countries because selective breeding in pigs for early maturity has increased aggressiveness and sensitivity to stress factors. This depends on various factors, like feeding heavy meat before journey, inadequate ventilation, summer season, distant journey etc. Use of tranquillizers has reduced aggression and stress in pigs, but the dose rate and injection techniques are very important. Careless injection can cause loss of meat due to sever tissue reactions such as gelatinous infiltration, hemorrhage and necrotic muscle changes at the site of injection. Losses up to 2.2 kg from this cause have been recorded. Besides, there is residual effect in meat tissue, if the animal is slaughtered shortly after the use of this drug.

Affections induced by transport

i. *Shipping (Transit) fever* – It is a catarrhal and fatal disease observed in cattle having a long journey by rail or sea without food during cooler months. This is related to virus and bacteria in respiratory tract. Myxovirus, *Pasteurella hemolytica, P. multocida,* Mycoplasma and Chlamydia has been held responsible for transit fever.

ii. *Transit tenancy* - It is seen in the similar conditions in cows and ewes with advanced pregnancy in warmer months of the year. This is associated with hypocalcaemia.

iii. *Salmonellosis* - It is precipitated in calves and lambs by transport stress and compounded by lack of food and water and by chilling.

iv. *Miscellaneous conditions* - These include heat shock, indigestion, abortion, post-parturient disorders, ketosis, foot diseases, enterotoxaemia, mastitis, gastric ulcers in pigs and infertility following transport.

Thus the pre-slaughter care and handling during transportation as well as in the lairage is having direct relation with the meat quality. It is also important to meet the welfare requirements to the slaughter animals as specified by the authorities. The faulty care and handling may lead to the conditions as specified in the text. The profitability and economic viability of the meat industry is dependent on the care and handling and weight loss or shrinkage has direct impact on the yield.

References

1. BIS (2005). Indian standards basic requirements for an abattoir (first revision). Indian Standards Institution, New Delhi. pp 4-24.
2. Gracey, J.F. and Collins, D.S. (1994). Pre-slaughter handling and Veterinary ante-mortem inspection. *In:* Reprint of 9th edition, Meat Hygiene, ELBS, The Bath Press, Avon. pp 132-142.
3. Mountney, G.J. (1970). Processing poultry. In: 2nd edition, Poultry Products technology, The AVI Publishing Company Inc, Westport Connecticut, London. pp 123-136.
4. Mountney, G.J. and Parnell, E.D. (1958). Proper slaughtering for good carcass quality. Poultry Processing and Marketing, 64(11): 14-15.
5. Sharma, B.D. (1999). Pre-slaughter handling, transport and dressing of poultry. In: 1st edition, Meat and Meat Products Technology including Poultry Products Technology, Jaypee Brothers Medical Publishers (P) Ltd, New Delhi. Pp 99-103.
6. Sharma, B.D. (2003). Organization, layout and management of slaughter houses. *In:* 1st edition, Modern Abattoir Practices and Animal Byproducts Technology, Jaypee Brothers Medical Publishers (P) Ltd, New Delhi. pp 11-25.
7. Singh, V.P.Singh and Pathak, V. (2011). Laboratory manual Abattoir practices and animal products technology, DUVASU, Mathura. pp 13-23.
8. Waskar, V.S. (2008). Management of an abattoir. In: Universal Meat Hygiene in Public Health care, International Book Distributing Co. Lucknow. pp 161-175.

Chapter 4

Ante-Mortem Examination

Ante-mortem examination includes all procedure or tests conducted by a competent person on live animals for the purpose of judgement of safety, suitability and disposition. It is an integral step to be performed by qualified veterinarian during conversion of animal to carcass for wholesome meat production. The animals are examined for cruelty due to overcrowding or suffocation or any other inflicted injuries and stress during transportation or otherwise, because it not only directly affects the quality of meat but also downgrade the carcass. Ante-mortem inspection ensures that only healthy animals are slaughtered and wholesome meat reaches to the consumers. A complete record of the ante-mortem inspection of all animals received in the abattoir should be maintained to ascertain that animal's health status at the time of slaughter. Antemortem examination not only ensures the health animals entry into slaughter house but also assist in postmortem examination. It is also important to make a decision on certain diseases based on symptoms because they may not show the postmortem lesions for final judgment. Ante-mortem inspection has twofold functions as it enables veterinarians to protect public health and to assess the welfare conditions in which the animal is placed.

The basic aim of ante-mortem inspection is to ensure only apparently healthy, normal animals are slaughtered for food and abnormal disease animals are segregated. In combination to postmortem inspection, it certifies that meat from animals is free from disease, wholesome and free from human health risk. Carefully performed ante-mortem and post-mortem inspection as well as hygienic dressing ensures safe, clean and wholesome meat production. There are three basic concerns of ante mortem inspection i.e. public health, animal health and animal welfare. Ante-mortem examination acts as first tracing point in quality meat production system because it filters the transmission of zoonotic diseases from animals to man and vice-versa.

Essentials in antemortem examination

i. To perform antemortem examination, adequate natural or artificial light of at least 540 lux or 50 foot candle is essentially required.

ii. Adequate identification of live animal as well as carcass after slaughter is a legal requirement. It can be achieved by using metal, plastic, nylon ear tags, ear tattoos, neck, tail, leg bands, freeze brands and marking aerosols and paints for cattle, sheep, goats and pigs. The recent innovation in this field is electronic identification.

iii. Animals destined for slaughter must be accompanied by adequate documentation along with individual identification. It assures the traceability of animals in meat production system.

iv. There should be an arrangement of properly designed and well-lit lairage pens alongwith isolation pen and a crush for individual animal examination.

v. There should be a room for veterinary services along with an office for record keeping.

vi. There should also be the competent staff for assistance in ante-mortem examination.

Objectives of ante-mortem inspection

i. Ante-mortem inspection facilitates the screening of animals based on health at reception. So only healthy animals gets entry to lairage where they thoroughly examined for detailed diseases status before slaughter.

ii. Ante mortem just before slaughter is performed to check that animals are properly rested and proper clinical information, which will assist in the disease diagnosis and judgment making and to ensure the quality meat production.

iii. It reduces contamination on the slaughter floor by separating dirty animals and condemnation of the diseased animals. It also prevents unnecessary contamination of building and equipment of the abattoir.

iv. To detect certain diseases whose identification *i.e.* either difficult or impossible during postmortem and are toxic or contagious ex: Rabies, tetanus, ephemeral fever, septic metritis and mastitis, sturdy in sheep and tuberculous meningitis in young cattle etc. Poor quality meat from febrile animals can also be prevented.

v. It also helps in implementation of disease control programme with more precision by tracing back the source of disease.

vi. It enables veterinarians to protect public health through prevention of communicable and zoonotic diseases.

vii. In general it accounts 50% of meat inspection and makes the post mortem examination much more efficient and less labour intensive.

viii. It ensures animal welfare and prevents inhumane handling of animals intended to slaughter.

ix. Provides guidelines for casualty or emergency slaughter.

x. To detect the animals suffering from scheduled or infectious diseases particularly anthrax, rabies and glanders which are communicable to man. It is notable that swine fever, foot and mouth disease and sheep scab were first detected at an abattoir.

xi. To prevent the slaughter of pregnant animals by early detection of pregnancy. It assures the legislations defining the prohibition of slaughter of pregnant animals or those have give birth within last 48 hrs and immature animals.

xii. Dead and moribund animals can be prevented to enter in the slaughter premises and supply of their meat to the human consumption.

xiii. Drug residue in the animals can be detected by knowing the history of animals at antemortem examination and their meat can be prevented for entrance in food chain.

Procedure

Animals at reception point are primarily screened by competent authority and passes to lairage house for rest and detailed examination. In antemortem examination animals are usually examined within 24 hrs of arrival in the slaughter house and repeated immediately before slaughter if the animal has been kept in lairage overnight. Antemortem examination must also be repeated if temporary condition of the animal precludes, such condition requires proper assessment of the health and proper information or diagnostic tests. However, poultry birds are generally examined on same day for ante-mortem reports in holding pens.

The procedure of ante mortem examination can be summarized as:

i. Animals intended for slaughter must be recorded with species, breed, sex, age and identification mark.

ii. Animals are examined in rest as well as in motion. The gait, posture, fatiguness are examined critically.

iii. Animals are examined for abnormal behaviour which may be evidenced in form of circling movement, abnormal gait or posture due to pain in the legs, chest or abdomen. Nervous diseases may be identified by seeing the symptoms of head pushing against the wall, charging various objects and acting aggressively, showing dull and anxious expression in the eyes. Confirmation abnormalities may be manifested by swelling, abscess, enlarged joints, enlarged udder for mastitis, enlarged jaw (lumpy jaw) and bloated abdomen.

iv. Animals are examined for abnormal discharge or protrusion from body such as discharge from nose, saliva from mouth, protrusion from vulva, rectum etc.

v. Examination is performed for evidence of cruelty to animals such as over trucking, over driving, overcrowding, suffocation, beating or other acts. Careless transportation is also manifested with brushes, torn skin, fractured bone, injuries etc.

vi. Physical parameters of animals' body such as temperature, respiration rate and pulse rate must be examined for any abnormalities. Animals showing fever must not be passed for slaughter as it affects meat quality.

vii. The lymph nodes such as scapular, poplitial and other superficial lymph nodes are palpated and examined for swelling and abnormalities. In case of abnormality animals are either rejected or passed with suspected note and instruction of careful postmortem examination can be issued.

viii. Diseases specifically important for antemortem examinations are Rabies, Anthrax, FMD, Tuberculosis, Actinomycosis, Actinobacillosis, Black leg, Tumors, Ringworm, Mange, Tetanus, Mastitis, Sheep scab, Cereous lymphadenitis, Pneumonish Swine fever, Gut edema, Swine Erysipelas, Atrophic rhinitis, White scour, Calf diarrhea, Salmonellosis, Listeriosis, Poisoning etc.

ix. Always avoid slaughter of pregnant animals or those have give birth within last 48 hrs, immature animals, animal under treatment or with a recent history of treatment, experimental animals unless or otherwise deemed necessary by veterinarian.

x. In case of any abnormality or suspect systematic examination should be conducted. Some of the examples deemed necessary in systemic examinations can be quoted as wings osculation for pneumonia, rumen palpation for bloat; genital organs for swelling, secretions and discharges etc.

Judgement of ante-mortem examination

There is only three fate of an animal presented for slaughter after ante mortem inspection.

i. **Passed / Accepted / Fit for slaughter/ Approval for slaughter:** Those animals/birds which are free from any symptoms of disease and normal are sent forward for slaughter.

ii. **Rejected / Condemned / Unfit for slaughter:** Animals with higher temperature (106^{0}F), dead animals, emaciated, immature or pregnant animals must be declared unfit and should not be passed. Animals with recent natural death should be rejected as perfect bleeding cannot be achieved resulting into poor quality meat. Animals showing symptoms of rabies, FMD, Black quarter, tetanus, generalized tuberculosis, white scour, calf diphtheria, hog cholera, Salmonellosis etc should not be passed for slaughter. Animals showing the symptoms of poisonings. Similarly birds with morbid conditions due to contagious diseases, heat stroke or traumatic injury which cannot be treated.

iii. **Suspect:** Suspect category of slaughter decision includes those cases in which judgment of either fit or unfit can not made at moment.

   a. **Slaughtered but may need a special detailed postmortem.** It is a category of slaughter decision in which animals are allowed to slaughter with the instructions that careful special detailed post mortem examination must be conducted before final decision. It is applicable to the animals showing evidence of localized conditions such as injuries, fractures, abscesses, benign tumours etc. It is also applicable to the animals showing symptoms of diseases such as actinomycosis, actinobacillosis, mastitis, sheep scab, gut edema, swine erysipelas, atrophic rhinitis, downers, leptospirosis, anaplasmosis and tuberculosis reactors, brucella reactor goats, anasarca, vesicular exanthema, vesicular stomatitis etc. This category includes the animals for emergency slaughter where a delay in slaughter would be contrary to the welfare of animal.

   b. **Delayed/Detained Slaughter:** The experimental animals, animals under treatment or with history of recent treatment or vaccination, febrile, fatigue, exited animals and animals carrying toxic residues are delayed for slaughter.

   c. **Segregated slaughter:** segregated slaughter decisions are made under special conditions such as dirty stock or animals suspected for some contagious diseases etc.

Ante-mortem examination and their judgements in food animals under specific disease conditions

S.No.	Disease/condition	Cause	Salient symptoms	Judgement	Specific reason
	a. Specific conditions				
1.	Septicemia	Massive invasion of bacteria in blood stream and failure of defense system leads to carry the organisms in different parts and organs of animal body.	High fever with shivering. Recumbent pasture and restricted movement. Associated with pathological conditions.	Unfit for slaughter	Poor bleeding, alkaline carcass, shorter shelf life.
2.	Emaciation	Associated with chronic disease conditions like Johne's, liver rot, swine erysipelas etc. Higher metabolic rate	Dejected and staring look, rough body coat, hides bound appearance. Condition always associated with oedema.	Unfit for slaughter	Less meat bone ratio and loss of protein in carcass
3.	Fever	Hyperthermia and/ or toxemia due to infection	Higher than normal body temperature, anorexia, depression.	Unfit for slaughter	-
4.	Still birth	Prolonged birth, fetal hypoxia, dystocia, infection of aborting agent like Brucella and Trichomonas etc.	Still birth or unborn animals	May be used in minced meat products and rarely as retail cuts	However, its use is unjustifiable and repugnant
5.	Malnutrition	Less availability or unavailability of feed and fodder	Ketosis, loss of body weight, less development of muscle mass, reduction in metabolic rate, serous fat atrophy.	Malnutrition followed by emaciation than unfit for	Lesser muscle mass, fat depot

				slaughter other-wise suspect.	
6.	Melanosis	Deposition of melanin in animal body and organs	Black coloured melanin deposition in skin, hair, horn and eyes.	Generalized condition leads to unfit for slaughter	Calves, sheep and goat shows bad appears
7.	Immaturity	Under age animals	Less muscle development, flabby body	Unfit for slaughter	Repugnant, higher proportion of bones and water, less calorie and palatability
8.	Oedema/dropsy	Deposition of fluid outside the blood vessels such as body cavities, lymphatic spaces, connective tissues due to toxemia	Oedema of thoracic cavity (Hydrothorex), oedema of abdominal cavity (Ascitis), oedema of subcutaneous and connective tissue (Anasarca)	Hydrothorax and Ascitis-suspect Anasarca- Unfit for slaughter	-
9.	Pneumonia	Infection due to bacteria or faulty drenching	Lungs are severely affected and shows inflammation	Suspect	-
b. Diseases					
1.	Rabies	Bites of affected animals	Neurological disorder, salivation, gating of teeth, neck spasm, tail switching	Unfit for slaughter (to be destroyed)	Notifiable disease
2.	Anthrax	Fatal diseases with the exception of hog. By *Bacillus anthracis* through inhalation,	Acute in most animals except swine in which it occurs in chronic form. Sudden death,	Unfit for slaughter (to be destroyed	Notifiable disease

		ingestion and skin penetration	high fever (42^{0}C), muscle tremor, mucosal congestion, characteristics inflammatory oedema of throat and face, bloody diarrhea and red dark blood discharge from natural orifices.		
3.	Foot and Mouth Disease (FMD)	Highly contagious disease of cloven footed animals caused by filterable virus	Depression, fever, loss of appetite, lameness due to vesicles with clear fluid in coronary bands and interdigital skin of foot as well as on dental pad and posterior portion of dorsal surface of tongue, profuse slobbering. Mouth lesions are not a prominent figure in sheep	Unfit for slaughter	Notifiable disease
4.	Haemorrhagic Septicemia (HS)	Acute and sub acute disease caused by *Pasteurella multocida* and *Pasteurella haemolytica*	High fever, rapid pulse, difficulty in breathing, painful edematous swelling on throat, pulmonary involvement, copious nasal exudate	Unfit for slaughter	Notifiable disease
5.	Rinderpest (RP)	Highly contagious viral disease	Rapid fatal febrile disease manifested with continuous high fever, mouth erosion	Unfit for slaughter	Notifiable disease but reported

			with gresyish yellow deposits, shooting dirrhoea and rapid emaciation		eradicated from India
6.	Johne's Disease (JD)	Chronic infectious granulomatous enteric disease of ruminants caused by *Mycobacterium paratuber-culosis* through ingestion of contaminated feed and water	Debilitating diarrhea with foul smell and gas bubbles, granulomatous enteritis, hide bound condition due to emaciation followed submandibular oedema till development of dirrhoea	Unfit for slaughter but in case of good animal condition 'suspect'	Notifiable disease. High bone and less muscle content
7.	Tuberculosis (TB)	Great white plague or pearl disease caused by *Mycoba-cterium tuberculosis* through inhalation, ingestion and direct exposure	Chronic inflammation of lungs, swelling of retropharyngeal lymph gland, marked emaciation, hide bound condition	Generalized-unfit Localized-Suspect	Notifiable disease
8.	Actinomycosis	Caused by *Actinomyces bovis* but route of infection is unknown	Chronic granulomatous disease showing lumps on upper and lower jawbones and termed as lumpy jaw condition	Suspect	-
9.	Actinobacillosis	Caused by *Actinobacillus lignieresii* but route of infection is unknown	Marked development of fibrous tissue causing enlargement and hardening of tongue (wooden tongue) and swelling around the jawbones	Suspect	-

10.	Black Quarter	Acute infectious disease caused by *Clostridium chauvoei* through ingestion of contaminated spores and wound infection	Severe inflammation of muscles followed by crepitating swelling on shoulder, neck, breast, loins or thigh. Incision on muscles releases sour smelling frothy dark fluid.	Unfit for slaughter (remove at once)	Gas in muscles with sour smelling frothy fluid.
11.	Tetanus	Acute high fatal infectious disease caused by neurotoxins of *Clostridium tetani*	Spasmodic and tonic contractions of voluntary muscles of face, neck, body, leg and tail especially of masseter muscles often causing lock jaw condition. Stiffness of muscles with muscle tremors, prolapsed of third eyelid	Unfit for slaughter (destroy at once)	-
12.	Mastitis	Disease of lactating animals with multi-pathogenic origin and complex events of bacterial infection, trauma and faulty management	Inflammation of teats, hot in touch and tender with thick, flaky and watery milk. In later stage very hard due to fibrosis.	Chronic-Suspect Acute septicemic mastitis- Unfit for slaughter	-
13.	Sheep Scab	Parasitic disease caused by sucking mite *Sarcoptes scabiei*	Crust formation on skin coupled with progressive emaciation. Absence of burrows showing the sign of papulo-vesicular eruptions with intense pruritis	Suspect	-

14.	Caseous Lymphadenitis	Chronic disease of sheep and goat caused by *Corynebacterium pseudotuberculosis* through wound	Enlargement of superficial lymph nodes with greenish yellow gelatinous pus	Generalized – unfit Localized- suspect	-
15.	Swine Fever (Hog cholera or Pig typhoid)	Highly infectious and contagious disease of pigs caused by Pestivirus through infected urine	Acute cases are common in young pigs while chronic in adults. Tendency of pigs to lie with back arched and uncurled tail, pneumonia, higher fever with foul smelling diarrhea, red or purple skin. Septicemia with multiple haemorrhages	Unfit for slaughter	In frozen pork virus may survive for over four years
16.	Swine Erysipelas	*Erysipelothrix rhusiopathia suis*	Characterized by different forms such as acute septicemia with high fever (40 to 42^{0}C), skin from (diamond skin eruptions), chronic arthritis and vegetative endocarditis. In advance stage skin may get necrosed and forms leather crusts	Acute- Unfit for slaughter Chronic -suspect	Due to septicemia
17.	Gut Edema/Bowel disease of swine	Toxin producing *Escherichia coli*	Sudden death, nervous sign, steady gait and swelling of eyelids	Suspect	-

18.	Atropic Rhinitis	Disease of pigs caused by inclusion body rhinitis virus (IBR)	Dished snout with wrinkling of skin. Distorted nasal septum with bloody nasal discharge, puffy eyelid	suspect	-
19.	White Scour	Disease of calves caused by *Escherichia coli* but other organisms may accompany	Large abscess in abdominal wall near umbilicus which becomes hard and swollen	Unfit for slaughter	-
20.	Calf Diptheria	*Fusiformis necrophorus*	Characterized by evil smelling diptheric patches, swollen tongue, yellowish or grayish patches on mucous membranes of cheeks, gums, tongue and throat.	Unfit for slaughter	-
21.	Salmonellosis	Salmonella group of organisms	Severe diarrhea with foul smell and shreds of mucous membrane from intestine and blood, fever, loss of appetite, dullness, dehydration	Unfit for slaughter	-
22.	Listeriosis	*Listeria monocytogenes*	Stiffness of neck, incoordinated movement of limbs and in advance stage circling movement, paralysis of muscles of jaw and pharynx as well as one side of face	Acute case- Unfit for slaughter Recovered- Suspect	-

c. Poisonings

1.	Arsenic poisonings	Dipping/spraying to control ectoparasites or through contaminated feed and fodder	Severe abdomenal pain, groaning, vomiting, salivation, foetid diarrhea, muscle tremor and coma	Unfit for slaughter	-
2.	Fluorine poisoning		–	Unfit for slaughter	
3.	Selenium poisoning		Peeling of skin	Unfit for slaughter Recovered animal-Suspect	

Diseases encountered in poultry birds during ante-mortem examination and their judgement

S.No.	Disease	Unfit for slaughter	Passes for slaughter as suspect
1.	Ornithosis	All affected birds	
2.	Ranikhet disease	Birds in acute stage	-
3.	Chronic respiratory disease	-do-	All others
4.	Infectious bronchitis	Birds in advanced stage	Birds with initial signs of disease or evidence of recovery
5.	Infectious laryngotracheitis	Birds in advanced stage with cyanosis	Recovered birds
6.	Infectious coryza	Acute stage of disease with debilitation	Birds with initial signs of disease or evidence of recovery
7.	Neural lymphomatosis	All affected birds	Highly affected birds
8.	Coccidiosis	Anaemic birds	-
9.	Infectious enterohepatitis (Black head disease of turkey)	Birds showing symptoms	Highly affected birds
10.	Fowl typhoid	All affected birds	Slight involvement and recovered birds
11.	Fowl pox	Birds in debilitated and febrile condition	-
12.	Fowl cholera	Birds with septicaemia	All others
13.	Botulism (limber neck)	All affected birds	-

Emergency slaughter

Emergency slaughter is required when an animal is in acute pain or is suffering from a condition where delay in slaughter would be contrary to animal welfare. However, it is mandatory that salvage of the carcass should not present any hazard to the consumer. Emergency slaughter conditions are applicable in cases of fractures, severe injuries, uterine prolapse, post-partum uterine haemorrhage in the bovine, acute respiratory distress and tympanitis in cattle, prolonged recumbency in cow and sow, pregnancy toxaemia in sheep etc.

Casualty slaughter

Casualty slaughter refers to situation where an animal is not in acute pain or immediate danger of death but affected with more chronic condition leads to unnecessary sufferings to the animals. Casualty slaughter is applicable in animal conditions like obturator paralysis and post-partum paraplegia following milk fever or benign superficial tumours etc.

PROFORMA FOR ANTE-MORTEM INSPECTION REPORT

1. Name and address of owner ....
2. Date and time of inspection ....
3. Identification of animal ....
   a. Species ....
   b. Breed ....
   c. Sex ....
   d. Age ....
   e. Behaviour ....
   f. Identification mark ....
4. General body condition of animal ....
   a. General condition of animal (Emaciated/ weak/good/very good) ....
   b. Posture and gait ....
   c. Reaction to environment (For hypersensitivity condition) ....
   d. Condition of hide or skin and hair (Photosensitization/eruption/haemorrhages/ mange infestation/orf/contusion/dermatomycosis/abscess/cyst/ wound/bruises) ....
   e. Body temperature ....
5. Systemic examination ....
   a. Head ....
      i. Jaw for Actinomycosis ....

ii. Eyes for Neoplasm ....

iii. Eyelids for oedema ....

iv. Conjunctiva for Septicaemia and jaundice ....

v. Nictitating membrane ....

vi. Ocular discharge ....

vii. Corneal opacity ....

viii. Horns for Neoplasm ....

b. Tail for gangrene ....

c. Digestive system ....

i. Salivation (Soapy/ stringy) ....

ii. Mouth ....

iii. Tongue(ulcers/vesicles/tongueworm/ actinobacillosis) ....

iv. Lips (For FMD lesions) ....

v. Gums (For FMD and Rinderpest) ....

vi. Anus (For diarrhoea and dysentery) ....

d. Genital system ....

i. External genitalia ....

ii. Pregnancy ....

iii. Oestrus ....

iv. Metritis/ retention of placenta etc. ....

v. Evidence of abortion/ parturition ....

e. Respiratory system ....

i. Nasal cavity and discharge ....

ii. Rate and nature of respiration ....

iii. Condition of lungs ....

f. Lymphatic system (Lymphadenopathy) ....

g. Skeletal system ....

i. Dislocation / fracture ....

ii. Arthritis ....

iii. Lameness ....

h. Muscular system ....

i. Hind quarter (For black quarter) ....

ii. Convulsions (Tonic/ clonic) ....

iii. Muscular spasm ....

i. Nervous system (undue furiousness/ circling/ataxia etc. ....

6. Any other condition or disease which affect the general health of animal or the meat quality ....

7. Presence of symptoms of any notifiable disease ....

8. Evidence of medication/ treatment given to the animal, if any ....

9. Judgement ....

a. Approved for slaughter ....

b. Condemned ....

c. Passed for slaughter under special precautions ....

d. Delay of slaughter ....

e. Emergency/ casualty slaughter ....

Date .... Signature of Meat Inspector

Place .... Seal...........................

Drug withdrawal period (NMPF, 2015)

Drug	Meat withdrawal time	Milk withdrawal time
Ampicillin trihydrate	6 days	48 hrs
Enrofloxacin	28 Days	-
Erythromycin	21 days	-
Ivermectin	35 days	-
Oxytetracycline dihydrate/ hydrochloride	5 days	96 hrs
Penicillin G (benzathine)	30 days	-
Penicillin G (procaine)	10-14 days	72 hrs post calving
Selenium (sodium selenite)	30 days	-
Tylosin	21 days	-
Vitamin E	None to 30 days	-
Cloxacillin (benzathine)	28-30 days	-
Novobiocin	-	72 days post calving
Chlortetracycline hydrochloride	01 day	-
Neomycine sulfate	01 day	-
Streptomycin sulfate	02 days	-
Sulfadimethoxine	07 days	60 hrs
Tetracycline hydrochloride	04 days	-
Dexamethasone		None
Oxytocin		None
Amoxicillin trihydrate	12 days	60 hrs
Cloxacillin	10 days	48 hrs
Anthelmintics		
Albendazole	27 days	-
Amprolium	01 day	-
Fenbendazole	08 days	72 hrs
Livamisole hydrochloride	02 days	-
Oxfendazole	07 days	-
Ivermectin	48 days	-
Morantel tartrate	14 days	None
Harmones		
Gonadotropine	None	None
Progesterone	None	None

References

1. Geoffrey, W. (1995). Black's Veterinary Dictionary, 18th Ed. Jaypee Brothers, New Delhi.
2. Gracey, J.F and Collins,D.S. (1994). Meat plant construction, equipments and operations. *In:* Meat Hygiene, 9th ed., ELBS, U.K. Pp 134-142.
3. National Milk Producers Federation (2015). Milk and Dairy Beef Drug Residue Prevention. Producers Manual of Best Management Practices. www.nmpf.org
4. Sharma, B.D. (2003). Ante-mortem examination of meat animals. *In:* Modern Abattoir Practices and Animal By-products Technology, First Edition, Jaypee Brothers Medical Publishers, New Delhi. Pp 30-34.
5. Sherikar, A.T., Bachhil, V.N. and Thapliyal, D.C. (2013). Ante-mortem inspection. In: Elements of Veterinary Public Health, Second reprint, ICAR, New Delhi, Pp 168-180.

Chapter 5

Post-Mortem Inspection

Post-mortem examination is a thorough examination or inspection of all relevant parts of slaughtered animals including carcass and organs by qualified veterinarian immediately after slaughter and evisceration to find out the possible changes and lesions that indicate unsuitability of the meat for food. *Postmortem examination* should be carried out as soon as possible after carcass dressing otherwise carcass gets set and the examination of lymph nodes becomes difficult particularly in beef and pork in winters. Detailed post mortem examination includes observation of all parts of *carcass*, dressing procedures, equipments and facilities to prevent contamination of edible parts. The basic motto of post mortem judgment is the safety, suitability and disposition of carcass for human consumption. Post mortem examination ensures safe and quality meat food to the consumers with greater shelf life. The carcasses and organs are examined for evidence of bruises, injuries, or discoloration and disease conditions. It also ensures contamination of carcasses from diseased parts ad animals. It is because post mortem examination emphasizes good hygienic conditions in production of meat and also during examination because knives and other instruments used for cutting and examining organs, glands and tissues are sterilized. Post mortem examination is a sequential thorough inspection which involves palpation of organs and tissues, incision where necessary and laboratory test in certain conditions.

Objectives of Post Mortem Examination

The basic aim of post mortem is to ensure the safe and fit food to the consumers. So the carcasses and organs are thoroughly examined after slaughter and dressing as well as before passing them to chilling section. Post mortem examination enables veterinarian to reach on a conclusion about a particular disease existence in carcasses and organs. So that proper preventive measures can be taken well in time to control disease right at farm level. Post mortem examination is also helpful to ensure proper slaughter and dressing practices such as bleeding, trimming etc. It is also helpful in adoption of proper disposal procedure for condemned meat and offal's. This is a systemic examination and performed in well defined sequences and involves all the systems of the body. Some of the major objectives of PM examination can be summarized as:

1. To ensure healthy meat to the consumers by detection and elimination of abnormalities and diseases from the carcass and organs including contaminations.
2. To check the overall quality of meat as well as efficiency of slaughter and carcass dressing.
3. To diagnose the diseases and conditions. So that control measures can be adopted for their prevention and eradication.
4. To ensure proper segregation and disposal of carcasses, parts or organs marked unfit for human consumption.
5. Protection of public health by rejection of meat which might be the source of food borne infection and intoxication.

General rules for post mortem examination

Post mortem examination is a key component of the slaughter business because it ensures quality. Quality enhances integrity and faith of the business. Some of the essentials for post mortem may be summarized as under:

1. The inspection should be performed as soon as possible after dressing of carcass otherwise carcass gets set and examination of lymph nodes and other abnormalities in carcass becomes difficult to diagnose.
2. There should be a specific schedule of slaughter and inspection. So that everyone should be there for inspection.
3. There are three main areas of post mortem inspection i.e. head, viscera and carcass. So head and viscera should remain identifiable with the carcass until the inspection is completed. There may be a failsafe method so that when a carcass is condemned the head, viscera and blood can also be retrieved for condemnation. There should be provision of detained room side by of inspection site.
4. There should be sufficient natural light along with artificial light of 540 lux (50ft candle) in intensity without any distortion. Natural light always considered better than artificial.

5. There must be one or more hand washing units with a supply of hot and cold water.

6. The post-mortem examination should be carried out in systemic and hygienic manner without omitting any part of the carcass, blood and organs.

7. Always use sterilized knives, saw, cleavers etc for post mortem examination. So there should be a facility of sterilizers for the complete immersion of these instruments. Sterilization of knives and other instruments can be achieved by dipping them in boiling water for 30 minutes or heating the knife for 10-15 minutes in oil, liquid petroleum jelly or glycerine at a temperature of 120^0C to 130^0C. But sterilization of anthrax contaminated knives requires special consideration and it will be better to dispose such knives.

8. Visual examination of carcass should be done properly followed by palpation and if necessary incise the part, carcass or organ but always avoid unnecessary cuts on carcass and glands.

9. The carcass of emergency slaughtered animals should not be passed for consumption before laboratory examination.

10. As per the recent government norm one veterinarian can inspect only 96 adult carcasses in a day.

11. The suspected cases of zoonotic diseases must be inspected with great and confirmation may be done by laboratory test if deemed fit.

12. In PM examination, lymphnodes are exposed and examined by palpation for size and consistency and if necessary, incised to observe colour and detection of lesions. It is because lymphnodes drains different parts of body and indicates real condition of a particular organ and part of the body. But proper knowledge of topography and normal appearance of lymph nodes (colour, shape, size etc.) in a particular animal is of paramount importance. Swelling, enlargement or discolouration of a lymph node indicates pathological conditions. Some lymph nodes which drain lymph from important muscles are of special interest in meat inspection and these are referred as meat lymph node. Meat lymph nodes in cattle and buffalo are pre-scapular, axillary, pre-femoral, ischiatic, popliteal while in pigs are pre-femoral and popliteal.

13. There should be the proper marking of fit and unfit meat in PM examination. Marking indicates the inspection of carcass/part/organ and provide guarantee to the consumers about its wholesomeness.

It also prevents substitution of sound meat/carcass/ organs with diseased ones and serves the ready means of identification of meat. Identification can be done using clip, paper or plastic tie-on-bands, stick-on-tickets, plastic studs, injection of small plastic or cellulose fastner holding paper or plastic. In Australia it can be performed by sticking gelatin strip.

The use of metal or hard rubber stamp is a common method of carcass identification. As per USDA or FDA rules, purple GL-1 vegetable dye is considered safe for carcass identification. In India, marking on carcass and viscera is generally done by using various types of dyes which are cheap, non-corrosive in nature. Marking of meat is done by using a stamp or branding or by labeling but commonly metal stamp dipped in a stamping ink is used. A solution of 1 to 2% fuchsine in acetic acid is used as stamping ink for carcasses. Alternatively, it can be prepared by using methyl violet 35 g, can sugar 450 g, ethyl alcohol 1363 ml and water 1636 ml. Sugar is first dissolved in water and methyl violet is added at the end. Stamping is generally done on head in live animals and on carcasses or viscera where it can retain for longer time.

Meat lymph nodes

Meat lymph nodes as discussed earlier are important in post mortem examination of carcass. The normal location, size, shape, colour, texture, consistency is utmost important to judge the condition of a particular part/carcass/organ. Since particular lymph nodes contain the drain of that organ/carcass part so it clearly indicates the normality and abnormality of that organ. The important lymph nodes for post mortem examination may be categorized as:

1. **Lymph nodes of forelimb:** there are number of lymph nodes in forelimb but prescapular and axillary has major role in PM examination. Prescapular lymph nodes are in pair on each side of outer surface of carcass embedded in fat. Location wise it is about a hand breadth in front of shoulder joint. Axillary lymph node is also termed as brachial lymph node and also in pair on each side of carcass between scapula and space between first and second rib about midway of vertebral column and sternum.
2. **Lymph node of abdomen region:** the major lymph node of abdomen region is prefemoral or precrural and present in pair on outer surface of each side of carcass. It is also embedded in fat and can be exposed by making an incision on edge of tensor fascialata about 18 cm down to apex of muscle.

3. **Lymph nodes of pelvic region:** ischiatic lymph node has major importance in post mortem examination. It lies on both side of the carcass at outer aspect of sacrosciatic ligament. It can be exposed by making a deep incision on vertical line midway between posterior part of ischium and sacrum.
4. **Lymph nodes of hind limb:** the major lymph node of hind limb is popliteal which accounts great importance in post mortem examination. It's paired lymph node and each one lies in deep of popliteal space in the round of carcass. It can also be palpated immediately above and behind the stifle joint in embedded fat.

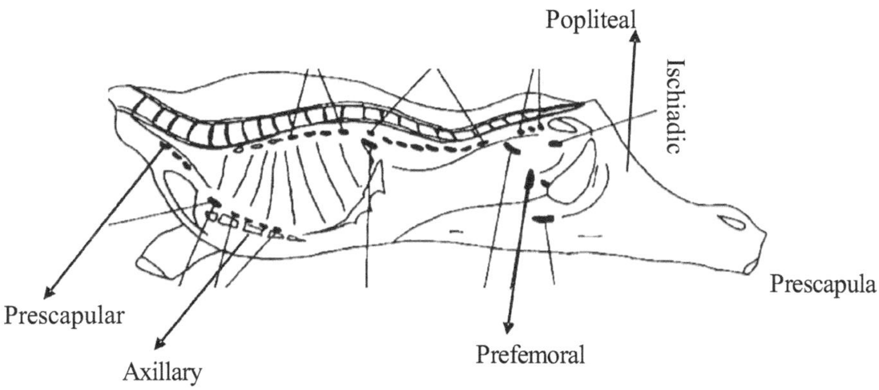

Figure 1 Lymph nodes of PM Value

In pigs prefemoral can be palpated in abdominal region same as in large animals. However, popliteal is more superficial and lies in midline equidistant from point of hock and anus.

Indication of lymph nodes in various conditions/diseases

Condition/disease	Observed changes
Normal	Normal colour of lymph node in most of the animal is white/grayish blue or almost black but pigs lymph nodes are lobulated and white in colour with the exception of reddish colour lymph nodes of head and neck region.
Anthracosis	Grey or blue but this colour is also common in lymph nodes of older animals
Congestion and imperfect bleeding	Red
Fatty infiltration	Yellow

Parasitic Eosinophilia	Green
Actinobacillosis	Abscess in parotid and submaxillary lymph nodes
Anthrax	*Pharyngeal form*- red and swollen mandibullar and retro pharyngeal lymph node *Septicaemic form*- engorged
Oedema	All lymph nodes appear edematous
Salmonellosis	Enlarge, edematous and haemorrhagic mesenteric lymph node
Haemorrhagic Enterotoxaemia	Red and swollen mesenteric lymph node
Tuberculosis (TB)	Presence of tubercular granulomas in bronchial and mediastinal lymph nodes but may be seen in any lymph node. In pigs- miliary tubercles in submaxillary, cervical, bronchial, mediastinal and mesenteric lymph nodes
Para tuberculosis	Pale, firm and enlarged mesenteric lymph node with prominent serosal surface
Pleuro pneumonia in pigs	Inflamed and haemorrhagic bronchial lymph node
Swine erysipelas	Swollen and haemorrhagic lymph nodes
Caseous lymphadenitis	Presence of central mass of laminated caseative necrosis surrounded by a wall of connective tissue in prescapular, prefemoral, popliteal, bronchial and mediastinal lymph node.

Post-mortem Principles

Careful post mortem examination is basically depends on four basic principles i.e visual perception, palpation, incision and laboratory test. However, the choice of principle to be adopted depends on conditions of carcass and suspect of diseases. Incision should always be avoided except where it deemed necessary.

1. *Visual perception:* First step in post mortem examination is to observe the carcass and visceral organs thoroughly by human senses. It should be examined visually for visible abnormalities which may include colour changes, atrophy, hypertrophy, neoplastic condition etc.
2. *Palpation:* In case of doubt in visual perception then carcass and/or organs being examined by palpation for changes in consistency, sliminess or gelation, cyst etc.

3. *Incisions:* Incision over carcass/organs is a last resort and it should be done when deemed necessary. It should be done to examine parasites, structural deformity or to observe any systemic disease etc.

4. *Laboratory tests:* In case of suspect and disease condition not clearly diagnosed at abattoir may be supported with laboratory tests. The carcass or part of carcass or organ should not be disposed before the findings of laboratory. The suitable masses or sample should be sent to the laboratory for accurate findings.

Order of Post-mortem examination

There should always follow a definite pattern of post mortem examination to get good results and to diagnose the disease or condition in carcass and/or organs. The pattern of post mortem examination for various animal carcasses may be summarized as:

System	Organs	Observations to be considered
Cattle/buffalo carcass		
General examinations	-	Verify the number, age and sex of animal. Examine the carcass exterior, cut surfaces of bones, pleura, perotonium and diaphragm for efficiency of bleeding, colour, cleanliness, odour, and evidence of bruises. Examination of injuries and bruises. Bruise of 24 hrs old - dark colour Bruise of 24-38 hrs old - Watery condition Bruise of 3 day + - Rusty orange colour and soapy to touch Observations on inflammation, abscesses and T.B. lesions in thoracic and abdominal cavities. Triceps brachii muscle for *Cysticercus bovis* If T.B. lesions are detected in viscera then main carcass lymph nodes must be examined.
Head examination	Outer covering and eyes	For deformity and disease conditions

	Gums, lips and tongue	FMD, necrotic and other forms of stomatitis, actinomycosis and actinobacillosis.
	Internal and external Masseter muscle parallel to lower jaw	*Cysticercus bovis*
	Retropharyngeal, Submaixllary and Parotid lymph nodes.	T.B. lesions, abscesses and actinobacillosis
Visceral organs	Lungs	Visual examination and palpation for pleurisy, pneumonia, tuberculosis, fascioliasis and hydatid cysts. Bronchial and medistinal lymph nodes for T.B. lesions. Palpation for tumors, abscesses.
	Heart	Pericardium for traumatic or tubercular pericarditis. Incision on heart ventricles for petechial hemorrhages, cysticerci and hydatid cyst on epicardium and endocardium. Myocardium for Liguatulae and Flabby condition. Flabby condition is an indicative of septic conditions.
	Liver	Visual examination for fatty changes, abscesses, telangiectasis, hydated cysts, actinobacillosis, *Cysticercus bovis*, linguatulae and larval stage of *Oesophagostomum radiatum*. Incision on thin portion of left lobe of liver for fascioliasis.
	Oesophagus, stomach and intestines	Serous surface for T.B. lesions, actinobacillosis and anterior aspect of reticulum for foreign body.
	Spleen	T.B. lesions, anthrax, hematoma and infarcts.
	Uterus	Septic conditions.
	Udder	Supramammary lymph nodes for T. B. lesions and abscesses.
	Kidney and Urinanary bladder	Defects, calculi and disease condition.
	Testicles	Outer surface, substance and superficial inguinal lymph node.

Calves		
General examination	Mouth and tongue	FMD and calf diphtheria.
	Abomasums	Peptic ulcers.
	Small intestine	Calf scour and dysentery.
	Liver, portal and posterior lymph nodes	Congenital T.B.
	Lungs, kidneys and spinal cord	Melanotic deposits.
	Umbilicus and joints	Septic omphalophlebitis.
	Hock joint	Synovial fluid consistency
	Renal fat	Colour and consistancy
Pigs		
General examination	Muscles, tongue and submaxillary lymph node	*Trichinella spirallis* by Trichinoscope.
	External massater muscle and route of tongue	*Cysticercus cellulosae*
	Skin	Erysipelas, swine fever, urticaria and shorty eruption.
	Tail	Necrosis
	Feet	Abscess
	Udder	Actinomycosis
	Submaxillary, bronchial and mediastinal lymph nodes	T.B and abscess
	Liver	Cirrhosis.
Sheep and Goat		
General examination	Carcass	Satisfactory bleeding and setting
	Head (lips, gums and nasal cavities)	Contagious ecthyma.
	Lungs	Hydatid cyst and nematodes
	Liver	Fascioliasis
	Bile duct	Fluke infestation
Equines		
General examination	Major lymph nodes	Systemic diseases, T.B. lesions, mullein test positive animals

	Thorough examination of mucous membrane, trachea, larynx, nasal cavity, sinus and their ramification	Suspected cases of glanders
	Spinous processes of thoracic vertebrae, supraspinous bursa, and first two cervical vertebrae	Fistulous conditions.
	Liver and lungs	Echinococcal cysts
	Muscles	Melanosis
	Axillary and subscapular tissues of white and gray horses	Melanosis.
Poultry		
General examination	First stage examination	Whole carcass examination after defeathering and washing of obvious disease, fractures, injuries, blood, blisters etc.
	Second stage examination	Body cavity of dressed bird is opened through transverse incision and visceral organs are drawn out and examined.
Systemic examination	Carcass	Diseases, bone abnormalities, wounds, muscular atrophy, tumors etc.
	Liver	Consistency, texture, lesions and colour changes.
	Spleen	Texture and abnormalities.
	Hock joint	Sinusitis

Note: The systemic examination in all animals is almost similar but some specific conditions as mentioned above should be examined specifically during post mortem examination.

Special conditions requires extended post-mortem examination

Carcass of buffalo/cattle is further examined if:

1. *Cysticercus bovis* (measly beef) condition is observed. In measly beef condition cysts may be seen in carcass, cheek muscle, tongue, diaphragm and heart. If more than ten clear or degenerated cysts are recovered accompanied by emaciation then total condemnation. Otherwise carcass/part/organ are passed with instructions of proper cooking.
2. Tuberculosis (T.B.) suspected cases are also requires further examination of carcass/parts/organs. In case of single T.B. lesion, carcass should be split and vertebrae, ribs etc are closely examined alongwith lower cervical and prefemoral lymph nodes. Generalized T.B. conditions require total condemnation. To declare Generalized T.B, any two of following organs and concerned lymph nodes should be affected i.e. lungs, spleen, kidney, uterus, udder, ovary, testicles, adrenal glands, brain, spinal cords etc. During declaration of generalized tuberculosis muscles, bones and joints should also be included. If local parts are affected with TB than local condemnation is generally recommended.

In pigs further examination is recommended when Trichinosis or T.B is diagnosed.

1. In case of Trichinosis, small pieces of tissues from diaphragm and muscle of larynx, abdomen and intercostals space are examined under Trichinoscope after pre-digestion with trypsin. Local condition requires local condemnation while carcass with heavy infestation recommended for total condemnation.
2. In generalized cases of tuberculosis in pigs, carcass and head are split; bone surfaces and spinal cord are examined. On observation of generalized T.B., total condemnation is recommended. If localalized head T.B. is declared than local condemnation of head alongwith associated lymph nodes are generally followed.

Post-mortem judgements

The final judgment in post mortem examination is based on total evidence observed by competent veterinarian on fate of carcass and its offal. The decision should be based on visual observations, palpation, incisions, smell, ante-mortem signs and results of laboratory tests, if any. The statement of judgment may be either of the following:

i. Fit for human consumption.

ii. Unfit for human consumption or total condemnation.

iii. Partial condemnation when affected organs are condemned and rest is passed for human consumption.

iv. Conditionally passed for human consumption as free bank system. Carcass/parts/organs may be approved for human consumption with conditions, distribution restricted to limited or small amount to a consumer with instruction.

In general, following conditions/diseases requires total condemnation of carcass:

i. *Diseases*: Generalized actinobacillosis and actinomycosis, black leg, generalized tuberculosis, generalized lymphadenitis, glanders, rabies, tetanus, acute salmonellosis, acute brucellosis, swine erysipelas, botulism, speticaemia, pyemia.

ii. *Conditions*: Bronchopneumonia, pleurisy, peritonitis, metritis, mastitis, arthritis, pericorditis, enteritis, meningo-encephalomylitis, generalized sarcocystosis, cysticercosis, trichinosis, advanced anaemia and emaciation, multiple tumors or abscesses or injuries, fevered carcasses, serious anomalies of colour, smell, consistency or taste.

iii. Still born or unborn carcasses with advanced anaemia and emaciation.

Post-Mortem Judgements in important conditions

Name of condition	Specific findings	Laboratory tests	Judgement
Imperfect bleeding	Generally seen if animal is moribund (dying) or very distressed. Characterized by dark colour meat due to capillary bleeding. Organs, particularly liver, lungs and kidneys are dark and congested and blood running can observe. The intercostals veins are easily discernible and full of blood. Carcass sets badly and decomposes rapidly. Tucked up condition of forelegs is often observed.	Malachite green test	Total Condemnation.

Bruising	Fresh bruise is actually reddish and haemorrhagic and remains same for about 10 hours. After 10 hrs and upto 24 hrs it remains blue or dark purple. 24 to 38 hrs bruise will show the watery consistency. The bruise of 3+days old shows rusty orange colour and soapy to the touch. Skin is not broken in a bruise as with a scrape or cut there is no risk of infection. However, meat appearance is greatly affected.	Bilirubin test	Extensive and severe bruising leads to total condemnation otherwise affected parts are condemned.
Abnormal odours	Abnormal odours may be seen due to male sexual odour, drug administration, diet, off odour absorption, catty odour due to lacquering and paint, ketosis, B.Q., gangrene and putrefaction. Diet with fish meal, drugs administered shortly before slaughter, e.g. linseed oil, turpentine, ether, chloroform, aromatic spirits of ammonia, etc. Absorption of the off odour durig storage like over-ripe oranges or citrus fruit. Catty odours in meat may be seen due to presence of mesityl oxide. It is common on exposure of paint thinners and solvents, in lacquers, adhesives, flooring compounds and plastic wrapping materials. Sexual odour is principally noticed in mature boars and male deer in rut. It is mainly due to presence of a steroid, androstenone in fat. Boar salivary glands on boiling in water give off a musty smell. Buck goat meat has an unpleasant smell and probably conveyed by hand during skinning and similar to the skin smell of buck. Carcass with acetonaemia or	Boiling test	Pronounced smell is liable to total condemnation

	ketosis gives peculiar sweet smell owing to the presence of acetone in tissues. The liver may be fatty with a strong smell of acetone. Specific disease, e.g. blackquarter which causes a cheesy smell, nasty smell in pigs, Specific type of smell is observed in gangrene and putrefaction of carcass/organs		
Fevered flesh	Characterized by dark coloured meat with small, scattered haemorrhages. Pleura, peritoneum and fat shows diffused redness with congested organs and lymph nodes. The carcass as a whole has a dull red appearance.	-	Total Condemnation
Emaciation	Characterized by wasting of muscular tissue with very less soft and wet fat which may turn to gelatinous mass in advanced cases. Carcass does not set and flesh is wet, soft and flabby. Freshly cut surface of muscles pit on pressure and are soft and sticky to touch. Pleura, peritoneum and brisket are considered wet areas in bovines while ewes' kidney fat gives a good indication.	Setting and dry out condition within 12 –24 hours. Water protein ratio estimation	Total Condemnation
Dropsy/ Oedema	Characterized by excessive accumulation of a clear fluid very similar to lymph in the tissues or serous sacs of the body. Local oedema is called inflammatory oedema which is mainly due to obstruction of vein or around an inflammatory area. Generalized oedema is a result of cardiac and renal diseases as well as chronic wasting diseases i.e. tuberculosis, Jöhne's disease, parasitic diseases etc.		If generalized, condition total condemnation

Haema-toma	Solid swelling of clotted blood within tissue due to physical injury.	-	Condemnation of affected parts
Inflam-mation	As a result of defense mechanism against injury caused by bacteria or their toxins, parasites, chemicals, heat or cold, or mechanical damage etc. Inflammation may be characterized as heat, pain, redness, swelling and disturbance of function.	-	Total condemnation in evidence of systemic infection otherwise condemnation of affected parts.
Jaundice or icterus	Characterized by yellow coloured body tissues particularly white tissues i.e. fat, skin of pigs, spinal cord and meninges, tendon sheaths and white of the eye. The colouration of body tissues is mainly due to deposition of bile pigments that have been absorbed into the bloodstream. Condition leads to liver cirrhosis, particularly in pigs, bile ducts blockage by calculi, tumours or parasites etc. Specific diseases which are responsible for destruction of blood corpuscles by infective organisms i.e. leptospirosis in pigs and red-water in cattle.	Bilirubin test	Total Condemnation
Necrosis	Characterized by death of a tissue/ organ/part whilst still in the animal body.	-	Condemnation of affected parts
Pyaemia	Pyaemia is a result of pus-producing (pyogenic) organisms in bloodstream and form multiple abscesses throughout the body. Abscesses are mostly seen in lungs, kidneys and liver.	-	Total condemnation
Gangrene	In gangrene, necrotic tissues are in vaded by putrefactive bacteria. It occurs most frequently in tissues liable to contamination, i.e. skin, lungs, intestine, vagina and uterus and in those tissues implicated in	-	Gangrene with evidence of toxaemia leads to total condemnation while affected

	penetrating wounds. In advanced cases tissues become livid, purplish or greenish and then brownish-black but often accompanied by emphysema and a foul odour.		parts are condemned in localized conditions.
Enteritis	Inflammation of stomach and intestinal tract. Dehydration, tucked up abdomen in chronic form.	-	Acute- Total condemnation Chronic- Total condemnation when systemic infection, otherwise condemnation of affected parts.
Anaemia	Pale mucous membrane. Enlargement of liver.	-	Total condemnation when emaciation
Malignant tumors	Uncontrolled growth in multiple organs. Dehydration and emaciation.	-	Total condemnation
Melanosis	Melanin deposition in different parts of body.	-	Total condemnation in generalized condition otherwise passed conditionally
Metritis	Inflamed uterine membrane. Purulent discharge from uterus.	-	Total condemnation in acute and septic otherwise local condemnation
Peritonitis	Inflamed peritoneum.	-	Total condemnation in acute, diffused septic otherwise local condemnation

Perico-rditis	Inflamed pericardium. Haemorrhages may be seen on pericardium.	-	Total condemnation in septic condition otherwise local condemnation
Pneum-onia	Inflamed lung tissues. Tucked up condition.	-	Total condemnation if gangrenous otherwise removal of lung
Rickets and osteody-trophia	Enlarged extremities of long bones with bending shafts. Bony swellings.	-	Total condemnation when carcass is emaciated and foul smelling otherwise passed conditionally
Poisonings	According to the poison involvement. Haemorrhages on vital organs.	Chemical testing for poison	Total condemnation

Post-mortem judgments in important animal diseases

Name of condition	Causative agent	Affected animals	Specific findings	Laboratory tests	Judgement
Actinobacillosis	*Actinobacillus lignieresi.*	Cattle	It typically affects soft tissues and usually spread through lymphatic and regional lymph nodes. Small nodules about 1 cm in diameter can easily be seen on lateral surfaces and dorsum of the tongue. Some nodules may erode through the surface, causing ulcers. In chronic form marked development of fibrous tissue is observed which causes enlargement and hardening of the tongue that typical condition is called 'wooden tongue'.	-	In generalized condition carcass and offals are condemned. Otherwise condemnation of affected organs.
Actinomycosis	*Actinomyces bovis.*	Cattle	Commonly known as 'lumpy jaw'. Characterized by osteomyelitis and affects bones of lower jaw but upper jaw is seldom affected. The bones becomes thick and enlarge and on cross section appear honeycomb like small abscesses and suppurative tracts.	-	Total condemnation in generalized condition. Otherwise condemnation of affected parts.

			Fistulae connect surrounding tissues and discharging into mouth or onto the skin of the jaw. Involvement of regional lymph nodes is not common.		
Anthrax	*Bacillus anthracis*	Cattle, sheep and pigs	Anthrax is a notifiable disease. Unclotted blood from natural orifices. Typical lesion is splenomagaly. Mucous membranes show swelling and extensive petechial lesions. Pale and friable kidney and liver.	Ascoli test	Total Condemnation. Disinfection of premises and disposal of the carcass – either by burning or by burying at least 2 metres from the surface with layers of 30 cm of lime above and below the carcass. PM is generally not recommended.
Blackquarter	*Clostridium chauvaei*	Cattle and occasionally in sheep, goat and deer	Infiltration of yellow gelatinous substance in connective tissues which may be haemorrhagic and gassy. Blackish-red muscle with oedematous appearance at the periphery of swelling and appears dry and spongy due to gas spaces in centre. Strong smell like rancid butter	-	Total Condemnation.

			or cheese observed in muscles. Enlarged and haemorrhagic lymph nodes.		
Bovine Viral Diarrhea (BVD)	BVD Virus	Calves and cattle	Ulcers in mouth. Abortion. Complicated with mucosal disease.	–	Total Condemnation.
Brucellosis	*Brucella abortus* in cattle, *Br. suis* in pigs and *Br. melitensis* in goats.	Cattle, pigs and goats	Abortion is a common feature. Pregnant uterus is predilection site and fetus is usually aborted during ^{7th} or ^{8th} month of pregnancy. Fetus generally appears oedematous with blood-tinged subcutaneous fluid. Cotyledons become necrotic, soft, yellow-grey covered with brown exudates. Characteristic clumps of pus between uterine membrane and fetal membrane. Bovine testicle may also be affected.	Abortus bang ring test	Condemnation of genital organs, mammary glands and associated lymph nodes.
Calf diphtheria	*Bacteroides necrophorus*	Young calves	Characterized by evil-smelling diphtheritic patches and ulcers in mouth, tongue, gums and pharynx. Intestinal lesions with septic bronchopneumonia.	–	Total Condemnation.

Caseous lympha-denitis	*Corynebacterium ovis*	Sheep and goats	Generally found in frozen imported lamb carcasses. Enlargement of affected lymph nodes with greenish-yellow gelatinous pus. Later it dries and become paler but in older lesions pus becomes laminated like layers of an onion.	-	Generalized condition- total condemnation. Otherwise condemnation of affected parts.
Foot and mouth disease	Most contagious animal diseases caused by seven major types are A, O, C, SAT 1, SAT 2, SAT 3 and Asia 1.	Cattle, pigs, sheep, goats, deer and hogs	Vesicles or blisters from pinhead to a half of walnut in mouth, tongue, cheeks, gums and dental pad. In pigs lesions may be seen on snout. Foot lesions are generally found at the junction of skin with the hoof and between the claws. In females on teats and skin of udder. Sometimes on muzzle, nostrils, inside the vagina and on the skin of pigs.	-	Total condemnation.
Glanders or farcy	*Burkholderia mallei*	Horse, ass and mule	It is a notifiable and contagious Mallein test disease. Characterized by enlargement of submaxillary lymph node and yellowish- brown blood-tinged nasal catarrh. In chronic glanders- lungs shows congestion, degenerated		Total condemnation.

			yellowish mass, shot-like grey nodules of pea size. Farcy is a skin form of glanders in which nodules resembles knotted cords. Cutaneous nodes suppurate, ulcerate and discharge a purulent material particularly on limbs and lower part of the belly.		
Jöhne's disease (paratuberculosis)	*Mycobacterium johnei.*	Cattle, sheep, farmed deer and goats	Disease in cattle is characterized by 3-4 times thickened than normal or thick ropes like intestinal mucous membrane with corrugations. It may also affect ileum, caecum, colon and rectum. Sheep and goat carcass shows caseation which is not found in cattle and deer. The mesenteric lymph nodes are enlarged and oedematous. Carcass is typically emaciated; dead white appearance of fat lacks lustre and tends to be wet and sloppy especially at brisket. Muscles pit on pressure.	-	Condemnation of intestine and mesentery However, decision is depending upon degree of emaciation and oedema and setting of carcass. Detain carcass for 12–24 hours to judge the set and wet condition. In Jöhne's carcass remains wet and does not set.
Leptospirosis	*Leptospira interrogans* can	Cattle, sheep, deer, pigs	Jaundice and abortion is main feature of Leptospirosis.	-	Total condemnation.

	affect all animals. *L. occid* in cattle, *L. hardjo* in sheep, *L. hebdomadis,* *L. australis* and *L. occid* in deer, *L. sejroe*, *L. occidi,* *L. icterohaemorr-hagica* and *L. ballum*; in pigs, *L. icterohaemorr-hagica*, *L. occid* and *L. canicola*.				
Listeriosis	*Listeria monocytogenes*	Cattle, sheep, goat and pigs	Almost all animals are affected by and cause abortion in sheep and cattle. Characterized by encephalitis, necrosis in liver, spleen, heart, mucosae of digestive tract and uterus.	-	Total condemnation.
Q- fever (Query fever)	*Coxiella burnetti*	Sheep and cattle	Abortion is main feature and highest risk is to fetal membrane.	-	Total condemnation.
Rabies	Rhabdovirus	All mammals	Rabies is a notifiable acute infective disease. Degenerative changes in brain.	Seller's staining and Negri Body detection	Total condemnation. PM is generally not recommended.

Salmonellosis (Paratyphoid)	*Salmonella occid*, *S. typhimurium*, *S. enteritidis* and *S. occidi suis*	Cattle, sheep, goats, pigs and reptiles	Multiple submucosal or subserosal haemorrhages and sometimes necrotizing fibrous enteritis.	-	Total condemnation when acute infection.
Scrapie	Virus-like particle (Prion)	Sheep and goats	It is a fatal notifiable disease. Characterized by slow progressive degeneration of central nervous system (CNS).	-	Total condemnation.
Strangles	*Streptococcus equi*	Horse	Characterized by abscess in lymph nodes of head, particularly in the submaxillaries and rarely in lungs, liver, spleen and kidneys.		Total condemnation in widespread condition otherwise head condemnation.
Swine erysipelas	*Erysipelothrix rhusiopathiae.*	Pigs	Acute infectious disease. Characterized by septiceimia, petechial haemorrgaes on lungs, idneys and serous coverings of stomach and intestines.	-	Total condemnation in systemic involvement Otherwise conditionally passed after removal of skin and affected parts.
Swine fever	Toga virus	Pigs	Notifiable disease caused by a virus. Petechial haemorrhages on larynx, trachea, lungs, kidney, heart, digestive tract and bladder. Swelling on associated lymph nodes.	-	Total condemnation.

Swine vesicular disease	SVD Virus	Pigs	Notifiable disease. Vesicular lesions up to 2 cm on the feet, lips, snout and tongue.		Total condemnation
Tetanus	*Clostridium tetani*	Sheep and cattle	Ante-mortem is important because no typical lesions in PM examination. However, it can be diagnosed by petechial haemorrhages on serous membrane of heart. Congestion and oedema on lungs.	Toxin-antitoxin neutralization test	Total condemnation
Tuberculosis	*Mycobacterium `bovis, M. tuberculosis, M. avium*	Cattle, sheep, goats, pigs, birds	Caseous and calcified foci on lungs. Pinhead or barley grain size caseous and calcified masses in liver. Pearls or grapes like caseous masses in pleurisy. Yellow granulation in ribs, vertebrae. Tubercles in spleen and peritoneum.	Ziel-Nielsen staining	Total condemnation and destruction of carcass and organs in generalized T.B. with emaciation. If localized condemnation of affected parts and lymph nodes.
Rinderpaste (R.P.)	Paramyxo virus	Cattle but sheep, goat and pigs may be affected	Necrotic foci with red erosions on mouth, muzzle and digestive tract. Soft grey plaques in mucous membranes of mouth cavity resembling sprinkled bran or	-	Total condemnation.

			soft cheese. Zebra markings in intestine.		
Haemorrhgic Septicemia (H.S.)	*Pasteurella multocida.*	Cattle	Clear yellowish fluid in subcutaneous tissues of head and throat. Petechial haemorrhages on whole body, organs and lymph nodes.	Bipolar organism in Leishman's stain	Total condemnation.
Sheep pox	Pox virus	Sheep	Eruption of vesicles and pustules around cheeks, eyes, lips, inner portion of thigh, belly and tail with degenerative crust.	-	Total condemnation.
Blue tongue	Orbivirus	Sheep, cattle and goats	Inflamed mouth cavity with ulcers. Erosion and necrosis of dental pad. Blue and enlarged tongue. Generalized oedema and necrosis of skeletal and cardiac muscles.	-	Total condemnation if emaciation and extensive lesions. Otherwise local condemnation.
Bovine Spongiform Encephal-opathy (BSE)	Prion	Cattle	Degenerative changes in central nervous system and vacuoles in brain.	-	Total condemnation.
Botulism	*Clostridium botulinum.*	Cattle, sheep and goats	Haemorrhages on gut, heart and brain. Toxins and carriage material in intestines.	-	Total condemnation.

Ascariasis	*Ascaris suum or Ascaris lumbricoides.*	Pigs	Long worms of yellowish-white in colour in small intestine of the pig but it may also be seen in stomach, large intestine and bile ducts.	-	Condemnation of 'milk spot' livers.
Trichiniasis	*Trichinella spiralis*	Pigs	Presence of Trichinae in musculature of pillar, coastal portion of diaphragm, tongue, larynx, abdominal and intercostal muscles. Numerous calcified white specks in meat and produces gritty sound on cutting.	Muscle biopsy	Total condemnation.
Dog Taeiniasis	*Taenia hydatigena*	Dogs	It is 5 m in long tapeworm generally occurs in small intestine.	-	In generalized condition organs and tissues condemnation like omentum, livers, haemorrhagic or degenerated 'tenuicollis tracks'. In mild cases only cysts removal.
Sheep and goat Tae iniasis	*Taenia ovis*	Sheep and goats	Tapeworm grows in dog intestine to about 1m long with very small head and contains 24–36 hooks. Its intermediate stage is found in sheep and goat known as	-	Condemnation of affected parts

			Cysticercus ovis. It is measuring 3–8 mm, ovoid in shape and contains single scolex. It's generally located in heart just under the epicardium but may also found in diaphragm, skeletal muscles, tongue, masseter muscles and oesophagus.		
Cattle Taeiniasis (Measly beef)	*Taenia saginata* *(Cysticercus bovis)*	Cattle	Adult worm found in small intestine of humans whereas the intermediate stage, *Cysticercus bovis*, is found in cattle. Its 4–10 m long tapeworm and their head have four elliptical suckers and no hooks, no arms. The predilection sites are the masseter muscles, heart, tongue, shoulder and diaphragm muscles. However, cysts can occur in any muscle as well as liver and lungs.	-	Presence of C. *bovis* of any stage is liable to condemn affected part and preserve rest of the carcass and offal at-7°C for 3 weeks or -10°C for 14 days. Passed conditionally with cooking instructions after cyst removal.
Pig Taeiniasis (Measly pork)	*Taenia solium* *(Cysticercus-cellulosae)*	Man, pigs, occasionally humans and rarely in sheep and dogs.	Tapeworm of man small intestine measuring 3–8 m length with a typical scolex having double row of 26–28 hooks. The intermediate stage is called *Cysticercus cellulosae* found in pigs. Predilection sites of cysts are deep	-	Total condemnation.

			muscles of thigh (Triceps brachi), muscle of heart, diaphragm, tongue, neck, shoulder, abdomen and intercostals. However, viscera can also be infected. Cysts number may be up to 3000 per 0.5 kg of muscle and can be detected after 8 weeks of infection. Cysts may be degenerated, caseated and calcified.		
Fasciolosis	*Fasciola hepatica*	Cattle and sheep	Common liver fluke of grayish brown colour, leaf-shaped, broader anteriorly than posteriorly. Anterior portion is with cone-shaped projection with a pair of broad 'shoulders'. Acute case is characterized acute swelling and congestion of liver with haemorrages and fibrin on liver capsule followed by necrotic liver tissue and immature flukes. Chronic fascioliasis in sheep exhibited distorted liver, enlarged, thickened and bluish bile ducts. Flukes may reach to number over 1000.	-	Condemnation of affected organs. Sheep with emaciation andoedematous condition leads to total condemnation.

			Sheep carcasses are often emaciated and oedematous while cattle liver shows cirrhosis and bile ducts becomes thickened, dilated and eventually calcified and condition is typical termed as 'pipy' or 'fluky' liver.		
Sarcocystosis	*Sarcocystis bovis*	Cattle	Frequently present in skeletal and heart muscles. Haemorrhages in muscle and brain.		Total condemnation in involvement of musculature and visible to naked eyes. Otherwise local condemnation.
Hydatidiosis	*Echinococcus granulosus*	Sheep, cattle and pigs	Tapeworm looks same as the organs. Predilection sites are liver in sheep and pigs while lungs in cattle. Clear fluid in central cavity. Connective tissue enlargement and covering of fibrous wall.	-	Condemnation of liver and lungs and destroyed.
Pimply gut	*Oesophagostomum* spp.	Sheep, goats and cattle	Pin head to pea size grayish white nodules in mucous membranes of intestines, colon and caecum.	-	Condemnation of intestines.

Post-mortem judgments in important poultry conditions/diseases

Coccidiosis	*Eimeria* spp.	Mammals and birds	It's a parasitic disease affects epithelium of the intestine and the bile ducts. Haemorrhages on duodenal mucosa with coagulated and necrotic mass.	-	Total condemnation in emaciated and oedematous condition.
Ascitis or dropsy	-	Poultry	Excessive fluid in body cavities. Green coloured putrefaction around vent.	-	Total condemnation.
Ornithosis/ Psittacosis	Chlamydia	Birds of parrot family	Enlarged liver and spleen, sacculities, pneumonia and pericorditis.	-	Total condemnation in active form.
Fowl typhoid	*Salmonella gallinarum*	Fowl, ducks, geese, Turkey, game and wild birds	Bronze coloured congested liver, brownish lung, congested spleen and jaundice of carcass.	-	Total condemnation.
Marek's disease (Fowl Paralysis)	Herpes virus	Domestic Poultry	Neoplastic leukaemia like disease. Small lymphoid tumors in viscera skin and muscles. Enlargement of bursa fabricious.	-	Total condemnation.
New castle disease	Paramyxovirus	Chickens, turkey, ducks, pigeons and wild birds	Notifiable infectious disease. Cyanotic comb and wattle. Inflamed air sac and trachea. Petechial haemorrhages on	-	Total condemnation.

			heart, proventriculus, ovary, gizzard and sternum.		
Gumboro (Infectious Bursal Disease)	IBD virus	Broiler chicken	Enlarged, inflamed and inspissated abscess in bursa.	-	Total condemnation.
Gout	Urates deposition in joints	Domestic fowl	White dry non purulent uric acid salt deposition in joints of feet and legs. Visceral gout may be seen in liver and heart.	-	Total condemnation in visceral gout. Otherwise local condemnation.
Avian in fluenza (Fowl Plaque)	*Myxovirus influenzae*	Domestic fowl, turkeys, geese, ducks, wild birds,	Purple and blue comb and wattle. Oedema of head and neck.	-	Total condemnation and destroyed at once.
Tuberculosis	*Mycobacterium aviam*	Poultry	Well marked emaciation with whitish yellow nodules on liver, spleen and intestines. Lungs are rarely affected. No calcification observed.	-	Total condemnation.
Pseudo Tuberculosis	*Yersinia pseudotuberculosis*	Rodents and birds	Necrotic nodules and enlargement of liver and spleen.	-	Total condemnation in generalized condition.
Lymphoid leukosis (Big liver disease)	*LL-RNA virus*	Chickens	Cancerous tumors on bursa fabricius. Secondary tumors in livers.	-	Total condemnation.

Myeloid leukosis	*Fowl sarcoma virus*	Fowl	Morocco leather like liver. Nodular discrete tumors in spleen, kidney and body cavity.	-	Total condemnation.
Bacillary White Diarrhea (Pullorum Disease)	*Salmonella pullorum*	Fowls	Enlarged liver with necrotic foci. Discoloured, shrunken and sometimes cystic ova. Enlarged kidney and heart with pericorditis and myocorditis.	-	Total condemnation.
Pasteurellosis	*Pasteurella anatipestifer*	Ducks	Petechial haemorrhages on heart, proventriculus, sternum, gizzard and peritoneum. Necrotic foci on liver, exudative pericardial sac.	-	Total condemnation in septecaemic condition. Otherwise head condemnation.
Overscalding	High temperature scalding	Poultry	Flesh with cooked appearance.	-	Total condemnation.
Aspergillosis	*Aspergillus* fungus	Mammals and birds	Milliary to large nodules on pulmonary system, particularly on bronchi, thorax and abdominal air sac.	-	Total condemnation.

References

1. Geoffrey, W. (1995). Black's Veterinary Dictionary, 18th Ed. Jaypee Brothers, New Delhi.
2. Gracey, J.F and Collins,D.S. (1994). Meat plant construction, equipments and operations. *In:* Meat Hygiene, 9th ed., ELBS, U.K. Pp 168-177.
3. Sharma, B.D. (2003). Post mortem inspection of meat carcasses. *In:* Modern Abattoir Practices and Animal By-products Technology, First Edition, Jaypee Brothers Medical Publishers,New Delhi. Pp 45-61.
4. Sherikar, A.T., Bachhil, V.N. and Thapliyal, D.C. (2013). Post-mortem inspection. *In:* Elements of Veterinary Public Health, Second reprint, ICAR, New Delhi, Pp 181-201.

Chapter 6

Animal Slaughter Procedures and Ritual Slaughter Methods

Slaughter is an act of killing or destruction of animals for food purpose and includes all processes and operations on all such animals in order to prepare it for being slaughtered. It is an expert act requires expertise and willingness. Slaughter is necessarily to be performed in a slaughter house recognized or licensed by authority empowered under law for the time being in force to do so. Only authorized animals are to be slaughtered for food purpose and restricted animals or animals prohibited for slaughter should not be converted into meat in any case. Animals in pregnancy, has offspring less than three months or under the age of three months, animals not certified by veterinarian for fitness should never be slaughtered. Slaughterman should also have a valid license or authorization issued by municipal or other authority. The persons below eighteen years of age and suffering from communicable or infectious diseases shall not be permitted to slaughter an animal.

General Rules of Slaughter

As per the provisions given in Prevention of Cruelty to Animals (Slaughter House) Rules, 2000 by sub-section (1) of section 38 of the Prevention of Cruelty to Animals Act, 1960 (59 of 1960), under the notification of the Government of India in the Ministry of Social Justice and Empowerment number S.O. 1165 (E) dated the 26th December, 2000 in the Gazette of India, Extraordinary, Part II, Section 3, Sub Section (ii) dated the 27th December, 2000 following rules should be followed during slaughter of an animal for food production:

i. The slaughter house shall have a reception area of adequate size sufficient for livestock subject to veterinary inspection. A veterinarian can thoroughly examine not more than 12 animals in an hour and not more than 96 animals in a day and shall issue a fitness certificate as specified by Central Government or State Government.

ii. There should be a separate isolation pens for watering and feeding arrangements for animals suspected to be suffering from contagious and infectious diseases, and fractious animals, in order to segregate them from the remaining animals.

iii. No animal should be slaughtered in a slaughter house in sight of other beast waiting for slaughter. To ensure this condition separate sections of adequate dimensions sufficient for slaughter of individual animals must be provided.

iv. No animal should be administered any chemical, drug or hormone before slaughter except drug for its treatment for any specific disease or ailment. In case of treatment, withdrawal period of drug must be considered for final decision.

v. There should be separate space for stunning of animals prior to slaughter, bleeding and dressing of the carcasses to ensure good quality meat.

vi. There should be a knocking section in slaughter house particularly for ritual slaughter. It is because knocking section and dry landing area in a slaughter hall help to escape an operator without allowing the animal to pass the escape barrier.

vii. A curbed-in bleeding area of adequate size should be in slaughter house. So that blood could not be splashed on other animals being slaughtered or on the carcass being skinned. The drain and collection of blood should be immediate and proper.

viii. There should be the provision of floor wash point for intermittent cleaning and a hand-wash basin and knife sterilizer for the sticker to sterilize knife and wash his hands periodically.

ix. Carcass dressing should not be done on floor and adequate means and tools should be provided to facilitate immediate disposal of hides or skins. There should also be the facility of immediately transport of hide and skin from a slaughter house either in a closed wheelbarrow or by a chute provided with self-closing door.

x. There should also be the provision of immediate disposal of legs, horns, hooves and other parts of animals through spring load floor chutes or sidewall doors or closed wheelbarrows.

xi. There should be the provision of viscera inspection, hand washing, tool sterilisation and floor washing as well as contrivances for immediate separation and disposal of condemned material.

xii. There should be the sufficient facility of identification, inspection and correlation of carcass, viscera and head.

xiii. There should be the provision of curbed and separately drained area or an area of sufficient size, sloped 33 mm per metre to a floor drain, where the carcasses may be washed with a jet of water.

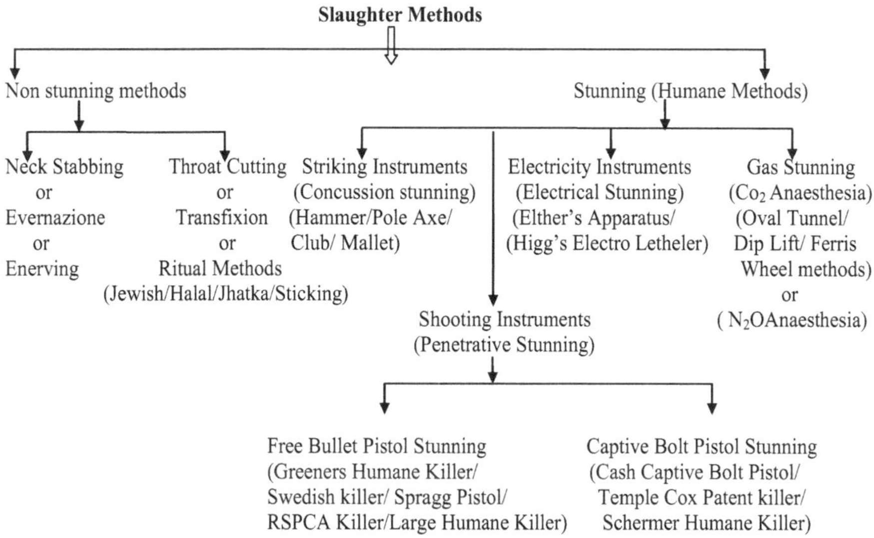

Neck Stabbing

Neck stabbing is also termed as Evernazione or Enerving is a most primitive method of animal slaughter. This slaughter method was initially followed by Tribal of South Africa, Mexico, Spain, and parts of Italy. In this slaughter procedure, short double edged knife (puntilla) is used to plunge on occipito-atlantal space at nape of neck and medulla oblongata is severed. Arctic Reindeers are killed by inserting curved one side sharp knife on occipito-atlointic space directed forward to destroy the brain. However, it's least effective method and animal shows reflex actions and sensations.

Ritual slaughter procedure

As per the definition of Federal Humane Methods of Slaughter Act, USA, ritual slaughter refers to "a method of slaughter whereby the animal suffers loss of consciousness by anaemia of the brain caused by the simultaneous and instantaneous severance of the carotid arteries with a sharp instrument and handling in connection with such slaughter".

However, slaughter of animals in the most parts of the world including India is carried out mainly by ritual or religious methods. In this slaughter method stunning generally is not allowed and the animal is bled directly using a sharp knife to cut the throat and sever the main blood vessels. It is resulted into sudden and massive loss of blood with loss of consciousness and death. However, many authorities consider that religious slaughter is unsatisfactory because animals are not rendered unconscious and suffer considerable discomfort and pain. To obtain good quality meat from animals by ritual slaughter procedures following recommendations may be incorporated:

i. Animals should be securely restrained, particularly the head and neck, before cutting the throat.

ii. Knife used to cut the throat, carotid and jugular blood vessels must be razor sharp and should be free from blemishes and damages. It is essential to ensure a swift, smooth cut across the throat behind the jaw and to ensure immediate and maximum gush of blood.

iii. Bleeding should be ascertained perfect because poor bleeding causes slow loss of consciousness and reduce meat quality.

iv. Animals should not be shackled and hoisted before bleeding because it induces severe discomfort and stress to animals. Animal hoisting should always be preferred after loss of consciousness.

v. Restraining equipments should be comfortable for the animal to minimize stress and align ness to the animals.

vi. Operator competence is of great importance in order to carry out satisfactory religious slaughter of food animals.

vii. Technique should be perfect and slaughterman should be skilled enough to avoid sufferings and cruelty to the animal.

1. Jewish/ Kosher/Kashrut method

Jewish ritual slaughtering procedure permits slaughter of land animals like cattle, sheep, goat, deer, all kinds of poultry etc. In Jewish slaughter method only healthy animals are liable to slaughter because they can produce *Kosher* (meat fit for Jews consumption) meat. Kosher is a very important aspect of Judaism because it is believe that kosher meat benefits the mind, body, and soul. Non-Jews often consume Kosher meat because of the special process involvement. *Shechita* (slaughter procedure) ensures the slaughtering of healthy animals and animals suffering with injury, pain and who is not able to stand on their own foot are always avoided. Eating of pigs, dead animals and blood is totally prohibited in Jewish method. Pig slaughter is forbidden because Jews believes that pigs are potent source of Trichinella and *Taenia solium*. Stunning of animals prior to slaughter is also forbidden in Jewish method. Meat unfit for human consumption is termed as 'Terefa'.

Jewish ritual slaughter method is controlled by Jewish Board of *Shechita* in Britain. It is a very difficult process and requires years of experience, a vast knowledge of biblical laws, and experience with the anatomy of the animals being slaughtered. To obtain license from *Rabbinical Commission, Shochit* (slaughterman) must have several years of experience and must be expert in slaughtering. To produce *Kosher* (fit meat), animals must be slaughtered and dressed according to Jewish ritual method specified in the *Talmud,* the body of Jewish law and legend based on the *Torah* which is the substance of God's revelation to man in the *Old Testament.*

Pre-requisites in Jewish slaughter

i. A person must be trained and certified by special rabbinic authorities to become a *Shochet*. It is essential to ensure Kosher meat products for Jews consumption.

ii. By law, Shochit must be an honest, kind and upright man. Cruel person cannot be a shochet.

iii. Stunning is against the laws of Kashrut because it might harm the animal and as per Jews law animal should be alive, healthy and have no injury are liable to slaughter.

iv. To make the meat kosher, animal must be alive, healthy and free from injury. Animals that lie quietly and cannot be made to rise must not be slaughtered.

v. *Shechita* must be foolproof because defect at slaughter in form of faults or disease lesions discovered in the carcass render the meat *terefa* (meat unfit for human consumption).

vi. *Chalef* (slaughtering knife) should be sharp without any notch or flaw and has been examined before the slaughter of each animal.

vii. Neck of animal should be fully extended in order to keep the edges of the wound open and to prevent pain and sufferings to the animals.

viii. The five rules of Jewish ritual slaughter in their traditional order are that the neck incision shall be completed without pause, pressure, stabbing, slanting or tearing.

Slaughter procedure

Jewish slaughter procedure allowed the slaughter of those animals that are properly restrained and animal neck should be fully extended. *Shochet* offer the prayer before slaughter and slaughter the fully conscious animal with a single, deliberate, swift action of a razor-sharp knife. The soft structures of neck region, anterior to the cervical spine i.e skin, muscle, oesophagus, trachea, both side carotid arteries and jugular veins must be severed. Shackling and other operations are generally performed on overhead rails. All the major blood vessels (twelve in number) from the fore quarter of carcass are removed prior to retail sale by the process called *porging*. Porging is normally practiced in only forequarter because hind quarter of carcass contains more than fifty major blood vessels which are very difficult to remove. As eating of blood is forbidden by Jews so they eat only forequarter meat and refuses hind quarter meat. *Shochit* also carries post mortem examination by making an incision posterior to the xephoid process and inserting the arm to detect any adhesions in the thoracic cavity (*searching*). Shochet is normally assisted by a sealer (*Shomer*) who is responsible for putting the kosher mark on the brisket and on edible offal. After completion of all operations carcasses are washed properly in order to remove blood and held in chill room for more than 24 hrs. Further, washing, curing (*meliha*) or broiling being carried out at the time of its consumption. As per Jewish law, carcasses are essentially consumed within three days of slaughter.

To restrain the animals for Kosher production, various types of restrainers can be used. In Britain, Dyne, Weinberg or North British Rotary type restrainers are common. In later, animals are entered and moves at 180^0 and head is cut with chalef. In USA, Royal Society for Prevention of Cruelty Act (RSPCA) restrainers such as Cincinatti-Boss Restrainers and Conveyor restrainers system are most commonly used. Following considerations must be adopted in Jewish slaughter procedure:

i. In standard condition, the length of blade of *chalef* should be twice the width of the animal's neck. *Chalef* blade should be razor sharp and free from any type of notch or flaw and enough.

ii. Thorough examination of animals prior to slaughter is essential part of Kosher production. It is essential to ensure the quality of meat and it provides a disincentive for Kosher farms to partake and animals hurt in any way, cannot be slaughtered.

iii. Restraining of animals for correct and painless slaughtering is essential and injury during restraining must be avoided.

iv. Cutting of skin, muscle, oesophagus, trachea, both side carotid arteries and jugular veins must be in a single swift quick incision. Pulling and tearing during cutting is never allowed. Cutting should be in such a way that after incision animal should die within 2 seconds.

v. Jews believes that blood contains the soul of the animal and forbid the eating of blood. So draining of blood after exsanguination should be complete.

vi. Examination of essential organs of the animal must be done carefully and defective organs must be discarded. Animal's lungs should be free from unwanted holes and signs of lung diseases. Lungs are inflated for examination of presence of holes.

vii. Removal of non-Kosher parts from the hind quarters of the animal: blood vessels and the sciatic nerves must be removed.

viii. Removal of whole fat surrounds the vital organs: the internal fat (Hebrew as cheilev) must be removed to make the meat Kosher.

Pros and cons of Jewish slaughter procedure

The proponents of Jewish slaughter method believe that Jewish slaughter method does not involve any act of cruelty because the knife is particularly sharp, the cut is made dextrously by a trained person and the severance of the carotid vessels is followed by a very rapid fall in blood pressure within the cephalic arteries. It is therefore suggested that the anoxia from the diminished blood supply to the brain tissues brings about almost immediate unconsciousness. It is also believed that bleeding of animal is more complete than in other method of slaughter. However, opponents advocated that it is a inhumane method because carotid arteries of cattle are severed transversely they tend, by virtue of their elasticity, to retract rapidly within their own external connective tissue coat, thus sealing off the cut ends. This automatic sealing of vessel leads to increase in blood pressure in anterior venacava and supply more blood to brain. They also believe that paler colour of the flesh of Jewish slaughtered animals is due to the violent respiratory efforts and depletion of oxygen and increase in proportion of oxyhaemoglobin in blood.

2. Halal / Mohammedans / Muslim or Islamic ritual method

Muslim or halal slaughter procedure is a most commonly used slaughter method. Slaughtering mandates and pattern of meat consumption are almost same in both Halal and Jewish slaughter methods. As animal welfare is a major consideration in both slaughter methods, eating of dead animals, blood and swine is forbidden. Dead animals are forbidden because decomposition of carcass may lead to generation of harmful chemicals to the consumers while blood contains harmful organisms, metabolism products and toxins. The reason behind prohibition of pork is religious as well believe that it is a vector for pathogenic worms to human beings i.e *Trichinella spiralis* and *Taenia solium*. Pork is also not considered for eating due to presence of incompatible fat to the human body fat and biochemical system. Other forbidden items in Halal procedure includes improperly slaughtered animals carcass, alcoholic drinks including all forms of intoxicants, carnivorous animals (lions, tigers, cheetah, dogs, cats etc.) birds of prey (eagles, falcons, osprey, kites, vultures etc.) and any food contaminated with any of these products. Sea food is controversial because certain group used fish meat of those fish which contains scales while others may like to have prawns, lobsters, crabs but prohibited Makrooh as halal. *Dhabihah* is an Islamic slaughter procedure for animals allowed to eat as a food. Islam has clear cut views on animal foods and clearly describes the eatable and non eatable food animals in their holy book "Quran". However, they are also giving relaxations for emergency and said that in case when no other food available then a Muslim is allowed to eat non-halal food. The rule states "Any action or method which will definitely lead to some harm damage or suffering is to be rejected or, any action which can be suspected to lead to a prohibited act is also to be rejected.

The Quran describes the procedure of carotid and jugular section as the 'cutting and draining of blood'. The act of slaughter (*Al-Dhabh*) is allowed in the name of God; therefore pronouncing the name of Allah is the usual practice. This is to remind the slaughterer that he is taking the life of a living creature. The Muslim method of slaughter is not controlled by a Central Board but is overseen by the local Islamic authority (*Muftis*) who decide whether or not particular acts and thoughts conform to the tenets of Islamic Law (*Shariah*). In some instances prior stunning with electricity or captive- bolt pistol is allowed.

Slaughtering procedure

i. As per the ritual, slaughterman in Muslim or Halal slaughter method offers prayer (Bismi) before going to slaughter an animal. He also directed the head of food animal towards Mecca. It is because Muslims are supposed to eat only those foods on which Allah name has been mentioned.

ii. Animals are slaughtered by a very very sharp knife by a deep swift cut done instantaneously and quickly to the blood vessels of the neck (the two carotid arteries which carry blood to the brain and head, the two jugular veins which bring blood from the brain back to the heart), the trachea (windpipe) and the oesophagus (gullet), but the central nervous system (the spinal cord) should be kept safe and intact (not cut). This deep, large cut through all the blood vessels of the neck causes acute blood loss and haemorrhagic shock which leads to almost immediate loss of consciousness.

iii. The intact spinal cord and medulla assures efficient bleeding. Intact spinal cord with safe nerve centres to the limbs, muscles and organs. So, the act assures huge amount of bleeding from the initial cut then blood loss is continuing with the squeezing pressure of these contractions and convulsions, leading to maximum bleeding-out and less retention of blood in the carcass, giving a better quality of meat.

Salient features of halal slaughter

1. Halal essentials includes slaughter of halal species only, slaughtering should be done by adult and sane Muslim only, name of Allah must be pronounced at the time of slaughter and slaughter method must be adopted to stab the throat and at least three of the four passages must be cut i.e carotids, jugular, trachea and oesophagus. The meat produced in this way is called *Zabiha* or *Dhabiha* meat.
2. Proper rest to the animals and provision of sufficient water to animals before slaughter and prohibition of sharpening the knife in front of animals are some other provisions mentioned in halal method.
3. Halal slaughter procedure is known for perfect bleeding. It is a fact because intact spinal cord and medulla oblongata produces jerk to the animal body and help in expulsion of blood from body.
4. The actual act of slaughter can be regarded as painless and humane if performed efficiently with the wound kept open. Rapid loss of blood in the act produces instantaneous insensibility and animal does not feel much pain.
5. In the actual slaughter method animal must not be slaughtered in the sight of other beast and those to be killed are to be fed and watered beforehand.
6. It is believed that the method is more economical because there is a little need of equipments and machinery.
7. It is believed that it is a quick, easy, practical and realistic method but machine slaughter is not permitted.

8. It is difficult to conceive a more painless and rapid mode of death; for a few seconds after the cut is made, the animal makes no movement in its body and then convulsed. The convulsive movements continue for about a minute and then cease. The interpretation of this fact is clear: the cut is made by a knife so sharp and so skilfully handled that a state of syncope with its associated unconsciousness follows instantaneously upon the severing of the blood pressure. The movement of the animal which begins at about 90 seconds are epileptiform in nature and are due to the blood-less state of the brain (cerebral ischemia with complete anoxemic). Sensation has been abolished at the moment of the initial syncope.' However, opponents believes that the ritual method of slaughter as practiced in Islam has been described as inhumane by animal welfare organisations in the U.K. and the U.S.A., who have stated that it "causes severe suffering to animals.

3. Jhatka /Sikh / Hindu method

Hindus and Sikhs have a simple method of slaughtering the animal for meat, often referred to as Jhatka. In real terms this means that the head of the animal is severed from the body with one blow. As the spinal cord is cut with one blow the death would in all likelihood be instantaneous. It is also considered painless method because animal gets unconsciousness immediately after slaughter.

The Sikhs Gurus have enjoined on then not to eat halal and suggested to partake of only Jhatka meat. In fact even before partition the Muslim dominated Union party that was in power in the undivided Punjab had entered into an agreement with the Sikhs. This agreement stated that Sikhs would be allowed to have their own Jhatka shops for meat. Thus Jhatka became the integral part of Sikhism. It is believe that Guru Gobind Singh also rejected eating of Halal meat and ordered to eat Jhatka meat from animals. In this connection the last Hukamnama (Religious Order) was issued by the Akal Takht in 1980.

The Hindus also will only partake of Jhatka and in festivals like Durga Puja, only Jhatka meat is served. After Independence this practice of separate Jhatka and halal meat shops has continued. The difference is not just confined to the manner of slaughtering the animals but also to what animals to eat. Muslims will not eat the meat of pigs as they are considered unclean and Hindus will not partake of Cow or beef.

Slaughter procedure

The proponents advocated that Jhatka method of animal slaughter is more humane because decapitation of the animal carried out by a swift single cut using a sword. The animal is allowed to bleed for 5-10 minutes but perfect bleeding does not takes place because medulla oblongata is partially destroyed. In this method of slaughter, animals has been killed by a single strike of a sword or axe to sever the head, as opposed to Jewish slaughter or Islamic slaughter in which the animal is killed by ritually slicing the throat. Jhatka slaughter method is practiced on sheep and goats as cattle are regarded as sacred by both Sikhs and Hindus and are not eaten. Jhakta slaughter involves instant decapitation. The head of the animal is held securely, or fastened to a rigid pole or other object. The hind legs are held away by hand. The head is severed with a heavy, sharp cutlass in a single stroke.

4. Sticking

Sticking is generally practiced in pig slaughter where a long pointed knife is inserted along the middle line of neck at the depression in front of sternum and pushing it forward to severe anterior venacava and carotid artery. It is not a common method for other meat animals.

References

1. Gracey, J.F and Collins, D.S. (1994). Meat plant construction, equipments and operations. *In:* Meat Hygiene, 9th ed., ELBS, U.K. Pp 86-108.
2. Mountney, G.J. (1970). Processing poultry. *In:* 2nd edition, Poultry Products technology, The AVI Publishing Company Inc, Westport Connecticut, London. pp 123-136.
3. Mountney, G.J. and Parnell, E.D. (1958). Proper slaughtering for good carcass quality. Poultry Processing and Marketing, 64 (11): 14-15.
4. Regenstein, J.M. and Chaudry, M. (2001). A brief introduction to some of the practical aspects of the kosher and halal laws for the poultry industry. *In:* Poultry Meat Processing by Alan R. Sams, CRC Press, Washington, D.C. Pp 281-299.
5. Sharma, B.D. (1999). Pre-slaughter handling, transport and dressing of poultry. *In:* 1st edition, Meat and Meat Products Technology including Poultry Products Technology, Jaypee Brothers Medical Publishers (P) Ltd, New Delhi. Pp 99-103.

Chapter 7

Humane Slaughter Method for Animals

Humane slaughter is an act of killing the food animals in such a way as to cause the minimum stress or distress to the animal. To achieve this objective animal must be rendered insensible instantaneously and remain insensitive to pain until there is a complete loss of brain responsiveness due to exsanguination. The unconsciousness in animals is induced by stunning procedures which are varying in number. The method of stunning primarily based on species, breed, age, sex, kind and mental state of animals. Stunning is essential to safeguard the feelings and anxieties of animals. It facilitates maximum bleeding from the animals because animal becomes unconscious after stunning. To make animal unconscious before bleeding is not only essential for animal welfare point of view but it is legislation in many countries. However, Jewish slaughter prohibited the stunning while halal slaughter restricts the stunning. Animal is so claver and sensible that he/ she can sight and smell blood, strange noises, movements, surroundings and feared by separation from fellow animals. All these conditions in animals ultimately induce stress and badly affect the carcass and meat quality. Induction of unconsciousness in animals by stunning also makes the slaughterman job easier and slaughter operations can be managed in well planned way.

Humane slaughter essentials

i. Slaughter and stunning procedure should be selected as per the demand of animal intended for slaughter. Cattle and buffalo are generally stunned by mechanical means, pigs by gas anaesthesia and poultry by electrical stunning.

ii. The stunning box should be of good design with non-slippery floor, fitted doors and adequate steadying of beast's head. There should be convenient place for stunner to work and stunning operation should be noiseless.

iii. Person authorized for slaughter and stunning should be well trained and have proper license from competent authority. Stunning instruments should be in proper working condition.

iv. Proper stunning is essential to render the animal insensible and insensibility should last until brain death supervenes.

v. Time between stunning and sticking must be as short as possible (less than 30 seconds to large animals, less than 15 sec. for sheep and goat and less than 10 sec. for calves in concussion stunning while it is 60 seconds in large animals) to ensure death by blood loss before the animal regains consciousness. In captive bolt penetrative stunning and electrical head only stunning prolonged time between stunning and sticking leads to muscles haemorrhages or blood splashing.

vi. Food animals shall be killed without unnecessary sufferings and stress which is essential part of animal welfare during animal slaughter and to obtain good quality meat from animals.

vii. Bleeding shall be as complete as possible to ensure the shelf life of meat and avoid contamination to carcass. It also enhances the aesthetic appeal of meat food.

viii. Slaughtering should be done out of sight of live animals awaiting slaughter which is an ethical requirement of humane slaughter.

Humane slaughter procedure

Humane slaughter is a two tier system in which animal stunned first to make them insensible followed by killing the animal by bleeding. Rest slaughter operations may follow the standard protocol specified by various authorities for clean meat production. The principles of HACCP, GMP, GHP and TQM can also be applied to cater the demand of today consumers. It is essential because today consumer is much more quality concern than before.

Stunning

Stunning is a process of producing unconsciousness or insensibility in animals prior to slaughter to ensure total freedom from sufferings to animals without alterations in meat and offal qualities. According to animal welfare considerations, stunning is a necessary step in slaughter operation. It also prevents injuries to staff engaged and helps in subsequent shackling and bleeding processes. As a safety measure, there should be a *dry land area* of about 3 meter in width to the opposing wall or bleeding trough fitted with upright bars of 5 cm diameter and 1.2 meter height in front of stunning pen. The restraining pens suitable for different animals must be arranged to get desired effect and for safety of operator. The choice of stunning method is dependant on various factors like:

i. Class of animals to be slaughtered and their body and mental status.

ii. Religious and legal requirements.

iii. Number of animals to be slaughtered and throughput management.

iv. Humane aspects in whole process of slaughter operation.

v. Intended line speed and number of animals to be slaughtered in a specified time frame.

vi. Capital and cost of maintenance involved in various slaughter operations.

vii. Efficiency of equipments and operations.

viii. Safety of personals engaged in different operations.

ix. Purpose of carcass utilization and effect of stunning on carcass and brain.

A. Mechanical stunning methods

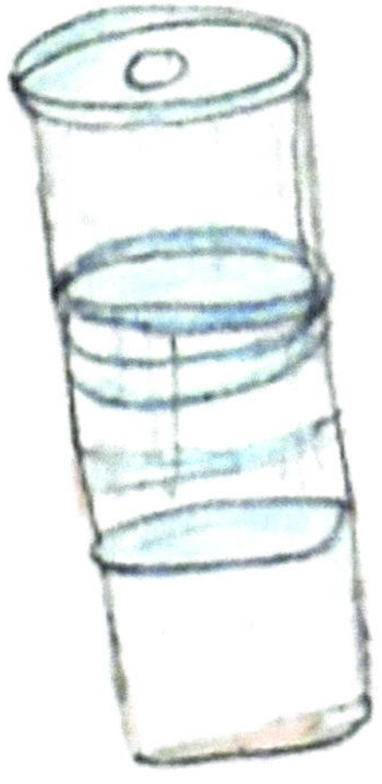

i. *Non-penetrative percussion or concussion stunning*: concussion stunning is generally performed by Hammer or Pole Axe or Club or Mallet on the head of small animals. It is a suitable stunning procedure for calves and sheep but not commonly applied in adult animals. In small animals it produces immediate insensibility which lasts within 30 seconds. Concussion stunning is a suitable method to obtain the brain for edible purpose. However, young calves with thin skull sometimes show intracranial haemorrhage. The point of strike in calves should be lower to the point in the middle of forehead where two lines drawn from medial canthus of eye to the base of opposite horn.

ii. *Penetrative stunning:* penetrative stunning produces instance and permanent insensibility by making a hole in head region where it strikes by force. However, it damages the brain and can not be utilize for edible purpose. There are two types of penetrative stunners are generally used i.e captive bolt stunner and free bolt stunner. Sometimes captive bolt stunners are further classified into mechanically operated and pneumatic stunner using blank cartridges. While a special type of water jet stunner can also be used to make the animal insensible. The percussion site at animal head is very important to produce the desired insensibility in a particular animal. Thus penetrative stunner can be classified as:

a. Captive bolt pistol stunner.

b. Pneumatic bolt stunner.

c. Free bullet pistol stunner.

d. Water jet stunner.

Head sites for percussive stunning in different animals

Animal type	Head site	Location
Adult cattle/Buffalo	Middle of forehead where two lines drawn from medial canthus of each eye to the base of opposite horn or horn prominence cross.	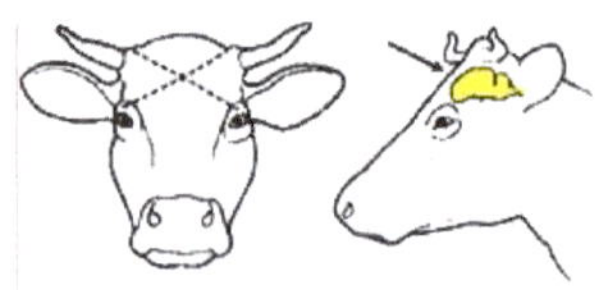
Calves	Lower to the middle of forehead where two lines drawn from medial canthus of each eye to the base of opposite horn or horn prominence cross.	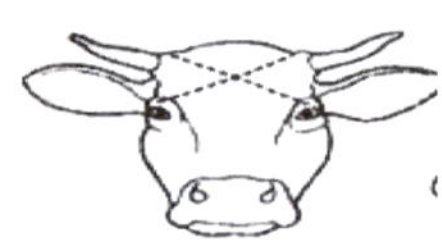
Bulls and old cows	13 mm side to the frontal ridge at middle of forehead where two lines drawn from medial canthus of each eye to the base of opposite horn or horn prominence cross.	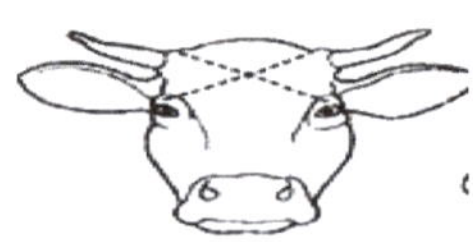
Hornless sheep and goats	Top of the head directed towards gullet	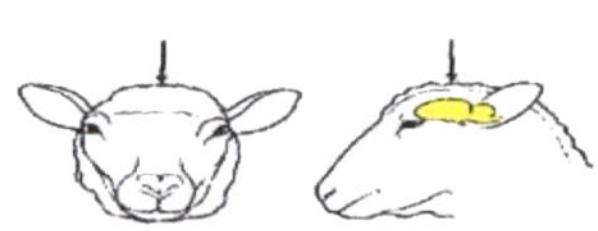
Horned sheep and goats	Top of the head behind the ridge connecting two horns and directed towards gullet	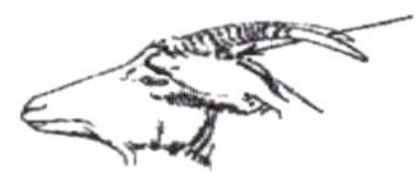
Pigs	Centre of the forehead 2.5 cm above the level of eye directed upwards into cranial cavity	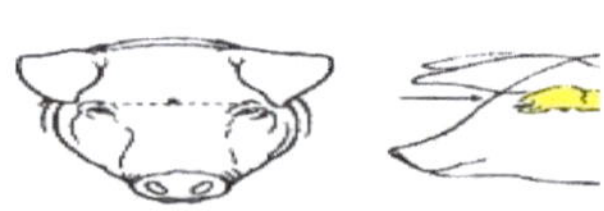
Horse	1 cm above the point where imaginary lines from eye to ear crosses at frontal surface	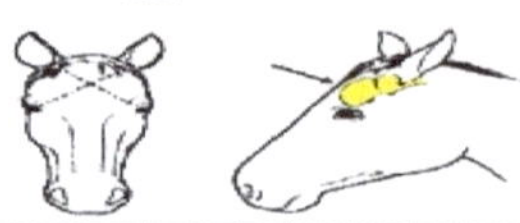

a. *Captive bolt pistol stunner:* captive bolt pistol stunner is a most commonly used in cattle and buffalo but can be applied in sheep and calves. This stunner is not suitable for bulls and pigs particularly in sow and boar due to presence of thick frontal bone. It is a suitable method for killing rate <250 animals/hr. In this pistol, a bolt is propelled forward on discharge of the blank cartridge and automatically recoils into the barrel. Use of correct strength of cartridge is important in captive bolt system. It induces immediate insensibility by acceleration concussion by destruction of cortex and deeper part of brain, alteration in intracranial pressure and sudden jerk. The insensibility is dependant on actual velocity of bolt and speed at which it strikes the brain. Normal effect can be produced in steers, heifers and cows with 55 miles/ sec while young bulls require 65 to 70 miles/sec but cartridge penetration in brain is not having any significance. However, strength of cartridge must match with the pistol robustness. There are two types of pistols are in use i.e cash active bolt pistol and temple cork pistol. Normally used cash instrument is working with 0.22 or 0.25 cartridges while horse require 0.64 blanks cartridge for proper stunning. The strength of cartridge used in different animals may be categorized as:

Type of animal	Strength of cartridge	Colour of cartridge
Small animals	1 grain or 0.065 grams	Green
Large animals	3 grains or 0.195 grams	Red
Mature bulls	4 grains or 0.260 grams	Red

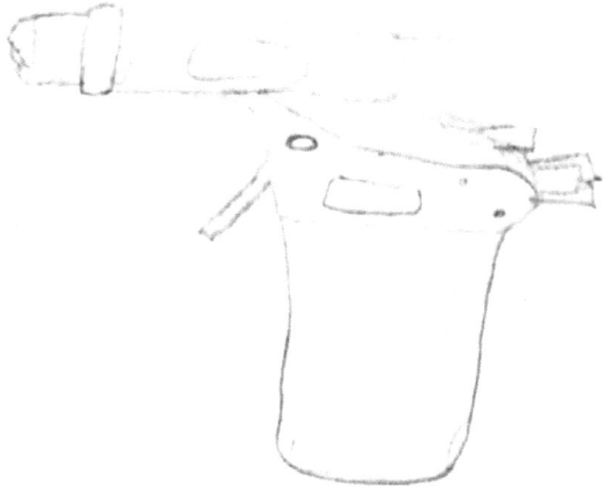

Captive bolt stunner

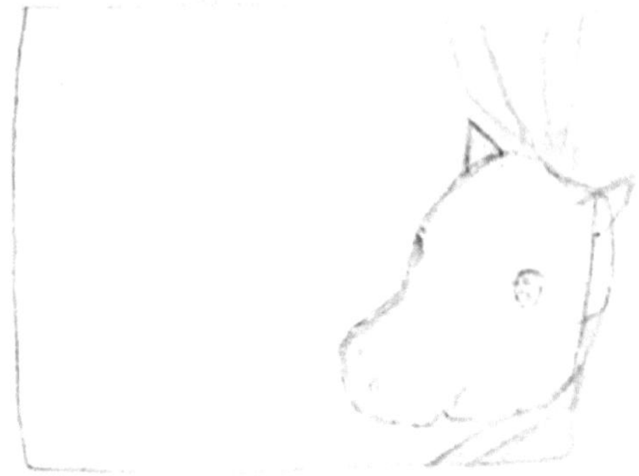

Animal restrainer for penetrative stunning

b. *Pneumatic bolt stunner*: pneumatic bolt stunner works on the principle of captive bolt stunner. But it is activated at high pressure (80 -120 psi). Proper pressure achievement is the key of success of pneumatic bolt stunner.

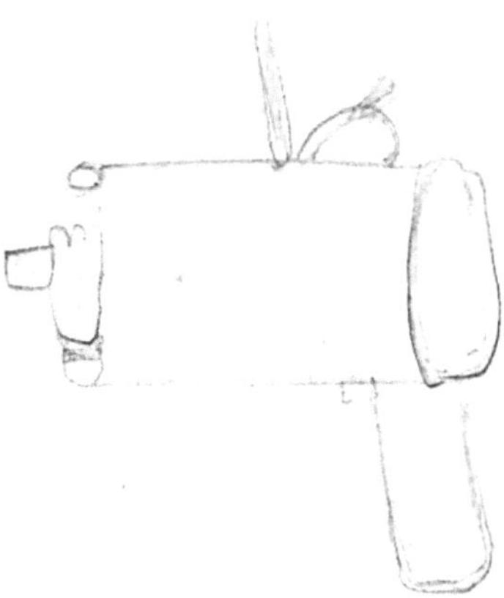

Pneumatic stunner

c. *Free bullet pistol*: free bullet pistol was older day device to stun the animals. It was also used to euthanize horse in military in Britain. In this technique hollow pointed type bullets or fragile iron plastic missiles or powdered iron bullets are fired through small bore rifle or gun on the points specified at head sites. The use of free bullet pistol for stunning is quite dangerous and always use with care to avoid accidents. Safety devices should be fitted with gun. It is hazardous to operator as well as to the animals and require license from competent authority.

d. *Water jet stunning*: water jet stunning is normally performed with fine water jet devised by Lamooji. It is usually a jet of 0.5 mm at pressure of 3500-4000 bar is applied to penetrate the skull.

Penetrative stunning devices cause destruction of brain tissues by penetrating bolt. So brain can not be utilized for edible purpose. It is also hazardous to the premises and operator if encountered the potential BSE organism. But it is a quite effective method for large animals stunning. The effectiveness requires good maintenance of instrument or pistol, site on head, velocity of bolt, size of cartridge for particular species and age, fitting of safety levers with pistols etc. There should always be a back-up pistol in hand for emergency. To minimize stress animal should be stunned within five seconds after its head is restrained.

For effective insensibility in large animals sometime hole in skull made by bolt of pistol in head is inserted with long, thin, flexible metal rod to destroy medulla oblongata therefore, minimising reflex muscular action that take place during sticking and dressing of the carcass. The process is generally termed as '*pithing*'. It is generally practiced before bleeding but does not affect bleeding in appreciable way. Pithing rods must be kept clean and disinfected between uses on each animal. The basic aim of pithing is to destroy motor centre of the brain so that reflex muscular action does not take place at sticking. But special care is required to minimize the conditions like slaughter spleen and BSE. It is because if pithing rod is longer than 0.6 meter it can damage greater splanchnic nerve resulting into dilatation of the splanchnic blood vessels. It ultimately causes congestion of liver, kidney and intestines leads to the enlargement and congestion of spleen and the condition is known as *slaughter spleen*. In another case if rod is not properly sterilized it may poses the hazards. Now this method is absolute in most of the countries after occurrence of Bovine Spongiform Encephalitis (BSE) like diseases.

B. Chemical /gas stunning methods

Chemicals are successfully used since long back to anesthetize the animals in various cases. The combination of gases or a single gas is also capable to induce effective anaesthesia in animals. The most commonly used gas for animal stunning is carbon dioxide (Co_2) but nitrous oxide (N_2O), argon-oxygen mixture can also be used to stun the animals. The effectiveness of gases as anaesthetizing agent is depending on induction time and respiratory distress. These two factors also decide the gas type and its concentration. Among carbon dioxide and nitrous oxide, previous gas is irritant and produces respiratatary distress at higher concentration while later has higher induction time.

Co_2 gas stunning: carbon dioxide is a most commonly used gas for stunning of animals and considered human method of anaesthesia because unconsciousness occurs prior to onset of excitation phase. Co_2 was first used to induce pre-slaughter anaesthesia in animals in 1904. Practically Co_2 anaesthesia is a satisfactory method for pigs stunning because pigs have tendency to lower down their head while passing in Co_2 chamber. However, Co_2 anaesthesia can also be used to induce unconsciousness in calves, sheep and poultry. Co_2 induces unconsciousness in animals by blocking the nerve endings and reduces the speed of nerve impulses. The most suitable gas concentration is 65-70 percent to induce pre-slaughter anaesthesia with exposure time of at least 45 seconds. Concentration and time of anaesthesia is an important factor in effective induction of unconsciousness in animals. If concentration is too low the pigs may not be properly stunned and if it is too high there is a tendency of pigs to become stiff. Similarly if exposure period is too long superficial congestion of skin occurs and when pigs are scalded the skin becomes bluish in colour. Bleeding of pigs should be done within 30 seconds of pig leaving the gas chamber. It is necessary to avoid the untoward effects of convulsive struggling and varying degree of excitement. Genetic factors play a large role in determining the aversiveness of Co_2 gas to pigs. Therefore, Co_2 stunning is probably very humane for pigs of a particular type of genetic make up and very stressful for others. Mixture of Co_2 and argon gas may create an improved gas stunning system for poultry.

Process of anaesthesia

Carbon dioxide gas is usually stored in cylinders or bulk tanks as a liquid under pressure. This gas is non inflammable and has a higher gravity than air, sinking to the bottom of any container and produces no hazards to the operator. Usually gas from storage tank is passed to analyser instrument and desired concentration is passed to gas anaesthesia chamber located down to the ground level. Pigs are usually passed in anaesthesia chamber with the help of trolley or lift.

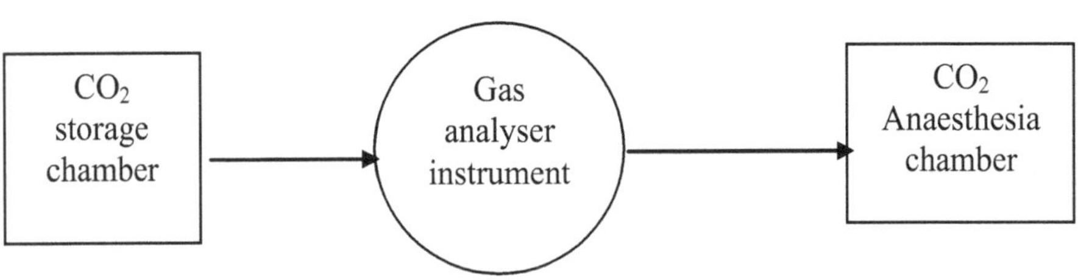

Methods of Co_2 anaesthesia

Method	Process	Structure	Capacity
Oval tunnel method	It is oval shaped Co2 gas tunnel sloping downward at an angle of 30^0 at entry point through which slot conveyor carries the pigs. Actual conveyer in tunnel is divided in ten compartments and animal is accommodated in each compartment. On exit pigs are shackled, hoisted to an overhead rail and bled.	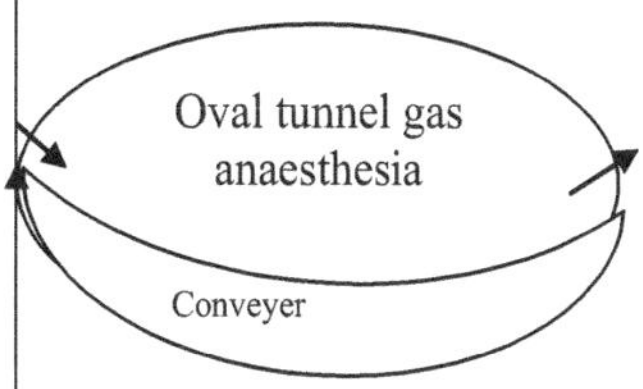	120-140 pig/hr but maximum weight bearing capacity is 113 kg and suitable for other species
Dip lift method	A cage measuring 213 cm length, 68 cm height and 53 cm width is used to held the animals. It descends vertically to the Co_2 pit where it remains for preset time in desired concentration. Then automatically returns to ground level and eject the unconscious animal for shackling and bleeding.	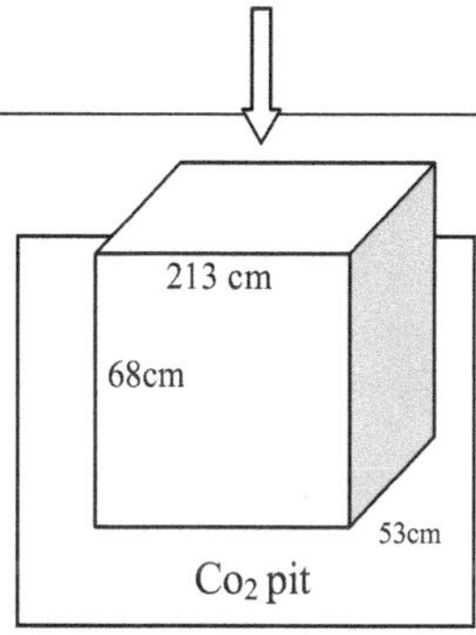	Throughput is small but can put any size of pigs, calves and sheep
Ferris wheel method	It is horizontally revolving three compartmental apparatus in which two compartments remains in gas chamber and one outside.	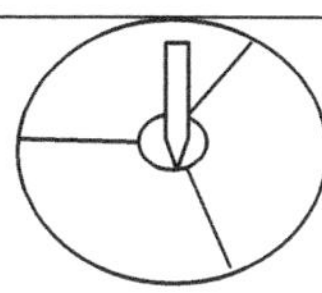	Suitable for pigs but can be used for small animals
Compact Co_2 Immobiliser	It is a compact design of Co_2 immobilizer divided into five chambers based on Co_2 concentration from higher to lower and animals are exposed serially in these chambers. First chamber is maintained with 10% Co_2 followed by 30% for 10 seconds, 60% for10 seconds and over 90% for 20 sec. at fourth and fifth chamber. After which pigs are discharged from unit.	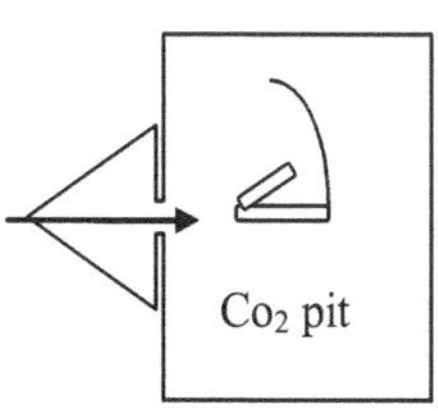	This system has a capacity of upto 300 pigs per hour.

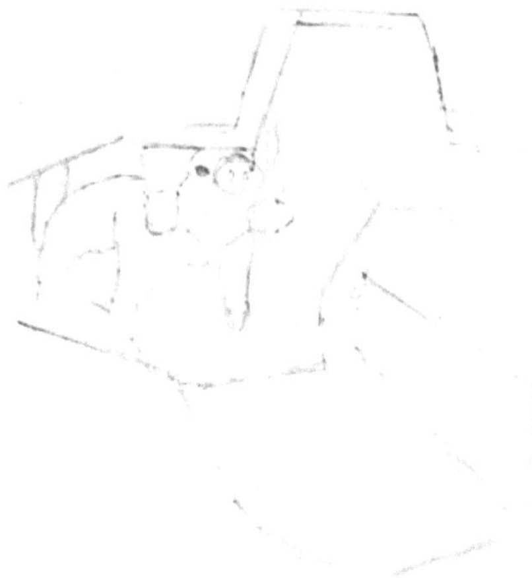

CO_2 gas stunning

Carbon dioxide anaesthesia is quite effective method for pigs because it produces less noise, labour intensive, produces relaxed carcass, easy dehairing and higher bleeding (0.75%). It produces less muscular haemorrhage and less breakage of bones due to less violent activity. However, installation cost is higher, animal undergo excitement and respiratory distress and dark chamber is not considered humane. There is a great chance of development of pale soft exudative (PSE) condition in pigs in compact chambers but overall incidences of PSE is lower in CO_2 anaesthesia than electrical stunning.

Carbon dioxide anaesthesia can also be used to stun the poultry but concentration requirement is 70 % for chicken with exposure time 1-3 seconds. However, turkey requires 73-77% percent CO_2 concentration with exposure time of 10 seconds to induce anaesthesia. Alternatively mixture of CO_2 and argon gas can create an improved gas stunning system for poultry and nitrous oxide (N_2O) can apply for stunning of pigs.

C. Electrical stunning

Electrical stunning is a method of animal stunning introduced in year 1930 to make the animal unconscious before slaughter. In this process an alternating current is passed through thalamus and cortex as well as chief sensory organs of brain which may lead to massive depolarization of neurons in the brain resulting into epileptiform seizure and animal rendered unconscious. Alternatively, current can also pass through heart of an animal. This method of stunning is most widely used for pigs but can also be satisfactorily used in sheep and calves. However, it is not considered satisfactory method for stunning of cattle/buffalo due to insulating effect of fine hairs on the animal head. The effectiveness of electrical stunning is depending on strength of electric current and their exposure time as well as placement of instrument on animal body. The strength of electricity is expressed in three units' i.e amperage, voltage and application time. It can collectively be express as electric energy in watt per second. The electrical energy requirement for bulls is 430 watts-seconds while for cow and horses is 285 watts-seconds, small stock (sheep, pigs and calves) is 198 watts-seconds and poultry is 100 watts-seconds.

Bleeding is better in electrically stunned animals because of increase in blood circulation, heart rate and vasoconstriction. It also induces smooth or rhythmic muscular contraction. Although, this method has some limitations like improper current may lead to paralysis in animals but animals' remains in conscious state. The condition is generally termed as *'missed shock'* condition or electrical curarization or motor paralysis. The time between stunning and sticking should be within 30 seconds and delay in sticking may lead to consciousness in animals and muscular haemorrhages or splash. So to reduce the chances of muscle haemorrhages prior resting, correct stunning and immediate bleeding may serve the purpose.

Important facts in electrical stunning

i. Electrical system is the most widely used stunning method for animals. In this method electric current is passed through the brain to produce instantaneous insensibility which is achieved by inducing a tonic/clonic epileptic fits before pain stimulus associated with the application itself is detected and transmitted to the central nervous system (15 milliseconds).

ii. The strength of the electric shock should be sufficient throughout the entire exposure. Fluctuation in current may lead to misleading results.

iii. The minimum period of application in production of electroplectic shock should be 7 seconds in low voltage system and below 3 seconds in high voltage system.

iv. The electrodes should be correctly positioned so that the current will pass through the thalamus and cortex in forebrain. Failing this, it may result to 'missed shock' condition. The right area of electrode placement in sheep is between eye and ears when in pigs below the ear and parotid gland.

v. The animal should be bled immediately within 30 seconds after unconsciousness, otherwise it may regain consciousness though still remain paralysed.

vi. Electrical stunning of cattle requires a two-phase stun whereas pigs and sheep are electrically stunned by use of a single-phase application of current. Due to the large size of cattle, a current is firstly applied across the head to render the animal insensible and second current is applied from the head to body to induce cardiac arrest.

vii. Electrodes must be cleaned frequently to insure good electrical connection between stunner and animal. The minimum cleaning schedule is once a day; and, for safety, the electrode wand must be disconnected from the power supply before cleaning.

viii. If head-only stunning is used, the tongs must be placed properly so that the current passes through the brain. Tongs may be placed on both sides of the head or one tong can be placed on the top and another tong on the bottom of head.

ix. The animals should be in low caloric intake or withdrawn in feed but ad-lib water should be supplied to facilitate easy passing of electric current.

x. Electrodes should be dipped in strong brine solution to reduce the resistance of hairs.

xi. Animals should be approached from behind and electrodes should be quickly and firmly applied on correct place of head and release after 10 seconds when animals fall down and loss conscious.

xii. It is a proven fact that current in between 50-80 volt for poultry leads to maximum blood loss and voltage higher than this causes less blood loss.

Electrical stunning equipments

i. *Manual equipments*: manual electrical stunning consists of a pair of electrode or tong connected with a power unit. Power unit supply the current to tong which supply electrical energy to forehead of

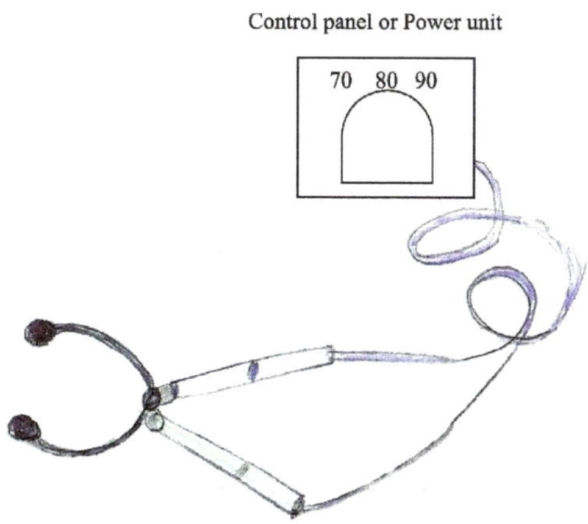

Electric tong for electrical stunning

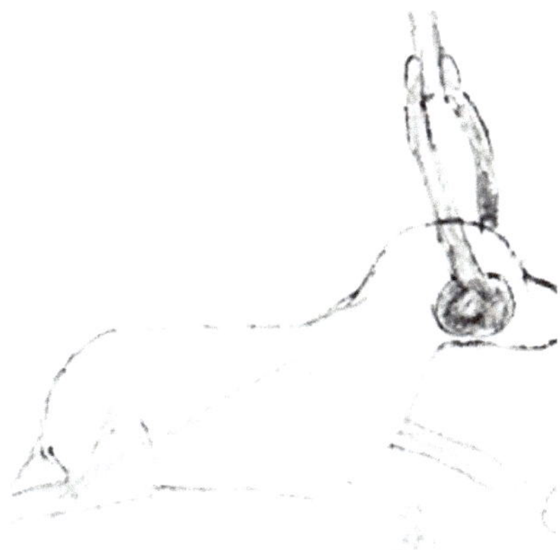

Placement of electric tongs in goat

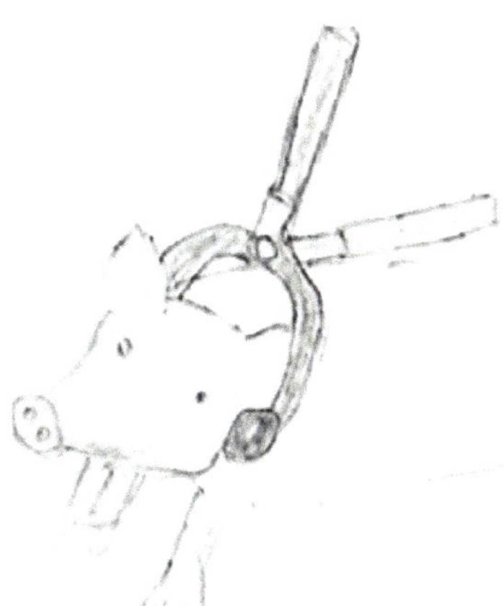

Electrical stunning of pigs

animal. Commonly used equipment is 'Elther's apparatus' but Higg's Electro Lethaler can also be used for the purpose.

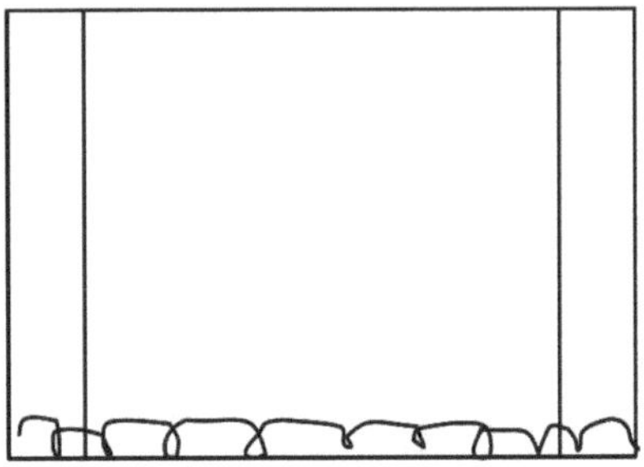

Automatic electrical grid

ii. *Automatic electrical grid:* automatic electrical grid is a type of water bath in which current is passed and poultry birds are exposed to this current for fraction of seconds. It can also be tried for pigs.

Methods of electrical stunning

i. *Low-voltage electrical stunning:* low voltage electrical stunning is used on sides of animal head. It is suitable method for poultry and pigs. The normal voltage used in method is 75 volt with 50 Hz main frequency and exposure time should be 7 seconds. To enhance effectiveness electrodes can be dipped in saline solution.

ii. *High voltage electrical stunning*: to ensure effective stunning in pigs and poultry, high voltage current of 300 volt for 2-3 seconds can be applied. However, high voltage system requires great care to both of operator as well as to the animals and birds. Faulty operation may lead to injury and shock to operator and vertebral as well as scapular fractures in pig and poultry on floor stunning.

iii. *Head to back or leg stunning*: in this system current is applied simultaneously to the head and/ leg. In this system brain anaesthetized and heart put on arrest. A minimum current of 250 V for 50 seconds is recommended for pigs and 375 V for lambs for about 23 seconds.

iv. *Automatic restrained conveyor stunning*: it is a suitable stunning technique for pigs in which pigs are stunned at 300 volt current at head region through electrodes suspended on hinged metal plates. Sheep may also be stunned by this technique.

Electrical stunning in poultry

i. *Manual stunning*: In small poultry units, hand electric stunning of 50-90 volt is performed. In manual system chicken weighing 2 kg requires 70 volt current for 2-3 seconds while turkey of 6-9 kg requires 90 volt for 10 seconds to become fully unconscious. Manual system is suitable for killing rate of 1000 birds/hr.

ii. *Automatic stunning devices*: in high throughput poultry dressing lines a current of 400-1000 volt is usually run in a grid and comb or parts of body touches the grid and desired unconsciousness occurs. This high voltage electric stunning leads to more number of cardiac arrests in birds.

iii. *Low voltage electric stunners*: low voltage electric stunners utilize a cabinet on conveyor line through which birds passes as suspended shackles. The current of 50-60 volt is passes for 5 seconds and birds remains unconscious for about 2-3 minutes.

iv. *Automatic poultry stunner*: automatic poultry stunner is generally used with the electric current of 70 volt for chicken and 50 volt for broiler through electrified water bath.

Sign of effective stunning in animals as noticed in various stunning procedures

Mechanical percussive stunning	Electrical stunning	Gas stunning
Loss of sensibility	Loss of sensibility	Loss of sensibility
Immediate animal collapse	Immediate animal collapse	Increased respiration followed by dyspnea
Muscular spasm	Limb flexion	Absence of corneal and palpebral reflex
Cessation of rhythmic breathing	Rigid legs extension	Muscle flaccidity with relaxed limbs and jaws
Protrusion of eye ball	Arching back of neck and spine	
	Downward rolling of eye ball	
	Muscular spasm	
	Muscle flaccidity	

To access the effectiveness of stunning body reflexes are generally used. The signs shown in above table can be measured in large and small animals. But signs in birds (chicken and turkey) stunned with electricity or gas are almost same as in other animals such as straight down head, limp and floppy tongue, flaccid and floppy head and body, absence of sensibility reflexes etc.

Effect of stunning on meat quality

i. Blood splashing in muscles due to unduly long interval between stunning and sticking and/or inadequate penetration of bolt in percussive stunning.

ii. Nonpenetrative stunning may produce the intracranial haemorrhages in animals and within frontal bones.

iii. Electrical stunning induces tonic and clonic muscle spasm and increases muscle glycolysis and lower pH in sheep. However, the technique may produce PSE condition in pigs.

iv. Head-to-back/leg electrical stunning produces very low incidence of blood splashing but petechiae may occur in connective tissues and fat.

v. High-voltage stunning may results in petechial haemorrhages throughout the loin and fracture of the bones.

vi. Use of tongs with 300 V in a restrainer- conveyor resulted in superior quality pig meat and lesser PSE condition as compared to automatic stunning with 680 V.

vii. It is generally accepted that CO_2 produces the lowest incidence of PSE and blood splashing and superior quality meat.

viii. In pigs: Electrical stunning sometimes leads to acute fall in muscle pH due to powerful activation of the glycolysis in the muscles and elevated release of catecolamines into the blood.

ix. In pigs: PSE incidence increases after use of electrical stunning whereas CO_2 stunning reduces incidence of PSE pork.

x. In comparison of electrical stunning and CO_2 stunning of hogs, it was found that pigs with similar genetic background (free from the Halothane gene) and with the same environmental exposure prior to stunning, electrical stunning resulted in twice the drip loss from the longissimus muscle with the same muscle pH and meat colour.

Exsanguinations or bleeding or sticking

It is an act of severing major blood vessels for rapid onset of anoxia resulting in the death of animal before the animal regains consciousness after stunning. The time taken to reach insensibility due to sticking depends upon the method of sticking, species and age of animal. The time taken to reach insensibility after bleeding is 20-102 seconds in cattle and buffalo, 12- 30 seconds in pigs and 2-7 seconds in sheep and goats. The bleeding in animals is considered perfect when removal of blood from the animal body is 50 percent It is essential to provide aesthetic meat to consumers because poor bled carcasses are dark in colour and not desired by most of the consumers. Good bleeding during slaughter enhances the shelf life of meat by reduction of microbial load because blood is a good medium for microbial growth.

There are two bleeding postures are generally preferred, horizontal and vertical. Bleeding when performed on floor or platform without hoisting on overhead rail is called horizontal bleeding while in vertical bleeding animal is hanged by hind legs on overhead rail for bleeding. Horizontal bleeding is a preferred posture for sheep and goats as well as for pigs because it yields 10 percent more blood in these animals than vertical bleeding. However, cattle and buffalo bled in vertical posture produces 40 percent higher blood than horizontal bleeding. On an average, animals' body contain about 3 percent blood on live basis and by all efforts only 50% blood can be removed. The amount of blood normally present in different animals is 13.6 kg in cattle and buffalo, 2.7 kg in calves, 1-2.5 kg in sheep and goats, 2.2 kg in horse, 3.0 kg in racoons and 3.6 kg in boars and sows. The standard bleeding time to obtain perfect bleeding is 5-6 minutes. In which 58.3 % blood is removed within 30 seconds, 76.6 % in 1 minute, 90% in 2 minutes and remaining blood comes in form of dribbling which is known as *drip blood*. For edible and pharmaceutical purpose blood should be collected in well hygienic manner with the help of hallow knife in a tube containing anti-coagulant. Normally drip blood is not used for edible purpose.

Bleeding methods

Animal species	Sticking/bleeding technique	Bleeding time (min.)	Superior bleeding posture	Comments
Cattle and buffalo	Bilateral severance of carotid arteries and jugular veins by making an incision across the throat caudal to the larynx. or Through incision on jugular furrow at the base of neck. Then knife is directed towards the chest to severe the branchiocephalic trunks and anterior venacava.	6	Vertical bleeding	Females yields more blood than males
Calves	Single incision at the side of neck to severe the jugular vein.	6	Vertical bleeding	Slow bleeding is desirable to produce white colour veal
Sheep and goats	Bilateral incision on jugular furrows close to the head to severe both carotid arteries and jugular veins by using straight knife containing 23 cm long and 4 cm wide unsharpened blade with sharp tip. Sometimes trachea, oesophagus and spinal cord is also severed at occipito-atlantal junction.	5	Horizontal bleeding	Thoracic inlet bleeding is superior
Pigs	Insertion of knife on midline of neck at the depression in front of sternum and is then pushed forward to sever the anterior venacava and brachiocephalic trunk at the entrance of chest. Sometime carotid artery is also pierced.	6	Horizontal bleeding	Electrical stunning yield more blood than non penetrative stunning.

Conditions associated with bleeding

i. Back bleeding or over sticking condition occur in neck bleeding technique of cattle, if knife is too far from chest than pleura may damage and blood is aspirated by thoracic cavity and accumulated in parietal pleura in posterior edges of ribs.

ii. Muscular haemorrhages or splash or over short meat or extravasation of blood condition observed when delay in between stunning and sticking takes place. It is occurrence of dark colour streaks due to collection of dark spots in internal musculature varying in size from visible to one fourth inch to half feet in length. It is mostly seen in muscular portion of diaphragm, muscles of necks, thigh and shoulder. Splash is mainly due to sudden infusion of capillaries which are in state of anoxia.

iii. Contamination of neck, head and blood with ruminal content when oesophagus is severed along with severance of carotid arties and jugular veins in sheep or knife withdrawal is at wrong angle after bleeding operation.

iv. In pigs bleeding, if knife pierce shoulder then blood and water from scalding tank enters into shoulder pocket beneath the scapula and produces cooked appearance to wall.

v. Imperfect bleeding produces dark colour meat which is not a desirable consumer attribute. Well bled animals can identify by seeing invisible intercostal veins whereas, prescapular lymph nodes are congested in poorly bled animals. Perfect bleeding condition can also be identified by Malachite green test.

To perform Malachite green test, 6 g of meat is added with 14 ml distilled water and allow standing for 15 minutes. Then 0.7 ml filter extract is collected and 1 drop malachite green reagent is mixed and add one drop of H_2O_2 and shake well till change in colour. Allow to stand for 20 minutes and see the observations. In perfect bleeding, solution become clear and blue in colour while imperfect or moderate bleeding shows cloudy solution with green colour. In case of marked bloody or total imperfect bleeding, solution appears cloudy with olive green colour.

References

1. Gracey, J.F and Collins,D.S. (1994). Humane slaughter. *In:* Meat Hygiene, 9th ed., ELBS, U.K. Pp 143-167.

2. Grandin, T. and Deesing, M. (2008). Humane Livestock Handling. Storey Publishing, North Adams, MA, USA.

1. Gracey, J.F and Collins,D.S. (1994). Humane slaughter. *In:* Meat Hygiene, 9th ed., ELBS, U.K. Pp 143-167.

2. Grandin, T. and Deesing, M. (2008). Humane Livestock Handling. Storey Publishing, North Adams, MA, USA.

3. Raj, B.M. (2004). Stunning and slaughter of poultry. *In:* Poultry Meat Processing and Quality, 1st ed., CRC Press, Washington. Pp 65-85.

4. Singh, N.P. and Bhatia, D.R. (1982). *In:* Proceedings of 3rd International Conference on Goat Production and Diseases. Dairy Goat J Publishing Co, USA.

5. Singh, V.P.Singh and Pathak, V. (2011). Laboratory manual Abattoir practices and animal products technology, DUVASU, Mathura. pp 13-23.

6. Waskar, V.S. (2008). Management of an abattoir. *In:* Universal Meat Hygiene in Public Health care, International Book Distributing Co. Lucknow. pp 161-175.

❑❑❑

Chapter 8

Slaughtering and Dressing of Meat Animals Including Poultry

Slaughtering and dressing of different kinds of animals and birds is an age old practice. Initially slaughtering was done by cutting the throat or stabbing the throat or breast. But today's world of progress and scientific evolution slaughter methods has undergone material changes. Scientifically there are two essentials of slaughtering i.e. humane slaughter to avoid unnecessary pain and sufferings to the animals and complete bleeding. Legislations require stunning of animals to render them unconscious before bleeding except in Jewish and Muslim slaughter. The animals subjected to slaughter must be clean which is generally achieved by cleaning. The premises and transportation vehicles should also be maintained in good hygienic and sanitary conditions. All the facilities required for slaughter animals and birds arranged well in advance. In commercial plants and export units, slaughtering and dressing is performed on overhead rails but for domestic use, booth and simple rails may serve the purpose due to low throughput. The requirements and systems of overhead rail are mentioned in chapter 1. Some of the requirements are listed in following table

Facilities and equipments required for slaughtering and dressing of carcasses

Slaughtering requirements	**Additional requirements for pigs and poultry**	**Dressing requirements**
Stunning instruments as per the need of animals.	Scalding tank or barrel for traditional system or tunnel for vertical scalding.	Sharp knife.
Sticking and skinning knives. Both side sharpened 15 cm knife for sticking and 15 cm curved skinning.	Pot, barrel or system for boiling water.	Small hatchet.
Sharpening steel or oil or water sharpening stone.	Bell scrapers.	Steel or whetstone for sharpening
Scabbard and belt for knives holding.	Solid scraping table or platform.	Rope or nylon cord.
Hand or electric operated meat saw and cleaver.	Thermometer for measurement of temperature of carcass up to 70°C.	Rubber bands.
Block or chain of sufficient strength to hoist animal for slaughter.	Singeing facility with blue flame.	Clean clothes or paper towels.
Dressing cradle, pritch plate or skinning rack.	Saw and clever should be sterilized at 82^{0}C before carcass splitting.	Resealable plastic bags.
Strong beams, tripod or track arranged on the height of 2.4 to 3.4 m from floor.		Large cooler with ice or refrigeration facility.
Spreader gambrel or metal pipes.		Ground pepper and cheesecloth.
Buckets.		Disposable plastic gloves.
Working platforms.		Clean drinking water.
Sterilization unit.		

Slaughtering and dressing of cattle and buffalo

Slaughtering and dressing steps	Description
Reception	At unloading dock with clean and sound animals.
Lairage	Resting and fasting of animals. Ante-mortem examination.
Isolation pan	If animals are sick or suspect.
Stunning	Captive bolt penetrating stunning or electric stunning.
Exsanguination or bleeding	By bilateral severance of carotid arteries and jugular veins by inserting the sticking knife carefully just above the breastbone at 45° pointed toward the head. Bleeding for at least 6 minutes in vertical bleeding posture hanging animal on one leg.
Horns and ears removal	Using sharp knife and saw.
Head skinning	Skin removal from head.
Foreshanking	Cutting of fore legs at knee/carpal joint.
Hind shanking and skinning	Removal of skin and cutting of hind leg at hock/tarsal joint.
Ripping, opening and loosening	*Ripping*: mid ventral line opening for hide removal. *Opening*: skinning of both sides of mid ventral line opening. *Loosening*: loosening of penis in male animals.
Rimming, removal of penis, tail and hind quarter skinning	Rimming: loosening of rectum and pushing into pelvic cavity. Removal of penis in male animal. Removal of tail in all animals. Skinning of hind quarter.
Skinning of forelegs, neck and mechanical dehiding	Skinning of forelegs. Skinning of neck. Mechanical dehiding by cutting the skin along the middle line from sticking wound to the tail. In high throughput plants by automatic hide puller using dressing cradle.
Head removal	Head removal by cutting neck muscles at occipital joint and hang the head on a hook.
Brisket cutting	Cutting of brisket by sharp knife at midline and pelvic cavity is severed along with abdominal cavity. Thoracic viscera, paunch and intestines are cleaned and inspected. In case of edible use of intestines, oesophagus and rectum is tied off during removal of hide.

Electrical stimulation	Electrical stimulation induces tenderness.
Evisceration and udder removal in female	Remove the viscera and disposed of properly. Udder in female is also departed.
Pluck removal	Pluck includes internal organs like larynx, trachea, lungs, heart and liver
Carcass splitting	Carcass splitting at downs the backbone (chine) with a saw or cleaver from the pelvis to the neck.
Carcass weighing	Weighing of carcass for dressing percentage and other parameters.
Post-mortem inspection	Thorough examination of carcass for safety and disease conditions.
Trimming	Loss of meat parts during fabrication of carcass cuts.
Carcass washing	Washing of carcass with spray.
Seal marking	Seal on carcase depicting passed for consumption
Carcass chilling	Chilling of carcase at 0-4°C with a core temperature below 7°C which is achieved within 28 to 36 hours.
Carcass deboning	Deboning of carcase at 10°-20°C.
Weighing and packaging	Weighing and packaging of carcass in suitable package.
Freezing storage	Freezing at - 30 to - 34°C with a core temperature below - 18°C

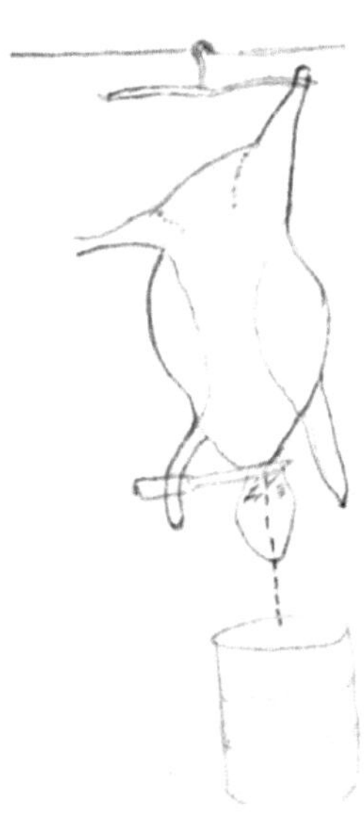

Sticking or bleeding

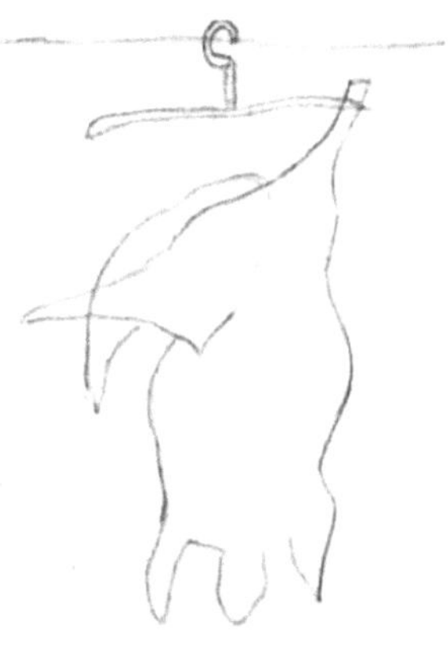

Leg removal

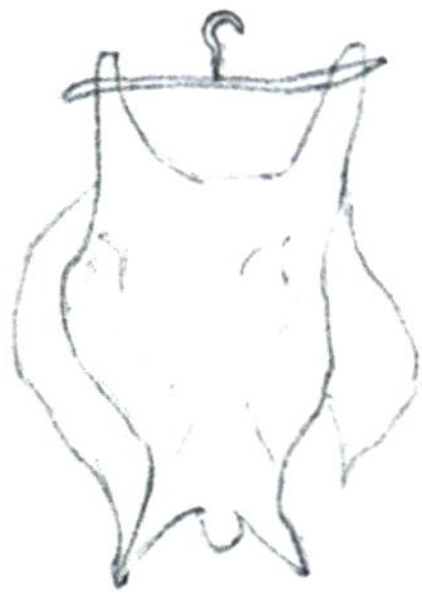

Dehiding

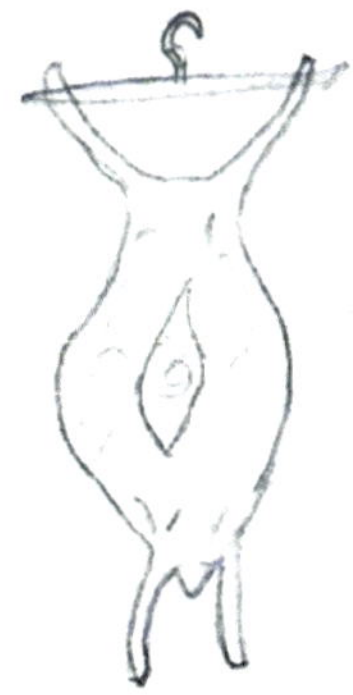

Evisceration or Paunch removal

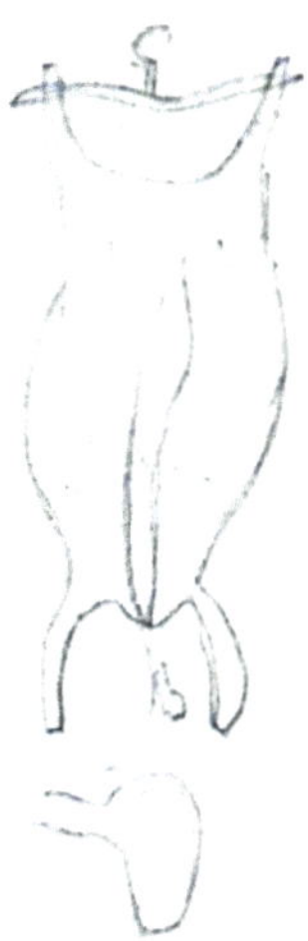

Evisceration

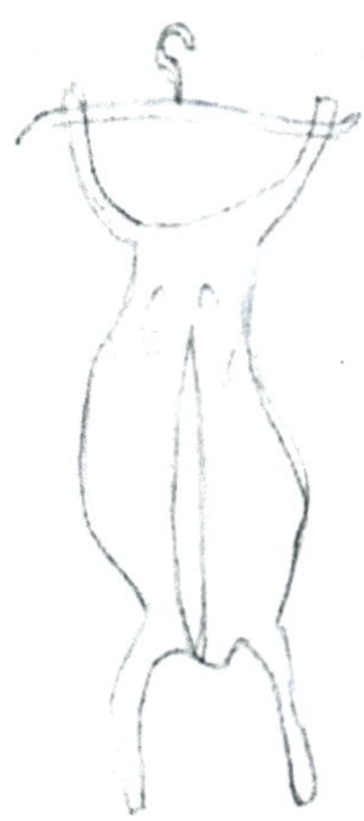

Dressed Carcass

Liver

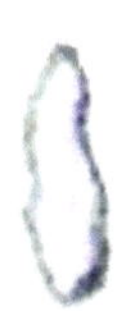

Tongue

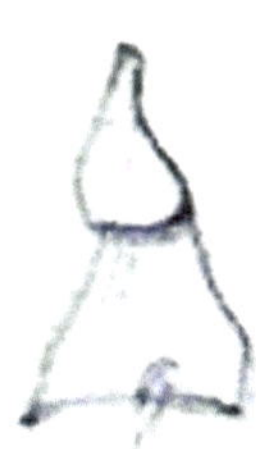

Pluck

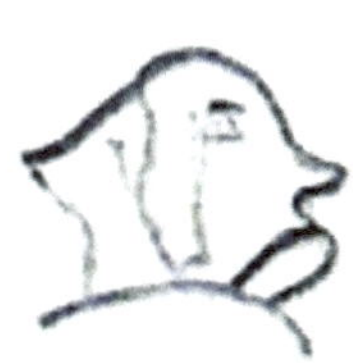

Head

Offals

Slaughtering and dressing of sheep and goats

Slaughtering and dressing steps	Description
Reception	Reception of sheep and goat on the unloading ramp in sound condition.
Lairage	Resting and fasting of animals. Ante-mortem examination.
Isolation pan	If animals are sick or suspect.
Stunning	Stunning **by** Co_2 anaesthesia or electrical stunning.
Exsanguination or bleeding	By making an incision in jugular furrow close to the head, severing carotid arteries and jugular veins for 5 minute in horizontal bleeding posture.
Head removal	Removal of head at atlanto-occipital joint.
Fore shanking and skinning	Sheep and goats are held back and cuts are made from the knuckles down the forelegs. The neck, cheeks and shoulders are skinned. The throat is opened up and the gullet (food-pipe) is tied off. Cutting of fore legs at knee joint.
Hind shanking and skinning	To remove the skin on hind legs, a cut is made to knuckles down to the tail root. Hind leg is cut at hock joint.
Skinning of hind quarter	After leg cutting sheep and goats are hoisted by a gambrel inserted into the Achilles tendons. Ripping is done down to midline and skinning proceeds over the flanks using special knives or the fists. Skinning of hind quarter is done on series of horizontal steel plates.
Testicle removal	Removal of testicles in male.
Skinning by fisting	Skinning by fisting.
Rimming	Loosening of rectum and pushing into pelvic cavity.
Carcass evisceration	Evisceration of the carcass by making a small cut at abdominal cavity just above the brisket. Viscera removal is carried out after withdrawn of omentum, tied of rectum and food pipe as well as splitting of breastbone. Kidney and its fat remains with carcass.
Pluck removal	Pluck removal which includes internal organs like larynx, trachea, lungs, heart, liver and spleen.
Carcass weighing	Carcass weighing for dressing percentage and other parameters.
Post mortem examination	To cheque the suitability, safety and disease conditions.

Trimming	Loss of meat parts during fabrication of carcass cuts.
Carcass washing	Spray washing of carcass with clean water.
Seal marking	Putting of seal on carcass depicting passed for consumption.
Chilling	Chilling of carcass at 0-4°C with a core temperature below 7°C which is achieved within 24 to 30 hours.
Carcass washing	Washing of carcass with spray.
Carcass deboning	Deboning of carcass at 10°-20°C.
Weighing and packaging	Weighing and packaging in a suitable package.
Freezing storage	Freezing at -30 to - 34°C with a core temperature below -18°C.

Slaughtering and dressing of Pig

Slaughtering and dressing steps	**Description**
Reception	Reception of pigs on the unloading ramp in sound condition.
Lairage	Resting (2-3 hrs) and fasting of animals. Ante-mortem examination.
Isolation pan	If animals are sick or suspect.
Stunning	Stunning by CO_2 anaesthesia or electrical stunning.
Sticking	By inserting knife in the midline of neck at depression in front of sternum and pushed forward to sever the anterior venacava and brachiocephalic trunk at the entrance of the chest.
Bleeding	Bleeding in horizontal posture for at least 5 minutes.
Scalding	Scalding in the hot water maintained at 60-63°C for 3-5 min or vertical scalding depending on facility available. Scalding is done to loosen the hair in the follicle.
Scrapping & Dehairing	Put the pig on overhead rail cut dew claws and toes. Dehairing is done manually or mechanically using bell scraper/ knife or hot resin adhesive or by rotating rubber-tipped paddles.
Carcass rinsing	Carcass rinsing with warm water.
Head and feet cleaning & gambrelling.	Cleaning of head and feet and gambrelling.
Singeing	Singeing is the removal of rudimentary hairs, shrinks and sets the skin, sterilizes the cuticles, decreases the

	number of adhering micro-organisms and leaves an attractive clean appearance. It is done with a hand-held gas torch or blow flame.
Carcass washing	Spray washing of carcass with clean water.
Head removal	Removal of head at atlas joint when carcass is open.
Brisket cutting	Opening of abdominal cavity.
Loosening of rectum	Evisceration of the carcass.
Evisceration	Viscera are removed by making a cut along the middle line through the skin and body wall from the crotch to the neck. Cut on pelvis and remove bladder and sexual organs and tied the rectum. Leaf fat is removed.
Pluck removal	Pluck includes internal organs like larynx, trachea, lungs, heart, liver and oesophagus.
Carcass splitting	Carcass splitting at downs the backbone (chine) with a saw or cleaver from the pelvis to the neck but head remains intact.
Carcass weighing	Carcass weighing for dressing percentage and other parameters.
Post mortem examination	To cheque the suitability, safety and disease conditions.
Trimming	Meat loss during fabrication of cuts.
Carcase washing	Spray washing of carcass using clean water.
Seal marking	Putting of seal on carcase depicting passed for consumption.
Chilling	Chilling of carcase at 0-4°C with a core temperature below 7°C which is achieved within 12 to 16 hours.
Retail cuts	Preparation of wholesale and retail cuts
Weighing and packaging	Weighing and packaging.
Freezing storage	Freezing at -30 to - 34°C with a core temperature below - 18°C

Slaughtering and dressing of poultry

Slaughtering and dressing steps	**Description**
Reception	Reception of poultry birds on the unloading ramp in sound condition.
Lairage	Resting (2-3 hrs) and fasting of animals. Antemortem examination.
Isolation pan	If animals are sick or suspect.
Stunning	Stunning with low voltage electric current (50 volts AC for 1 minute) or using water bath running with current for high throughput.
Exsanguination or bleeding	Bleeding is carried out in inverted cone shaped apparatus protruding head outside. Most preferred method is modified kosher method by severance of jugular vein just below the jowl but trachea and oesophagus remains intact. Bleeding time is 1.5 to 2.0 min.
Scalding	Scalding in hot water maintained at 50-55°C for 1.5 to 2.0 min (Semi or soft scalding) for broilers or 55-60°C for 2 minutes for spent birds (sub scalding) or 63°C for 2-3 minutes for turkey and other large birds (hard scalding). It is done to loosen the feathers and at least 750 ml of water is required per bird.
Defeathering	Defeathering manually or by feather plucker.
Singeing	Singeing over a blue flame for 5-10 sec.
Carcass washing	Spray washing of carcass to remove dust, dirt and other contaminations. At least 0.5 litre water is required for washing per bird.
Head, feet and glands removal	Pulling of head and removal of feet at tarsometatarsal joint and oil glands.
Evisceration	Hanging of carcass on hock joint for shackling and evisceration. It is done by making a slit opening from the tip of the breast bone and abdominal cavity is opened with transverse cut. A circular cut around the vent is also made to drawn out the viscera outside. Another slit opening at neck region to remove crop and neck.
Post mortem examination	Post mortem examination to ensure safe meat to the consumers.
Giblet and offal removal	Removal of inedible offals and collect, cleaned and pack giblet. Giblet includes gizzard without mucosal layer, heart without pericardium and liver without gall bladder placed in abdominal cavity.

	Inedible offals like trachea, lungs, oesophagus, crop, intestines, gall bladder and kidney's removal.
Carcass weighing	Weighing of carcass to find out dressing percentage and other data.
Chilling	Chill the carcass in slush ice for 30-45 minutes to achieve 4°C core temperature. Alternatively air chilling technique can also be adopted. Excess water removal by draining for 10 min.
Grading	Grading of carcass on the basis of confirmation, degree of fleshing, bruises, cuts and other quality attributes.
Packaging	Packaging of dressed carcass with giblets in abdominal cavity. Packaging is done in Polyethylene bags or by shrink packaging.
Storage	Storage at 2°C for 7days or at -18 to -20°C for 4-6 months

Slaughtering and dressing of rabbits

Slaughtering and dressing steps	**Description**
Reception	Reception of rabbits on unloading ramp in sound condition.
Lairage	Resting (2-3 hrs) and fasting of animals. Ante-mortem examination.
Isolation pan	If animals are sick or suspect.
Stunning	By hard, sharp pull on head backward to dislocate the neck or by struck a hard, quick blow by blunt stick to the skull behind the ears.
Exsanguination or bleeding	By decapitation or complete removal of head from body.
Hanging on one hind leg	Hang the rabbit with one hind leg.
Fore feet deskinning and fore shanking	Fore feet skinning and fore shanking at stifle joint.
Hind leg deskinning and hind shanking	Removal of skin from hind leg and hind shanking at hock joint.
Tail removal and skin pulling	Tail removal and pulling of skin down and forward over the body.
Evisceration	Evisceration and removal of intestinal tract and lungs by a cut from the lower part of abdomen near anus to the mid-point of the lowest rib.

	Liver, kidneys, and heart remain with carcass. Carcass removal from the hanger and hind feet cutting at the hock joint.
Post mortem examination	Post mortem examination to ensure safe meat to the consumers.
Carcass washing	Spray washing with cold water of temperature not more than 5^{0}C to remove hair and soil or debris.
Carcass weighing	Weighing of carcass to find out dressing percentage and other data.
Chilling	Chill the carcass with 4°C core temperature.
Packaging	Packaging of carcass in plastic cartons and trays.
Storage	Storage at 2°C for 7days or at -18 to -20°C for 4-6 months
Carcass washing	Spray washing with cold water of temperature not more than 5^{0}C to remove hair and soil or debris.
Carcass weighing	Weighing of carcass to find out dressing percentage and other data.
Chilling	Chill the carcass with 4°C core temperature.
Packaging	Packaging of carcass in plastic cartons and trays.
Storage	Storage at 2°C for 7days or at -18 to -20°C for 4-6 months

References

1. Gracey, J.F and Collins,D.S. (1994). Meat plant construction, equipments and operations. *In:* Meat Hygiene, 9th ed., ELBS, U.K. Pp 86-108.

2. Grandin, T. and Deesing, M. (2008). Humane Livestock Handling. Storey Publishing, North Adams, MA, USA

3. Sharma , B.D. (2003). Slaughtering and dressing of meat animals. *In:* Modern Abattoir Practices and Animal By-products Technology, First Edition, Jaypee Brothers Medical Publishers,New Delhi. Pp 35-44.

4. Smith, T.W. (2016). Slaughtering and dressing rabbits. *In:* Domestic Rabbit Biology and Production by L. R. Arrington and K. C. Kelley and Raising Rabbits, USDA Farmers' Bulletin No. 2131.

❑❑❑

Chapter 9

Evaluation and Grading of Live Animals and Carcasses

Levitical Law of Old Testament initially authorized meat animals for food of man who had to part the hoof and chew the cud. So man started eating the animals and their edible parts of animals who consume grass and other arable crops. Examples were cattle, buffalo, sheep, goat, pigs, horses, deer, reindeer, yak, camel etc. Now poultry have become major meat producing species while rabbit, guinea pigs, various game animals and birds provides substantial meat. Advancement of knowledge on quality and safety enforced the man to evaluate and grade the live animals and carcasses for values decision in marketing. *Evaluation* of live animals and carcasses is necessary to produce high priced and palatable lean with least amount of fat and bones. The other factors decides the grades of live animals and carcasses are quantity and quality of meat, dressing percentage, quality and yield of by-products, meat-bone ratio, cuttability etc. These parameters are basically decided on the basis of animal species, sex, breed, body condition and health status of animal. *Grading* is segregation of live meat animals into a group based on relatively high degree of uniformity in certain specified attributes associated with market valuation and performance. The basic objective of grading animals and carcasses are to estimate the value of animals and carcasses, uniformity maintenance, profit earning and to facilitate slaughter and inspection operations.

General considerations in judging of live animals for meat

Criteria	Quality
Body frame	Compact
Neck	Short and thick.
Shoulder bone	Should not be visible.
Wings of pin bones, tuber coxae and sacrum	Should not be visible.
Hind quarter	Massive.
Hind leg	Round and thick.
Ribs	Should not be visible.
Barrel	Round shape.
Fatness	Normal and according to species and breed.

Criteria for evaluation and grading of animals and carcasses

Criteria	*Assessment formula*
Meat yield =	$\frac{\text{Total weight of meat and meat cuts}}{\text{Cold carcass weight}}$ 100
Dressing percentage=	$\frac{\text{Carcass weight}}{\text{Live weight}}$ 100
By-product yield=	100 - dressing percentage
Meat-bone ratio=	$\frac{\text{Weight of meat recovered from carcasses}}{\text{Weight of bone}}$
Carcass cuttability=	$\frac{\text{Weight of retail cuts excluding meat trimmings}}{\text{Weight of carcass}}$ 100

Points to be considered during meat animal judging

i. *Type* and conformation term is generally applied in judging of meat animals. *Types* means all characteristics of animals raised for specific purpose i.e. meat, milk and drought type. *Conformation* refers to form and shape of animal.

ii. Judge of live animals and carcasses must be well aware about animals' anatomy, location of high priced wholesale cuts, ability to compare the qualities for logical decisions.

iii. Systemic evaluation and grading should be done on the basis of initial observations on standing and moving positions, confirmation assessment on degree of fleshing, finish from side, front and rear.

iv. Animal must be examined and palpated if required on top of shoulder, ribs, back, loin, rump and round.

v. Animal must be judged on normal characteristics like animal type, breed, sex, age and weight, physiological characteristics such as general condition, musculature, musculature fat ratio, gestation, stage of lactation, overall appearance and health characteristics includes general health (icterus, anaemia etc.), disease condition, parasitic infestation, abnormities and overall fitness.

vi. Animals must be segregated and graded according to the meat production quality. So that slaughtering and dressing operations as well as inspections can be facilitated.

vii. The dressing percentage in the range of 45-50 percent in sheep and goats, 50-60 in cattle and buffalo, around 70 percent in poultry and around 80 percent in pigs is considered optimum.

viii. Dressing percentage is mainly decided by animal species like ruminant and monogastric animals and slaughter factors like skin, hide, horns and feet in cattle and buffalo, skin, fleece, horn and feet in sheep, skin, hairs, horn and feet in goats, feet and feather in poultry as well as presence of genitallia in females etc. It is also affected with the body condition like emaciation, dehydration, bruises, grubs etc.

Judging and grading of cattle and buffalo for meat

There are two basic criteria are implied for judgment of animals for meat production in cattle and buffalo i.e age and confirmation.

Criteria of judging	**Quality**
Age	*Veal*: young calves of 1-3 months of age.
	Calf: animals ranging 3-10 months of age.
	Beef/ carabeef: mature animals over 1 months of age
Conformation	*Back*: long, straight and good depth.
	Body: rectangular.
	Head: short and broad between eyes.
	Rump: long and broad.

Ribs: barrel.

Thigh: thickly fleshed.

Legs: straight and short.

Tail: coarse.

Skin: mellow with fine hairs.

Fat: less fat on brisket ad flank.

Hide: no extra hide on throat, dewlap and sheath.

USDA quality grading system of beef /buffalo

Grades	Qualities
Prime	Top most grades. Good musculature, full brisket, flank and cod or udder.
Choice	Good musculature, marked fullness of brisket, flank and cod or udder.
Select	Slightly developed musculature, slightly full brisket, flank and cod or udder.
Standard	Thickly muscled shoulder, thick well rounded back and wide loins.
Commercial	Less developed musculature, moderately brisket, flank and cod.
Utility	Slight full brisket, flank and cod.
Cutter	Mature animal with only thin fat covering.
Canner	Inferior to minimum specified standards.

Judging and grading of sheep and goat for meat

Sheep and goats are mainly judged for meat on the basis of type, conformation and finish. Finish is the fatness. Thigh and loin are high value cuts of sheep and goats.

Body parts	Qualities
Fore head	Broad.
Neck	Thick and short.
Legs	Short.
Body	Deep wide blocky body, symmetrical confirmation.
Flank	Full and firm.
Chest	Wide.

Back	Thick and wide.
Loin	Thick and wide.
Rump	Long.
Stifle	Bulging.

Grades	Quality based on confirmation
Prime	Thick musculature, symmetrical, wide and thick body, slightly discernable ribs and backbone, small bones.
Choice	Slightly thick musculature, slightly wide and thick body, moderately prominent rib and backbone, thin fat covering on back, ribs, loin and rump.
Good	Slightly thin musculature, lack in symmetry and moderately narrow body, prominent shoulders, hips, backbone, ribs.
Utility	Inferior quality characteristics than specified to good grade.

Judging and grading of swine for meat

USDA grading of swine is mainly based on general appearance, form, finish, quality and expected dressing percentage.

Criteria	Quality characteristics
General appearance	Corresponding length, depth and width, arch strength, well developed back, loin and rump, full body, neatness of head and neck.
Finish	Fairly high and uniform.
Back and loin	Good length, moderately wide, uniform arch.
Ham	Wide, plump, smooth, firm and trim at base.
Belly	Neat, trim, firm and smooth.
Legs	Medium length.

USDA grades

Grades	Quality
Grade-I	Long and wide musculature, moderately full and thick back and loins, moderately long and slightly thick bellies, slightly thick and full shoulder, thick and plump ham.
Grade-II	Slightly short and moderately wide musculature, full and thick back and loins near edges, slightly short and

	moderately thick bellies, thick and full shoulder, thick and plump ham.
Grade-III	Short and wide musculature, very full and thick back and loins, short and thick bellies, thick and full shoulder, thick and plump ham.
Grade-III (medium grade)	Long and narrow musculature, lack in fullness and thin back and loins, long and moderately thin bellies, moderately thin and flat shoulder, ham is slightly thin and less plumpness.
Utility or Cull grade	Long and narrow musculature, thin back and loins, long and thin bellies, thin and flat shoulder, thin and flat ham.

Grades based on musculature

Grades	Muscling scores
U.S. No. 1	Thick musculature.
U.S. No. 2	Thick musculature.
U.S. No. 3	Average musculature.
U.S. No. 4	Thin musculature
U.S. No. 5	Thin musculature.

Grades based on sex

Grades	Characteristics
Boars and sows	Old breeding animals.
Barrow	Male pig castrated early in life.
Stag	Male pigs castrated on development of boar characteristics.
Gilt	Young females not yet produced young one.

Judging and grading of poultry for meat

The meat quality in live poultry is assessed by seeing the deformities, body confirmation and breast meat quantity.

Parameter	Quality
General	Poultry birds should be according to the traits.
Deformities	Poultry birds should be free from severe crooked toes, leg and foot abnormality, crossed beak and severely crooked back.

Body conformation	Shoulder: width across the shoulder.
	Back: full length.
	Body: deep.
	Ribs: spring.
	Keel: wide.
	Breast: well muscled and fully developed.
Fleshing	Well fleshed.
Fat covering	Ideal.
Discolouration	Bruises not permitted in thigh and breast.

Grading of poultry

Grades	Characteristics
USDA-A	Free from defects, bruise and well structural and muscular development.
USDA-B	Slight variation from USDA -A. like slight alteration in structural and muscular development.
USDA-C	Moderate variation with slight defects, bruise other than the thigh and legs, less musculature and structural development.
Cull grade	Thin musculature, high bone development, bruises and other deformities.

Considerable points in assessment of fatness in meat animals

i. In good fat animals flank region grasp in double fold while in poor animals little more than a double layer of skin can be felt.

ii. Degree of fatness on barrel can be adjudged by placing thumb and finger on either side of the last rib.

iii. Fatness in meat animals can also be adjudged by placing finger tip on backbone above hip where rump and loin is separated.

iv. Cod fat or dug fat in heifer can be examined by holding the tail and passing the right hand between the back legs.

Score card for judging of meat animals

Parameter	Standard qualities	Maximum score
General		
Form	Top line straight, underline deep, low and well spring ribs	10
Condition	Muscle development and degree of finish	10
Weight	As per age and trade requirement	10
Quality	Fine hair, mellow skin, uniform finish, higher muscle and sufficient firm	10
	Total	40
Head		
Face	Broad and short	1
Muzzle	Broad, wide jaw and large nostrils	2
Horns	Fine texture if present	1
Ears	Medium in size	1
	Total	5
Forequarter		
Ribs	Well barrelled with thick flesh	8
Chest	Large girth and full crop	4
Shoulder	Well muscled, smooth and neat	3
Shoulder vein	Full	2
Neck	Thick and short	2
Brisket	Wide and well forward	1
Legs	Straight with fine shank	2
	Total	22
Hind quarter		
Back	Even, smooth and straight	10
Loin	Broad and thick	8
Thigh	Well muscled	4
Rump	Even, long, wide with smooth tail head	3
Hip bones	Well covered and smooth	2
Pin bones	Well apart and prominent	2
Flank	Full and in level of underline	2
Legs	Short, straight with fine bones	2
	Total	33
	Grand Total	100

Carcass evaluation

Carcass evaluation is basically a detailed examination of carcass for prediction of yield, processing, palatability characteristics (tenderness, juiciness, and flavour) and overall quality. Evaluation of carcass helps in protection of consumer's preferences, lean meat yield calculation, assessment of meat quality parameters, estimation of cutability and taste appeal of meat cuts and enhancement of overall meat marketability. Grading of carcasses in different countries has their own grading pattern and detailed specifications to suit their market and consumer requirements. Most of them have been adopted from USDA and modified as per the local needs.

Beef carcass evaluation and grading

In United States Department of Agriculture (USDA) grading system of beef carcass evaluation, first step is determination of class or sex group. Class determination of beef carcasses is based on evidences of maturity and sex condition at the time of slaughter. In addition to class, the bovine species is subdivided into kind. The differentiation between veal, calf, and beef carcasses is made primarily on the basis of colour of lean, although such factors as texture of lean, character of the fat, colour, size, and ossification of the bone and cartilages, and the general contour of the carcass are also given consideration. The evaluation of beef carcass can be broadly categorized as: quality grading system and yield grading system.

Quality grading of beef carcasses

Quality grading of beef can be obtained on the basis of *objective evaluation* and *subjective evaluation. Objective evaluation* is mainly based on class or sex and also on kind while *subjective evaluation* is performed on the basis of physiological maturity, marbling, muscle firmness and dark-firm and dry (DFD) conditions.

Objective evaluation of beef carcass

i. *Class determination:* Class determination is an important criterion for quality grading and evaluation of carcass. Quality parameters like tenderness, colour, texture etc. are mainly decided by class of beef.

Class	Identical quality characteristics	Grading pattern
Steers	Typically rough and irregular fat deposits in cod region. Relatively small pizzle eye (white disc) located caudal to aitch bone and severed at proximal portion of penis.	Prime, choice, select, standard, commercial, utility, cutter, canner
Bullocks	Disproportionate heavy rounds, noticeable crests, thickly fleshed chucks, and large prominent pizzle eyes. Noticeably small jump muscle or round muscle adjacent to the hip bone. Typically rough and irregular scrotal fat. Dark and coarse textured lean. Well developed skeletal (bone and cartilage) maturity.	Prime, choice, select, standard, utility
Bulls	Disproportionate heavy rounds, noticeable crests, thickly fleshed chucks, and large prominent pizzle eyes. Noticeably small jump muscle or round muscle adjacent to the hip bone. May be covered with fat. Typically rough and irregular scrotal fat. Dark and coarse textured lean. Advancement in developed skeletal (bone and cartilage) maturity.	Not eligible for quality grading
Heifers	Characteristic smooth, uniform fat deposit in udder region. Absence of pizzle eye, a slightly larger pelvic cavity, and a straighter aitch bone. Bean-shaped bald spot on gracilis muscle. Less heavily muscled.	Prime, choice, select, standard, commercial, utility, cutter, canner
Cows	Characterized by large pelvic cavity and nearly straight aitch bone. Slightly prominent to very prominent hips. Fused sacral vertebrae and appears as a single bone. Most bones looks hard, white, and vertebrae is associated with cartilage. Complete ossification of aitch bone except for buttons. Slightly prominent to very prominent hips. Fused sacral vertebrae and appears as a single bone. Most bones looks hard, white, and vertebrae is associated with cartilage. Complete ossification of aitch bone except for buttons.	Choice, select, standard, commercial, utility, cutter, canner

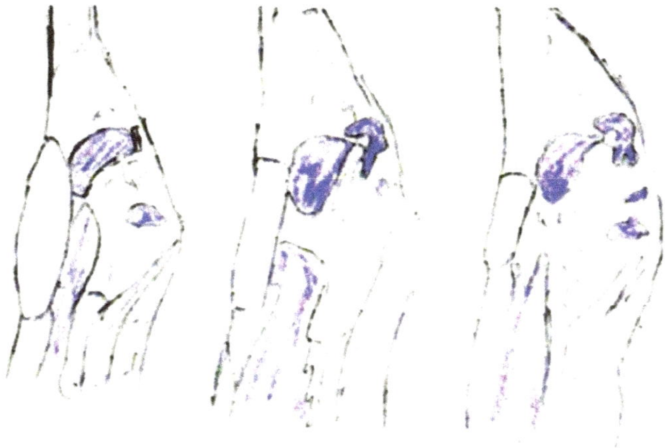

ii. *Kind determination*: kind in carcasses of veal, calf and beef can be differentiated on the basis of general carcass contour, lean colour and texture, fat colour, size and characteristics and ossification of bone and cartilage.

Kind	Identical quality characteristics
Veal	Colour of lean is grayish pink to dark grayish pink. Lean is smooth and velvety in texture. Slightly soft and pliable fat. Narrow and very red ribs.
Calf	Lean colour is grayish red to moderately red. Flakier fat. Light red wider ribs.
Beef	Evidence of advanced maturity. Lean colour is moderately red (young beef) to very dark red (mature beef). Flaky fat and flat ribs. Ossified cartilage in sacral and lumbar regions.

Subjective evaluation of beef carcass

Grading is a segregation of different cuts of animal's body to rank them as per standards. Carcass is basically evaluated on the basis of conformation (morphology of animals), quality (neat) and finish (fatness of animal). In detail *conformation* describes build, shape and outline (contour) of animal and its different primal cuts (wholesale cuts). It is also dependant on shape and size of bones and muscles and the fat covering and attributable to breeding and care of the animal. *Quality* is the character muscle or lean meat (without bone) in presence of intermuscular and intramuscular fat (marbling) in meat. It is decided by firm texture, refinement of head, hide, hair, bone. Quality decides eating desirability like tenderness palatability, colour, juiciness, odour, water holding capacity, etc. *Finish* refers to the fatness and includes fat on outer surface of carcass, inside of abdominal and thoracic cavities and also of inter and intramuscular fat. Finish is mainly dependant on breeding and to a large extent of kind and quality of the animal, age and sex of the animal and methods of handling. All there factors are basically decided by physiological maturity, marbling and muscle firmness.

i. *Physiological maturity*: physiological maturity is dependent on physiological age rather than chronological age. It is an important criterion to decide eating quality such as tenderness, juiciness, and flavor which alter with the advancement of age. There are two main considerations or indicators in assessment of maturity groups:

   a. *Skeletal maturity*: skeletal maturity is mainly judged on the basis of bone characteristics, ossification of cartilage. As age advances cartilage ossifies and bone whitens and becomes harder, flinty-like and white. The pattern of cartilage ossification in vertebral column started from sacral followed by lumber and thoracic with advancement of age. Skeletal maturity can also be assessed by seeing appearance of split chin bone and shape of rib.

   b. Colour and texture of lean: it is normally measured at rib eye muscle at 12th rib cross sectional area. Colour of lean changes from light grayish red in veal carcass to dark red in beef. It is due to accumulation of myoglobin. Texture of ribeye muscle is fine in young animal carcass and course in old animal carcass.

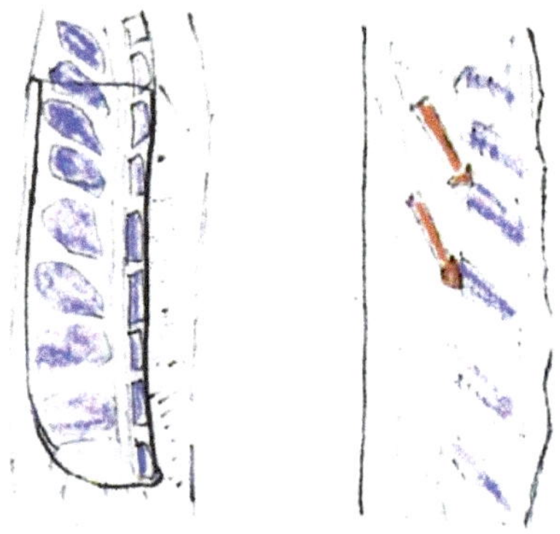

Fig: Left: Mature carcass – bones have red color and buttons show no ossification. Right: Immature carcass – bones are whiter and buttons (indicated by arrows) are completely ossified.

Based on physiological maturity carcass can be classified into five groups:

Maturity groups	Characteristics of carcass
A	No ossification on the cartilage buttons at the end of chine bones. All vertebrae of the spinal column have evidence of cartilage and sacral vertebrae are clearly separated. The split chine vertebrae are soft, porous and very red in colour whereas rib bones have slight flatness and red in colour.
B	Ossification in bones and cartilages of sacral vertebrae.
C	Ossification in bones and cartilages of lumber vertebrae.
D	Ossification in bones and cartilage of thoracic vertebrae.
E	Split vertebrae devoid of red colour, very hard, flinty with entirely ossified cartilage at the end of all vertebrae along with wide, flat and flinty rib bones.

ii. *Marbling score*: marbling is generally refers to intramuscular fat in meat. It is estimated on lean cut surface of rib eye muscle at the 12th rib interface. Marbling is an indicator of eating quality particularly tenderness and palatability. However, enhancement in marbling also increases caloric content. Extent of marbling is decided by length of time on feed, type of feed and genetic capacity for laying down this fat deposit. For grade decision both physiological maturity and marbling is considered together. High grade like USDA Prime and Choice indicates higher marbling while lower marbling score in USDA Select and Standard. Amount of marbling in the eye muscle is divided into ten degrees from higher to lower as:

a. Abundant
b. Moderately abundant
c. Slightly abundant
d. Moderate
e. Modest
f. Small
g. Slight
h. Traces
i. Practically devoid
j. Devoid

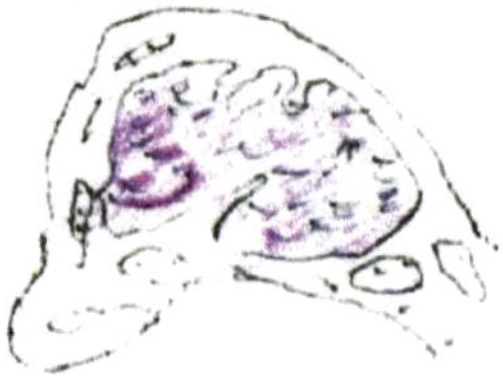

U.S. Prime

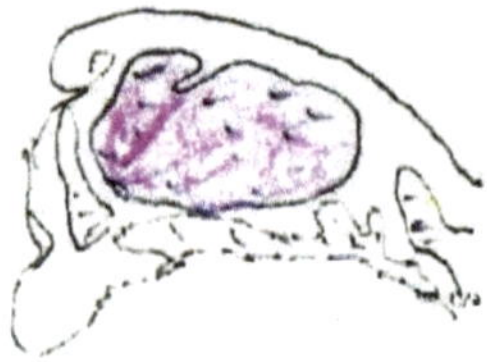

U.S. Choice

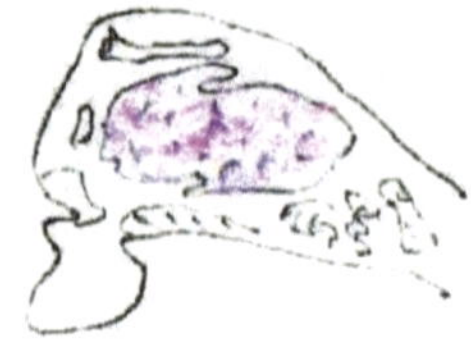

U.S. Select

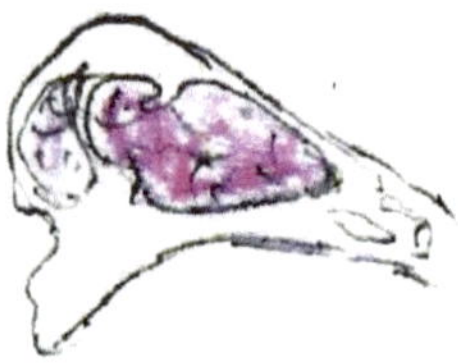

U.S. Standard

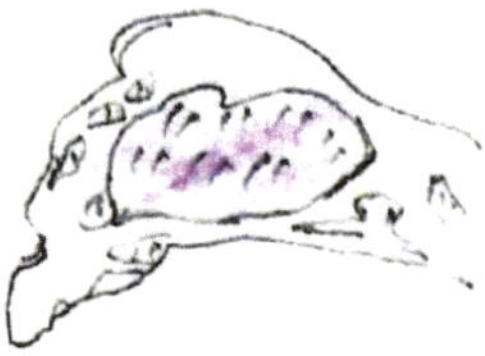

U.S. Commercial

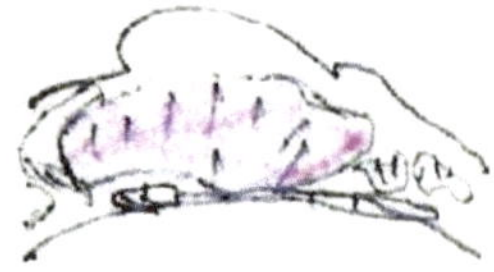

U.S. Utility

USDA standards are mainly relying on physiological maturity and marbling for beef carcass grading. On these basis beef carcasses may be classified in six distinct grades- prime, choice, select, standard, commercial and utility.

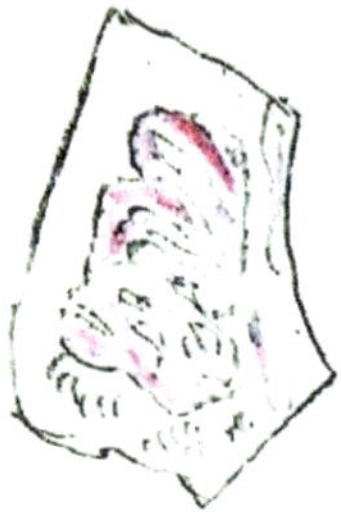

Moderately abundant

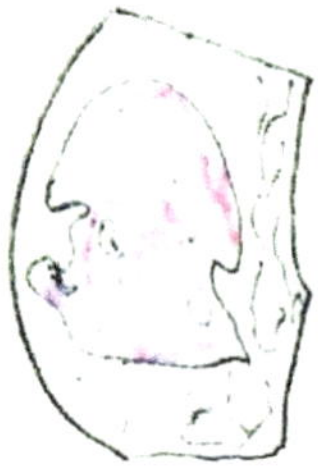

Slightly abundant

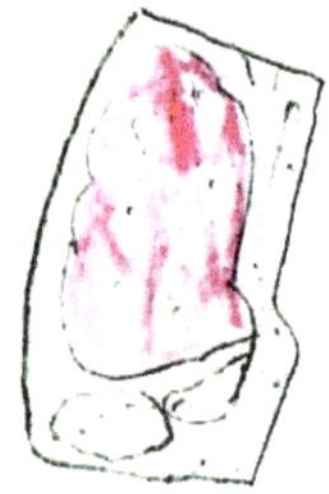

Moderate

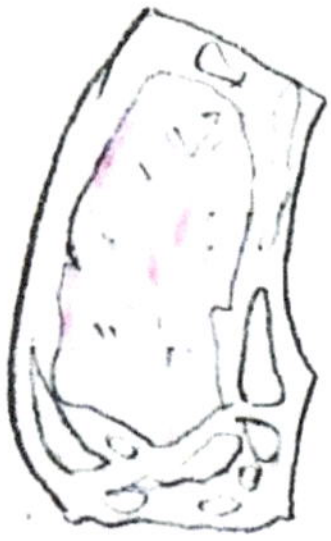

Modest

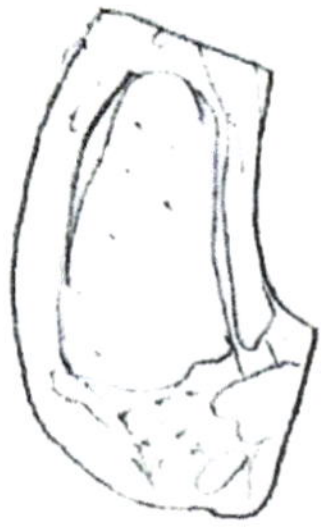

Small

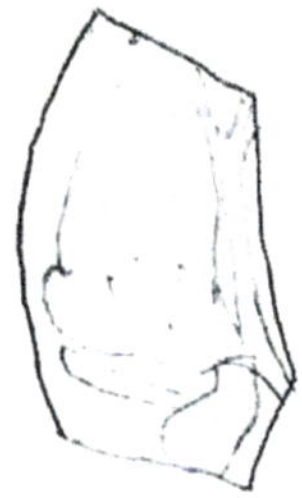

Slight

iii. *Muscle firmness*: muscle firmness is determined by rib eye cross section. On the basis of lean firmness carcase may be divided into four main quality grades. However, superior firmness is not advantageous.

Prime grade	Moderately firm
Choice grade	Slightly soft
Select grade	Moderately soft
Standard grade	Soft

iv. *USDA quality grading system:* USDA quality grading system is followed for grading the carcass for consumers' acceptance. It is utmost important to evaluate the carcase for dark firm and dry (DFD) condition. If DFD condition is found then final quality grade of carcasses may be reduced as much as one full grade for Prime, Choice and Select grades; half grade for Standard and Commercial grades but this condition has no importance in Utility, Cutter and Canner grades.

Yield grading of beef carcasses

Yield grade is a numerical value from 1 to 5 and representative of percent boneless, closely trimmed retail cuts from the high value parts of the carcass such as round, loin, rib and chuck etc. It is used to determine the cutability of the carcass. These four whole sale cuts make up about 75% of the weight, but about 90% of carcass value. Yield grade is dependent on following factors:

i. *Amount of external fat thickness:* external fat thickness is determined by thickness of fat over the cut side of the cross sectional rib eye muscle at the 12th rib. It is most important factor to determine the yield grade. Normally it is 0.3 inch and every 0.1 inch increase in fat thickness, the yield grade increases ¼ of a grade.

ii. *Percent of kidney, pelvic and heart fat:* percent kidney, pelvic and heart fat is determined by percent hot carcase weight.

iii. *Area of the rib eye muscle:* rib eye muscle area is determined by measuring the square inches area by using a dot-grid or planimeter of the longissimus muscle at 12th rib cross section.

iv. *Hot carcase weight:* hot carcass weight is determined just prior to cooling.

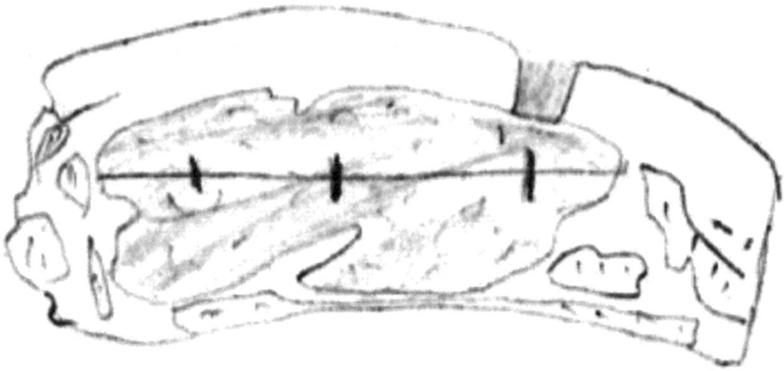

Yield Grade = 2.5+(2.5 x adjusted fat thickness in inches) + (0.20 x kidney, pelvic and heart fat) +(0.0038 x hot carcase weight in lbs) - (0.32 x rib eye area in square inches)

Cuttability (percent closely trimmed boneless retail cuts from round, loin, rib and chuck) = 51.34 - (5.784 x adjusted fat thickness in inches) - (0.462 x % kidney, pelvic and heart fat) - (0.0093 x hot carcass weight in lbs.) + (0.74 x rib eye area inch)

Evaluation and grading of buffalo carcasses

In India, Bureau of Indian standards (BIS) -IS: 2537 are generally followed to evaluate the Buffalo or Cara-beef carcasses. For grading, carcasses are evaluated on the basis of conformation, finish and quality. On these basis buffalo carcasses are graded into six distinct grades.

Grade	Characteristics
Prime	It is a top quality meat, produced from young and well fed bovine animals. The carcasses and wholesale cuts of prime grade are thick fleshed, blocky and compact. The fat covering is dependant on age as carcasses of young animals are slightly thin while mature animals carcasses are moderately thick. Carcasses are uniform in colour which may vary from light red to dark red. The chine bones are soft and vary in colour from red to tinged with white.
Choice	High quality meat with less fat. Moderately thick fleshed, blocky and compact carcasses and wholesale cuts.

	Moderately abundant fat covering in carcass which mainly dependant on age of animal. Uniform coloured carcasses and wholesale cuts of light red to slightly dark red in colour. Chine bones are soft and red to tinged white in colour.
Good	Carcasses and wholesale cuts are moderately thick fleshed, slightly compact and blocky in appearance. Fat covering of the carcass is soft or slightly oily and ranges from thin in young animals to slightly thick in more mature animals. Colour of meat varies from light red to slightly dark red. Chine bones are soft and vary in colour from red to tinged white.
Commercial	Carcasses are fairly wide and vary from angular and slightly thin fleshed in young carcasses to slightly thick fleshed and irregular in contour. Patchy or wasty thin fat covering in young animals to moderately thick in mature animals. Young animals' fat and meat is moderately soft or oily while firm in mature animals. The rib eye muscle in young animals is soft and watery, whereas coarse in mature animals. Meat colour varies form light dark red to dark red which is double toned or shady. Chine bones of young animals are red while hard and white in mature animals.
Utility	Utility grade contains meat of age animals with lack of natural tenderness and juiciness. Carcasses and wholesale cuts are thinly fleshed, angular and irregular in confirmation. Fat covering varies from very thin in young animals to moderate in mature animals. Fat is usually soft but practically no marbling. Lean usually soft and watery in younger animals but fairly firm and coarse in mature animals. Meat colour varies from light red to very dark red with double toned or shady appearance. Bones are usually hard and white.
Cutter and Canner	Lowest grade. Meat is usually less tender, less nutritious but wholesome. Meat is generally utilized by curing, canning or in sausages and other meat specialties.

Raw Meat (chilled/frozen) Grading and Marking Rules (1977) specify the buffalo grades to as choice, good and commercial. They considered *choice* as grade of choice and carcass with deviation in uniformity, fleshness at hip and thigh are graded as good grade. Lower qualities than described above are graded as *commercial grade*. However, a *special grade* is also mentioned in rule in which exporter and importer may decide any grade with the mutual understanding for the sake of business.

Score card for judging of beef or buffalo carcass

Quality parameters	Quality characteristics	Highest Scores
General		
Conformation	Compact, well fleshed, small bone	15
Finish	Smooth, uniform covering of firm creamy fat	10
Quality	Flesh with marbling, fine grain, good colour	5
Internal fat	Suet in proportion to general finish	2
Weight	As per trade requirements	5
Soundness	Well dressed, free from bruises and scores	3
	Total	40
Hind quarters		
Loin	Well fleshed but not excessively fat	15
Rump	Full, uniformly fleshed from head to tail	5
Round	Full, extending well down hock	12
Flank	Full with thick meat	2
Leg	Fine bone, fat extending well down shank	2
	Total	36
Fore Quarters		
Ribs	Well fleshed, deep, good eye muscle, smooth finish	15
Shoulder	Compact well covered	2
Neck	Short and thick	2
Brisket	Short and well fleshed	4
Shank	Fine bone	1
	Total	24
	Grand Total	100

Evaluation and grading of sheep and lamb carcasses

USDA grading pattern of sheep and lamb carcasses is broadly classified as quality grading system and yield grading system. Overall it is essential that sheep and goat carcasses must not have greater than 1% kidney and pelvic fat in the carcasses.

Quality grading system

To grade the sheep and lamb carcasses properly, it is essential to know their sex condition or class and their maturity group or kind. So that correct set of standards and grades can be identified and implemented because they are decided by kind and class in sheep and lamb carcasses.

Kind determination

Kind determination is mainly dependant on maturity of lamb and it is an important factor in quality grading system. Kinds in case of sheep and lamb carcasses may be classified as:

Kind of sheep and lamb

Class	**Age (months)**	**Parts of the carcass examined**				**USDA grades**
		Break joints or spool joints	**Rib bones**	**Colour of flank muscle**	**Lean texture**	
Lamb	3-14	Characteristic 'break joint' on at least one of their front shanks.	Round to moderately flat with redness on surface.	Slightly dark pink to slightly dark red.	Fine	Prime, choice, good, utility, cull
Yearling mutton	14-24	Spool joints on both front shanks or one spool joint and one imperfect break joint, or imperfect break joints on both front shanks.	Moderately wide and tend to be flat with slight redness to no redness on surface.	Slightly dark red to moderately dark red.	Slightly course	Prime, choice, good, utility, cull
Mutton	>24	Always have spool joints.	Wide, flat, and ribs appears in colour similar to mature bone.	Dark red to very dark red.	Course	Choice, good, utility, cull

Break joints: break joint is a epiphyseal cartilaginous area of cannon bone. A perfect break joint has all the ridges of joint intact and is well defined. In an imperfect break joint, a portion of ridges may be missing or damaged because of an imperfect break. In younger animals break joint is not ossified while in older sheep the epiphyseal area ossifies and fuses to the diaphysis of metacarpal. Break joint in young animals can be easily broken on pressure application while it is not possible in older animals.

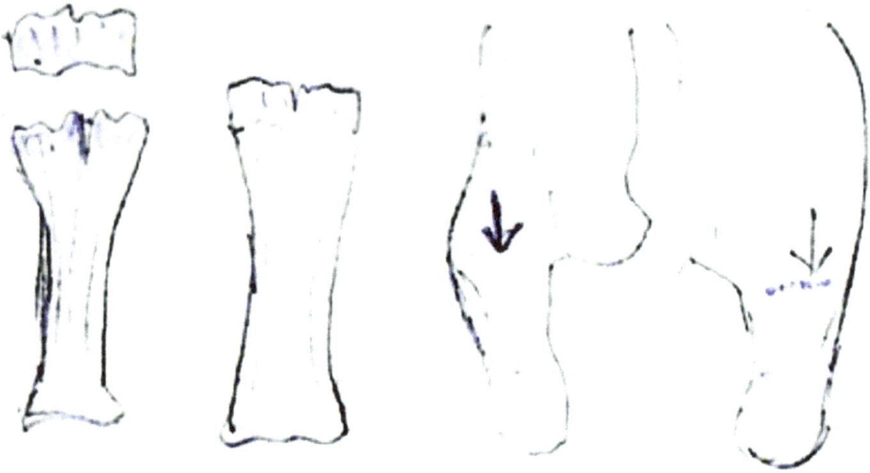

Fig: Left: The bone on the left shows a break joint, bone on the right shows a spool joint. Right: Illustration of a break joint on a lamb carcass.

Maturity grades

USDA grading of sheep and lamb carcasses on the basis of physiological maturity broadly showing two grades: Grade A and Grade B. The classification is mainly based on bones include the break joint(s) and the shape of ribs. In Grade-A carcasses ridged surface of break joint(s) is quite red, moist, and porous while it is progressively less red, drier, and harder with advancing maturity in the B group.

Break joints- Immature & mature

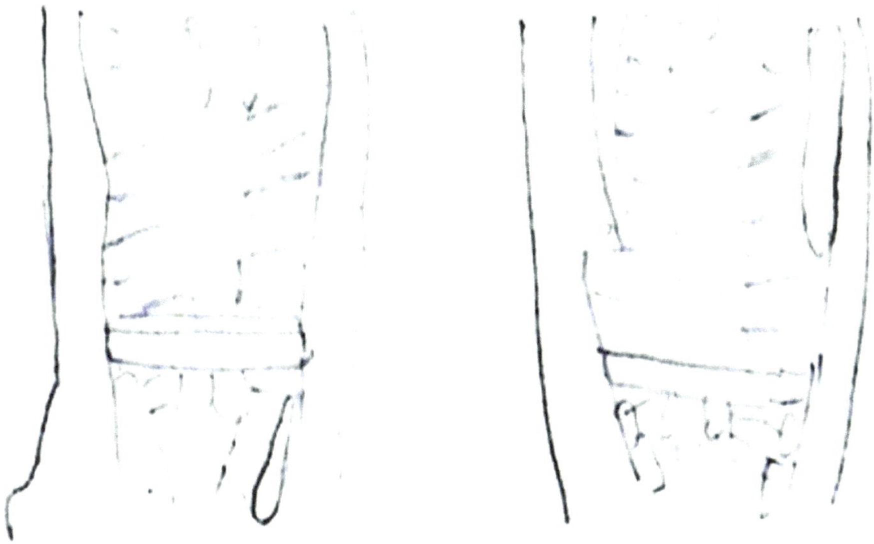

Rib shape-left: Immature Right: Mature

Class determination

Class determination is mainly based on sex or gender classification. Gender is not of much value in quality grading of sheep and lamb carcasses. However, carcasses from rams with buck like appearance are discounted with ½ grade in young lambs to two grades in mature lambs. On the basis of gender classification sheep and goat carcass may be divided into following classes:

Class	Characteristics
Ewes	Ewes contains udder while it is removed in mutton but in lambs and yearlings udder is relatively long, smooth fat deposit.
Wethers	Wethers contain cod fat which is rough, irregular and present in form of small fat deposits.
Rams	Wide configuration with heavy shoulders and thick necks. More scrotal fat and overall fat is irregularly shaped.

USDA quality grading

USDA quality grading is basically determined on the basis of conformation, lean score, lean firmness and fat coverings. *Conformation* is the thickness of muscle and fullness of carcass and determines in terms of carcass width and thickness in relation to the carcass length. *Lean score* or quality is evaluated on the basis of quantity of fat streaking on inside flank muscles, firmness of the lean flesh, and external fat. The quality grades of lamb carcasses are U.S.D.A. Prime, Choice, Good, and Utility.

Rib eye cross section area measurement

To access the lamb carcasses for ribeye muscle and actual fat thickness it is ribbed between 12th and 13th rib. Lamb carcasses are quality graded prior to ribbing but yield grading performed after the carcass is ribbed. The area on both right and left eye muscle is measured because they sometimes differ in area. It is usually do not differ by more than 0.1 or 0.2 square inches. Area may be measured directly on the carcass with a grid or from a tracing of the right and left eye muscle by a compensating planimeter.

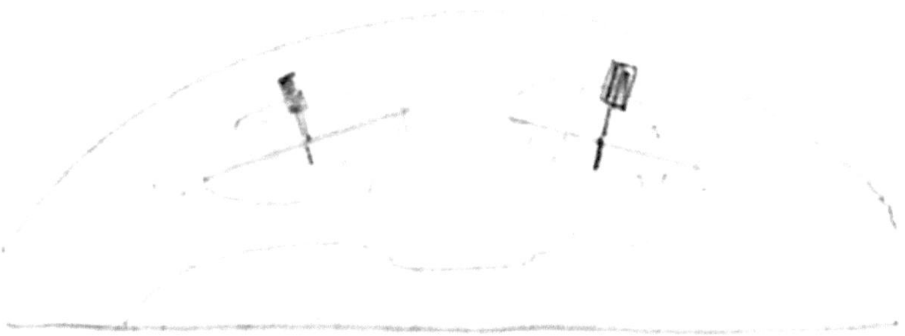

12th Rib Fat Thickness Measurement

Yield grading system

Yield grading system for sheep and lambs is initially decided by percent closely trimmed, boneless retail cuts obtained from leg, loin, rack and shoulder and carcass cuttability. These four wholesale cuts represent 80% of the carcass weight and approximately 90% of carcass value. But now it is determined by subcutaneous fat level or external fat and is poor predictor of carcass cuttability. The other considerations of yield grade determinations are -adjusted fat thickness over the rib eye at the 12th and 13th rib interface, subcutaneous fat thickness at the midpoint of the rib eye and fat deposition over the other parts of the carcass. As the amount of external fat increases, the percent of retail cuts decreases. Each 0.05 inch change in adjusted fat thickness over the ribeye muscle between the 12th and 13th ribs changes the yield grade by one-half a grade.

Yield grades: based on external fat there are five yield grades denoted by numbers 1 through 5 in which 1 represents the highest degree of cutability.

USDA Yield Grade	Adjusted fat thickness at the 12th rib(in inches)
1	0 to 0.15
2	0.16 to 0.25
3	0.26 to 0.35
4	0.36 to 0.45
5	0.46 or greater

Yield Grade = 0.4 + (10 x adjusted fat thickness in inches)

BIS standards for sheep and goat carcass grading

On the basis of BIS, IS2536: 1995, sheep and goat carcasses can be divided into six grades based on conformation, finish and quality of the carcasses or cuts. The fleshing characteristics are also of importance in sheep and goat carcass grading.

Grades	Characteristics
Prime	Highest grade practically ideal in conformation, finish and quality. Carcasses and cuts are compact and blocky with short, thick and plump legs, broad backs, thick and well fleshed loins, ribs and chucks, well proportioned breasts with full thick flanks. Carcass fat is firm and of excellent quality. Interspersed fat covering with strips of pink flesh but outer covering of fat is smooth, moderate in depth and evenly distributed over the back and sides. Interior fats are plentiful but not excessive or wasty. Lean is firm, all parts are fine grained and cut surfaces are smooth and velvety in touch.
Choice	Carcasses are good in conformation, finish and quality. Short and stocky legs, thick loins and ribs, full fleshy shoulders and thick breasts. Body fat is good in quality and outer fat covering is smooth and well distributed over loins, ribs and shoulders. Lean is moderately fine grained, firm and of proper colour.
Good	Carcasses are good in conformation, finish and quality but inferior to prime and choice. Well proportioned plump carcasses but slightly less in breadth or depth across the backs, hips or shoulders. Carcasses are showing slight paunchiness or tanginess with long tapering shanks and longer body. Whole body fat is good in quality. The outer fat covering is smooth and even over the back and hips but diminishes sharply towards

	the shanks and flanks. Plentiful unevenly distributed interior fat. Lean is moderately firm and fine in grain.
Commercial	These carcasses have fair conformation, finish and quality.
	They are angular or rangy in conformation with moderately long thin necks and shanks and relatively narrow hips, back and shoulders.
	They have moderately long tapering legs with little plumpness. Depth of flesh on Ribs and loins are lacking.
	They have excessive quantities of fat. The outer covering of fat is moderately thin but it is not evenly distributed. Whereas, interior fats are relatively scarce. The kidneys are partially covered with fat.
	The lean flesh is soft, spongy and moderately fine grained.
Utility	Low grade carcasses are lacking in quality and finish.
	Carcasses contain high percentage of bone to flesh.
	Carcasses are poor in conformation and back bone contour is plainly visible form neck to tail.
	Bluish tinge fat with lesser quantity of exterior and interior fat.
	Coarse and fibrous dark coloured red lean.
	Carcasses are angular and all bones are prominent and disproportionately long and narrow.
Cull	Lowest grade carcasses with high bone to flesh ratio due to use of old aged animals.
	Exterior and interior fat is scanty.
	Dark, soft, coarse and watery lean.

Raw Meat (chilled/frozen) Grading and Marking Rules (1977) specify the sheep and goat grades to as choice, standard and special. They considered choice as grade of choice and carcass with deviation from choice characteristics like uniform fleshing and carcass with deficient trimmable fat, bone and rib prominence are considered for standard grade. However, a special grade is also mentioned in rule in which exporter and importer may decide any grade with the mutual understanding for the sake of business.

Score card for judging of sheep and goat carcasses

Indicators	**Quality characteristics**	**Highest score**
General		
Weight	As per trade requirements	10
Conformation	Compact, well fleshed legs and loin	10
Condition	Well fleshed with smooth covering of white fat	10

Quality	Sappy and food colour flesh	10
	Total	40
Body characteristics		
Carcass	Well dressed, clean, free form cuts and bruises	10
Shoulders	Well fleshed and neat but smooth in finish	7
Ribs	Well fleshed, well barrelled and short	6
Loins	Broad and long eye muscle with correct cover of fat with optimum kidney fat	20
Legs	Thick, plump and extending well down the shank with uniform fat covering.	15
Neck	Short and neat	2
	Total	60
	Grand total	100

Evaluation and grading of pork carcass

Pork carcass evaluation and grading is determined by class or gender, carcass length, dressing percentage, major carcass cuts, loin eye area, back fat thickness, meat colour, firmness and marbling etc.

Class determination

Class determination is important to know the quality of pork meat because it decides the parameters as mentioned above for carcass quality assessment.

Class	Characteristics	USDA Grades
Barrow	Presence of a small pizzle eye near penis located dorsally from the aitch bone. Gracilis muscle ventral to aitch bone is relatively small and partially covered with fat.	US 1,2,3,4 and utility
Gilt	Absence of the pizzle eye. Gracilis muscle is considerably larger; bean shaped, and has very little fat covering. No mammary development.	US 1,2,3,4 and utility
Sow	Characteristics same as gilt. Presence of developed mammary tissue associated with lactation or advanced stages of pregnancy. Heavier than gilt.	US 1,2,3,4, utility and US cull
Stag/Boar	Characteristics same as barrow. Larger and more prominent pizzle and than	Not eligible for grading

barrows because of sexual maturity.
Heavier muscled and larger bones and joints of shoulders.
Skin over shoulder is thicker and lean is darker compared to boars.

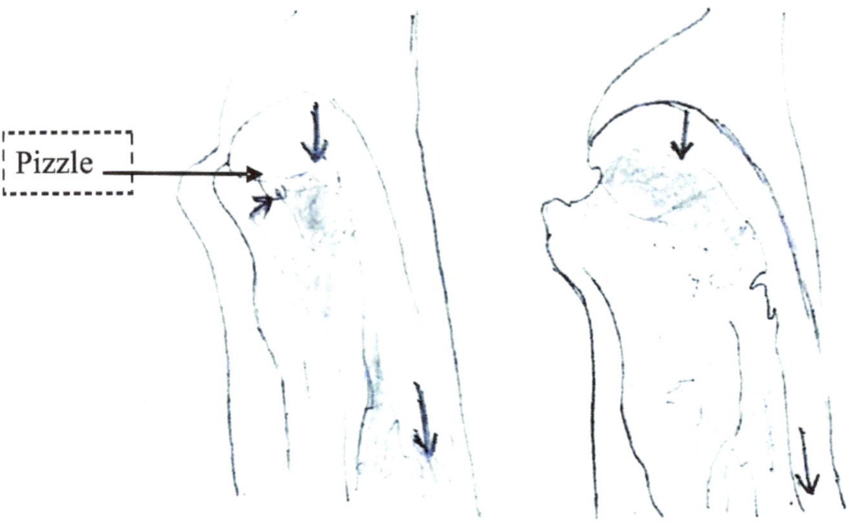

Carcass length measurement

Length of pork carcass is measured with a metal tape or may be estimated on the hanging carcass from the cranial edge of the first rib adjacent to the backbone to the cranial edge of the aitch bone or pubic symphysis. Both side measurement of carcass length and average measurement is generally recommended.

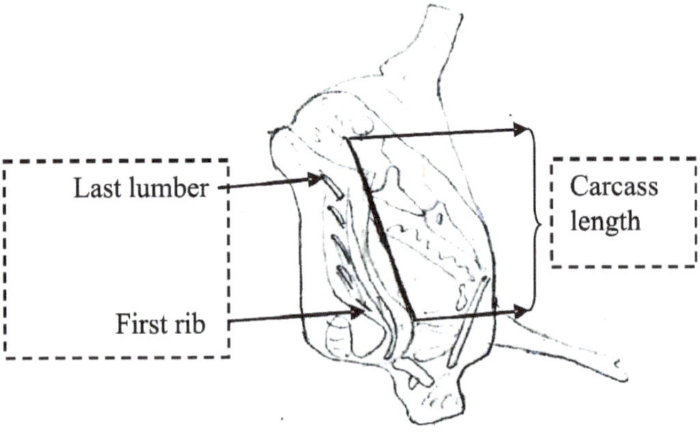

Back fat thickness

Backfat thickness of pork carcass is generally measured at two locations. One at last rib to determine pork carcass for U.S.D.A. grade and second measurement is taken at the 10th rib which is used to calculate percent muscle in pork carcasses. It is usually measured with a metal ruler and the measurement is made to the nearest 0.1 inch.

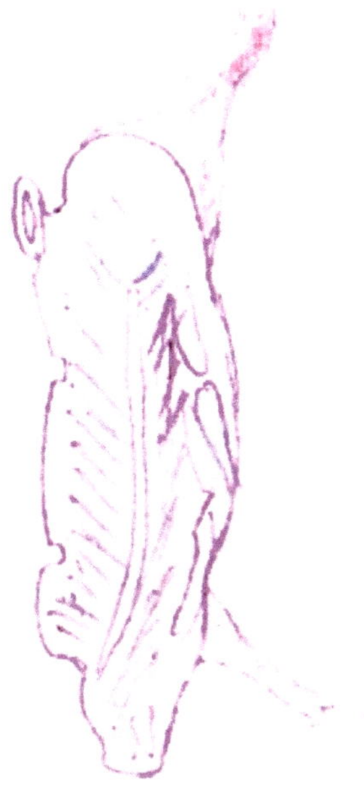

Ribbing

Ribbing refers to portioning of carcass in between 10th and 11th rib to expose the loin eye muscle and at 10th rib interface for backfat. However, for commercial purpose unribbed carcasses are usually considered for pork carcass grading.

Back fat thickness at 10th rib

The depth of subcutaneous fat including skin is generally measured in tenths of inches at 10th rib interface. It is more accurate measurement of subcutaneous fat than average backfat thickness because it is not influenced by variation in carcass splitting and trimming.

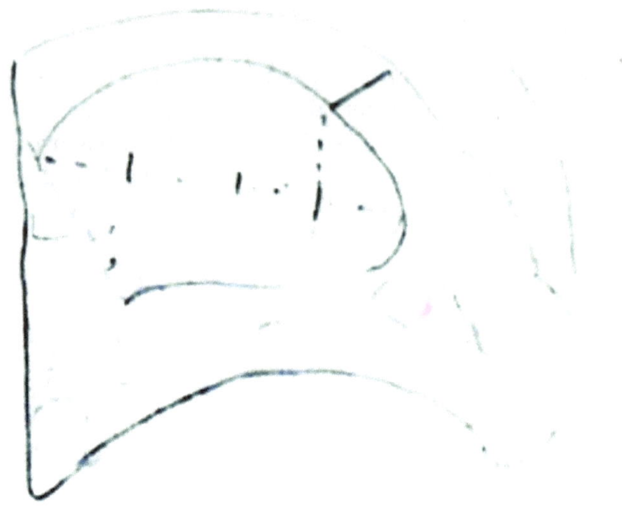

Back fat Measurement at the 10th Rib

Loin eye area

Longissimus or eye muscle area is estimated in square inches on cross section of muscle at 10th rib interface. It is determined most frequently with a plastic grid. It can also be measured by tracing eye muscle with a compensating polar planimeter.

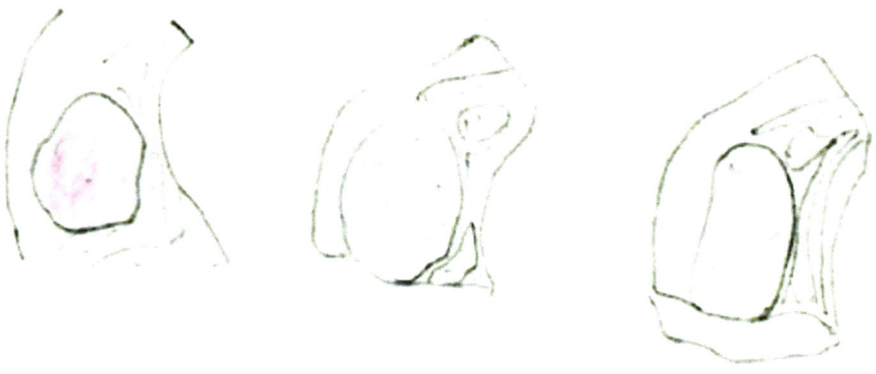

A- Loin eye area B-large loin eye area C-Small loin eye area

Grading of pork carcass

Generally barrow and gilt carcasses are graded on two considerations like Quality indicating characteristics of lean and fat and cuttability grade or expected yield of the four lean cuts (ham, lion, picnic shoulder, and Boston shoulder).

i. *Characteristics of lean:* based on lean quality pork carcass can be categorized as acceptable and unacceptable. To qualify for *acceptable category* lean quality is assessed at 10th rib interface either on ribbed carcass or on wholesale loin. Lean should have slight degree of feathering, firmness of lean in eye muscle, degree of marbling and colour should be greyish pink to moderately dark. The values helps in scoring the lean numerical basis from 1 to 5. The *unacceptable* lean will be considered if its quality is below minimum quality standards and with pale soft and exudative (PSE) condition.

ii. *Cuttability grade*: cuttability grade is a numerical representation of percent yield of bone-in, closely trimmed lean cuts such as ham, loin, boston and picnic shoulder. It is determined on the basis of last rib back fat thickness and muscle score.

   a. *Last rib back fat thickness:* it is most important factor in determination of yield of lean cuts and amount of external fat. External fat quantity is indirectly proportionate to the lean cut, as the amount of external fat increases, the yield of lean cut decreases. To measure the external fat, skin is also included so that if carcass is skinless then 0.1 inch is added to the measure. External fat is measured at a point along the back fat opposite the last rib perpendicular to the skin surface.

   b. *Muscle score:* muscle score is primarily determined at the ham, ham-loin junction and loin. Generally there are three muscle scores are used in standards-Thick (3), Average (2) and Thin (1). These are often sub-divided into five groups like 1.0, 1.5, 2.0, 2.5 and 3.0

Cuttability Grade = (4.0 x last rib fat thickness) - (1.0 x muscle score)

USDA grades for barrow and gilt

USDA Grade	Yield of bone-in, closely trimmed lean cuts i.e. ham, loin, Boston butt and picnic shoulder (%)	Backfat thickness in inches	Muscle status
US-1	>60.3	1.3-1.6	Thick
US-2	57.4 - 60.3	1.6-1.9	Moderately thick
US-3	54.4 - 57.3	1.9-2.2	Slightly thick
US-4	< 54.4%	>2.2	Thin

Alternate grading system for pork carcass

Some packers are using alternative system of grading for pork carcasses in which premium or a discount grid is used to measure the fat thickness across one axis and weight down the other axis. The price per 100 lbs of carcass weight is determined by identifying the point where carcass weight and fat measure meet on the grid. This will give the percent premium or discount which will multiply by the base carcass price. The salient features of alternative system of pork carcass grading are given below:

i. Carcass weight and carcass length along with back fat thickness is used as a guide for grading pig carcasses.

ii. The table given below shows the normal length range for given weight. The final grade is determined subjectively.

iii. Carcass weight is based on chilled shipper style carcasses.

iv. The back fat thickness is measured at the level of 1st rib, last rib and last lumbar, which is equal to the measurement of back fat thickness at the 7th rib level.

Grade wise correlation of carcass weight, length and backfat thickness

Carcass weight (kg)/ length (cm)	**Grade wise average back fat thickness (cm)**				
	US1	**US2**	**US3**	**Medium**	**Cull**
Barrow and Gilt					
< 55 /70	3.0 - 3.75	3.75 - 4.75	>4.75	2.0- 3.0	< 2.0
55-75/ 70-76	3.25 - 4.25	4.25 - 5.25	>5.25	2.5 - 3.25	< 2.5
75-95/ 77-84	3.5 - 4.5	4.5 - 5.5	>5.5	2.75 - 3.5	< 2.75
>95/> 85	3.75 - 4.75	4.75 - 5.75	>5.75	3.0 - 3.75	< 3.0
Sow (BFT grade)	3.75 - 5.0	5.0 -6.25	>6.25	2.75 - 3.75	< 2.75

Poultry grading system

Poultry carcasses are evaluated for grading on the basis of conformation, degree of fleshing, bruises, cuts and other quality attributes. The quality attributes and grades are basically dependant on the kind, class and type. The kinds and classes of live, dressed, and ready-to-cook poultry is mentioned in U.S. class, standards, and grades and are applicable in all segments of poultry industry.

Kind: Kind refers to different species of poultry such as chicken, duck, turkey, geese, guineas and pigeons.

Class: Class refers to certain physical characteristics which are essentially same. Class is basically associated with sex and age i.e. fryers or hens.

Type: As per standards and specifications dressed chicken can also be classified as dressed chicken (chilled) and dressed chicken (frozen).

USDA kind standards for chicken carcasses

Category	Age	Quality
Cornish game hen	5-7 wks	Young immature chicken
Broiler or fryer	9-12 wks	Tender meat. Soft, pliable, smooth textured skin. Flexible breastbone cartilage.
Roaster	12-20 wks	Tender meat. Soft, pliable, smooth textured skin. Moderately flexible breastbone cartilage.
Capon	Surgically unsexed male <30 wks	Tender meat. Soft, pliable, smooth textured skin.
Stag	Male < 40 wks	Tough and dark meat. Course skin. Hard breast bone cartilage. Maturity level is in between roaster and cock.
Hen or fowl	Female > 40 wks	Less tender meat than roaster. Non flexible breast bone tip.
Cock or old roaster	Male >40 wks	Tough and dark meat. Course skin. Hard breast bone tip.

USDA kind standards for turkeys

Category	Age	Quality
Fryer roaster turkey	Young immature <16 wks	Tender meat. Soft, pliable, smooth textured skin. Flexible breastbone cartilage.
Young hen turkey	Young females of	Tender meat. Soft, pliable, smooth textured skin.

		Moderately flexible breastbone cartilage.
Young tom turkey	Young males of 21- 30 wks	Tender meat. Soft, pliable, smooth textured skin. Moderately flexible breastbone cartilage.
Yearling hen turkey	Mature females of 64 wks	Reasonably tender-meat. Reasonably smooth-textured skin.
Yearling tom turkey	Fully matured males of <64 wks	Reasonably tender-meat. Reasonably smooth-textured skin.
Hen or Tom	Mature or old >64 wks of either sex	Tough meat. Course skin.

USDA kind standards for ducks

Category	Age	Quality
Broiler or frying duckling	Young duck < 8wks	Tender-meat. Soft bill and windpipe
Roaster duckling	Young duck< 16 wks	Tender-meat. Moderately hard bill. Easily dented windpipe.
Mature or old duck	Ducks > 26 wks	Tough meat. Hard bill. Hard windpipe.

USDA kind standards for guineas

Category	Age	Quality
Young guinea	Young guinea	Tender meat. Flexible breastbone cartilage.
Mature or old guinea	Mature or old guinea	Tough meat. Hard breastbone.

USDA kind standards for pigeons

Category	Age	Quality
Squab	Immature pigeon	Extra tender meat.
Pigeon	Mature pigeon	Tough meat. Course skin.

Indian kind standards (ISI-1975) for chicken

Category	Age
Broiler or fryer	8-10 wks
Roaster	12-20 wks
Stag	Male < 40 wks
Stewing chicken or Fowl	Female > 40 wks
Cock or roaster	Male > 40 wks

Class (indication of age) standards

Class	Young	Mature
Chicken comb	Pliable, resilient, wrinkleless with sharp points.	Round, wrinkled, coarse, with thick points.
Ducks bill	Pliable and moderately hard.	Hard.
Plumage	Fresh with glossy appearance.	Faded and worn.
Fat	Brighter colour arranged in smooth layers. Feather tract shows no lump.	Darker coloured. Heavy feather tract with lumps.
Breastbone	Pliable and soft breast bone cartilage.	Hard and bony cartilage at the end of keel.
Pinbones	Pliable.	Pliable less.
Shanks	Small, smooth with scales.	Large, rough with scales.
Oil sac	Small and soft.	Enlarged and hard.
Chicken and turkey spurs	Small, undeveloped and corn-like.	Length enhances with age, curved and sharp.
Ducks and Geese wind pipe	Vulnerable to dent.	Hard and bony.
Meat	Tender, fine textured and translucent.	Hard, coarse textured and dark.
Drumsticks	Underdevelopment and vulnerable to dent.	Round, full and firm.

Class (indication of sex) standards

Class	Males	Females
Head	Large and coarse.	Small and fine.
Plumage	Long and pointed feathers. Long and curved tail feather. Brilliant in colour. Male duck have a curl in the tail feathers.	Short and blunt feathers. Short and straight tail feathers. Modest in colour.
Body	Large and angular. Deep from keel to back. Bones including shanks are longer, larger and coarser.	Round with Fine bones.
Skin	Slightly course. Large feather follicles. Less fat under skin. Heavy feather tracts and back.	Smooth. Well distributed fat in between feather tracts.
Keel	Well muscled, long and taper at base.	Short and round.
Legs	Long thigh and drumstick.	Short thigh and drumstick.

USDA Grades for poultry carcasses

Quality parameter	Grade-A (No.1)	Grade-B (No.2)	Grade-C (No.3)
Conformation	Normal	Practically normal	Abnormal
Breast bone	Slightly curved. Dent: Chicken- 1/8", turkeys 1/4"	Slightly crooked	Crooked
Back	Normal but slightly curved.	Moderately crooked	Crooked or hunched back
Legs &wings	Normal	Slightly misshapen	Misshapen
Fleshing	Well fleshed, moderately broad and long breast	Fairly well fleshed	Thin fleshed, underdeveloped narrow breast.
Fat coverings	Well fat coverings. Moderate fat covering in chicken and turkey fryers and young toms. Normal abdominal fat.	Enough fat coverings on legs and breast. Excessive abdominal fat in hens or fowl.	Very less fat covering on back and thighs. Small fat on feather tracts.
Defects	Slight	Moderate	Serious

Exposed area on flesh	Breast ¼″ and legs 1".	Not more than 1/3.	Limitless.
Discolorations	¾″ of total area	11/4"	Limitless.
Disjointed & Broken bones	1 & no broken	2 & no broken or 1 with 1 non protruding broken.	Limitless.
Tears	Free	Free	Free
Bruises, scratches and callouses	Slightly	Moderately	Limitless.
Shanks	Slightly scaly	Moderately scaly	Seriously scaly
Missing Parts	Wing tips and tail.	2nd wing joint and defective back.	Wing and defective back.

Indian Standards for dressed chicken

Quality parameters	Grade -I	Grade-II
Conformation	Free from deformities except slightly curved or dented breast bones and slightly curved backs.	Acceptable appearance with dented, curved or crooked back and misshapen legs or wings.
Fleshing	Rounded well fleshed with moderately long and deep breast.	Substantially fleshed with short and narrow breast.
Fat covering	Evenly distributed fat in skin and between heavy feathers.	Sufficient fat under skin, breast and legs.
Defeathering	No pin feathers, diminutive feathers and hairs.	Occasional protruding pin feather or diminutive feathers.
Cuts and tears	No cuts and tears on breast and legs.	Very few cuts and tears.
Discolouration	No discolouration except lightly shaded discolouration.	Presence of discoloration due to bruising without clots. Moderately shaded discolouration of skin or flesh such as blue back.
Freezer burn	Occasional pock marks not exceeding 0.5 cm in diameter on carcass due to drying of the inner layer of skin.	Few pock marks with no single area exceeding circle of 1.5 cm in diameter due to drying of inner layer of skin.

References

1. Cuthbertson, A. (1968). PIDA dissection techniques. *In:* Symposium on methods of carcass evaluation. EAAP, Dublin; 1968.
2. Sharma, B.D. (1999). Pre-slaughter handling, transport and dressing of poultry. *In:* Meat and Meat Products Technology including Poultry Products Technology, Jaypee Brothers Medical Publishers (P) Ltd., New Delhi. Pp 99-103.
3. Sharma, B.D. (2003). Evaluation of dressed carcasses. *In:* Modern Abattoir Practices and Animal By-products Technology, First Edition, Jaypee Brothers Medical Publishers, New Delhi. Pp 62-68.
4. Singh, V.P. and Pathak, V. (2011). Evaluation of animal carcass. *In:* Laboratory Manual of Abattoir Practices and Animal Products Technology, DUVASU, Mathura. Pp 30-46.
5. USDA (1965). Poultry grading manual. Agriculture Handbook no. 31. U.S. Department of Agriculture-Consumer and Marketing Service- Washington D.C. Pp 2-25.

❑❑❑

Chapter 10

Cutting and Fabrication of Carcasses of Different Animals

Meat cutting and fabrication is a skilled process in which separation of carcass into wholesale primal cuts is done to facilitate meat trade requirements, consumer preference and easy handling to the butchers. The person engaged in cutting and fabrication of carcass cuts must be skilled and expert in their job. He/she must have the expert knowledge of carcass configurations and location of retail cuts in animal carcasses. To obtain good quality retail cuts, carcass should be essentially chilled and temperature of meat cutting room should be 15-20°C with relative humidity of about 80%. Meat cutting room should be fully synchronized for better utilization of carcass. The equipments required for meat cutting should be of stainless steel and quite sharp. Cutting and fabrication of different cuts should be in accordance to standard specification by trained butchers. As a thumb rule sharp knife should be used for cutting of muscular parts of carcass and manual or mechanized saw should be used for separation of bony parts and for disjoining at joints limited force should be applied. Various cutting systems are prevalent worldwide like American cutting method, British cutting method, French cutting method, Australian cutting method etc. However, all these cutting methods are modifications of United States Department of Agriculture (USDA) standards. In India, Bureau of Indian Standards (BIS) recommended carcass cutting and fabrications procedures and cuts are generally accepted.

Salient features

1. Beef/buffalo carcasses are generally subjected to halving or splitting into two halves or sides. So each side of beef carcass consists one fore and one hindquarter which are equally matched.
2. *Ribbing or quartering* is generally adapted to produce fore and hindquarters. The separation of sides is done between 12th and 13th rib, where 13th rib remains with hindquarter.

3. Beef/buffalo carcasses are generally separated into thymus, mediastinal tissue and heart fat before shipment.
4. Diaphragm is usually separated, if not, the tendinous portion is trimmed down to lean muscle tissue. But diaphragmatic muscles and gullet may or may not be removed from the carcass.
5. Generally lamb and mutton carcasses are exported in form of entire un-split dressed carcass but heart, liver and lungs, spleen and caul fat is removed.
6. Veal carcass is generally remains unsplit without hide. The heart fat is usually trimmed but diaphragmatic muscles and gullet may or may not be removed from the carcass.
7. In *Packer Style* hog jowl remains intact with carcasses but head, liver, heart, lungs and kidneys are removed along with leaf fat, lumbar, pelvic and heart fat.
8. Portioning or separation of chilled carcass into various commercial parts is referred to as the cutting operation or fabrication of carcasses of food animals.
9. Always cut right angles to the grain and separate out high and low muscle pieces, high and low degree fat parts.

Desirable factors in carcass fabrication

1. Cutting and fabrication should be neat and generally performed in chilled carcasses with 7^{0}C internal temperature.
2. Buture should be expert enough and cutting technique must produce identical cut in all the carcasses. The variation in size and shape is permitted only to the extent of ± 3% which is generally refers as ± 3% dexterity or accuracy. Value ratio in cutting and fabrication should be 9:5.
3. Always a standard procedure should be adopted to produce identical cuts with their valuation.
4. Cutting room should be maintained in good environmental conditions and provision of hygiene and sanitation must be provided. The temperature of cutting room should be 15-20^{0}C with the relative humidity of 80%.
5. All equipments such as knives, saws, cutting table ad other machinery should preferably of stainless steel. Electrically or mechanically operated equipments may be used to enhance the efficiency.

6. Three basic principles of carcass cutting or fabrication like cutting of muscular portion with knife, bony structure with saw and breaking or disjoining with far less physical effort should always be followed.
7. There should be a synchronized working atmosphere in cutting room in which cuts and trimming should pass through a separate outlet, fresh cuts should be immediately packed and passed for chilling, fat should be transferred to rendering unit and cuts like ham, shoulder if requires should be passed to curing room.
8. In modern plants in-line operations of cutting and fabrication of carcasses are generally performed and cuts are cryovaced to extent the shelf life.

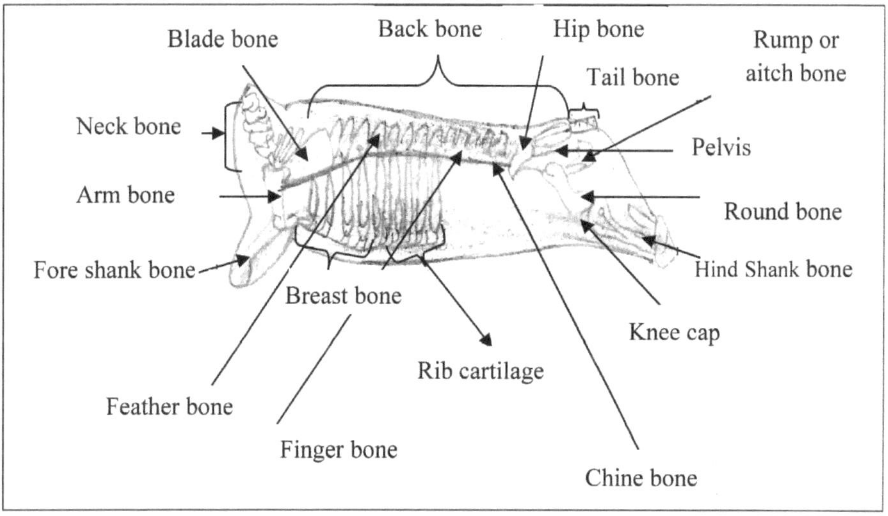

Bone structure of beef/buffalo

Cutting and fabrication of beef/buffalo carcasses

The process of dividing of chilled carcass into various commercial parts is referred as the cutting operation or fabrication of carcasses of food animals. Different cutting styles are generally followed in various countries. In US, Middle West, and South West countries, Western or Chicago cut is generally followed for beef carcass fabrication. However, Eastern sea bound states are applying Eastern or New York style of cutting beef. In Chicago and New York style 13th rib usually attached with the hindquarter while in Boston method 11th, 12th and 13th rib remains with hindquarter. In Philadelphia method of cutting all ribs are left in forequarter. In India, beef and buffalo carcasses are split into two halves or sides. The right side of carcass is called kidney close side or tight side whereas, left side is known as kidney free side or open side.

1. *Ribbing or quartering*: It is process of separating the beef/buffalo sides into forequarter and hind quarter by making cut between the 12th and 13th rib, leaving the 13th rib on the hindquarter *(Chicago style).*

2. *Wholesale cuts of forequarter:* forequarter of beef or buffalo carcasses contribute around 51 percent of whole part of the animal carcass. Cut wise forequarter contains rib (9.0%), plate (9.5%), shank (4.0%), brisket (4.5%) and chuck (24%). Rib and plates are placed together while chuck, brisket and shank complex are placed on the table with rib side down.

   i. *Rib and Plate:* rib and plate portion is separated from chuck, brisket and shank by making a cut in between 5th and 6th ribs. To separate upper rib from the lower plate, a straight and parallel cut to the backbone is made by joining two points at loin and chuck ends. These points are located at a distance of 8 inches from their respective protruding edges of chine.

   ii. *Shank*: the shank portion of beef or buffalo carcasses is obtained by making the cut parallel to the underline and just dorsal to the prominence (lateral condyle of humerus) on lower extremity of humerus.

   iii. *Brisket:* to remove the brisket, cut is continued through the breastbone and lower ends of ribs from the point of shank and parallel to back bone. Alternatively, brisket can also be obtained by making a cut perpendicular to 4th rib at a point about 4 cm proximal to the olecranon process of elbow.

   iv. *Chuck:* the remaining portion of forequarter is called chuck. It is large thick square cut of forequarter.

3. *Wholesale cuts of hindquarters:* hind quarter cuts of beef and buffalo carcass contribute 49 percent to whole carcass. In which flank shares 4.0%, loin 17.5%, round 23.5% and kidney knob 4.0%.

   i. *Flank*: to obtain flank cut, incision is made from a point immediately ventral to the aitchbone and following the natural seam until the thick muscle of the flank is reached and then a straight cut is made to a point about one and a half inches below eye muscle.

   ii. *Round:* round cut removes a half of femur and about the size of a silver dollar. Round cut is usually separated from loin by making a cut at a point about one and half inches anterior to the aitch bone and parallel to the rib end of loin. As per the choice, separation of rump from round can be done by making a cut immediately parallel and ventral to aitchbone.

iii. *Loin:* the remaining portion of hindquarter except kidney knob is called loin. Loin cut can further be divided into anterior and posterior section at anterior tip of hip and between the lumbar and sacral vertebrae. The posterior third portion containing the hip bone or ilium is known as sirloin and the anterior portion containing five lumbar and one thoracic vertebra is known as shortloin.

iv. *Kidney knob:* kidney knob cut can be obtained by separation of kidney along with adjoining fat. However, very little fat on tenderloin still remains after separation of kidney knob.

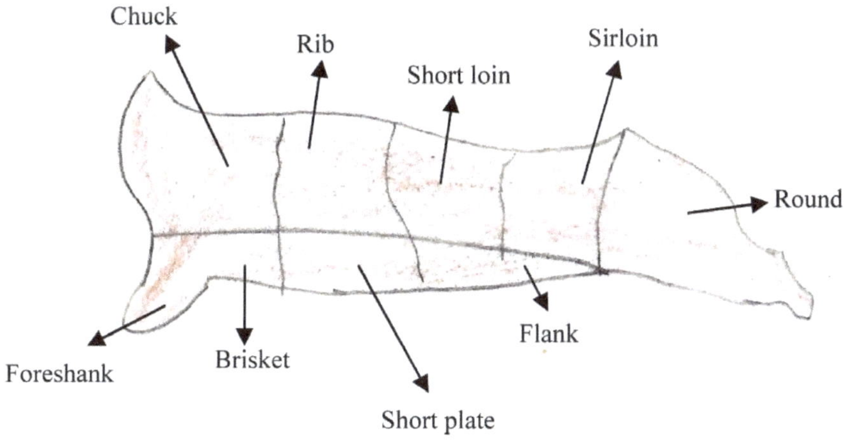

Wholesale cuts of beef/buffalo

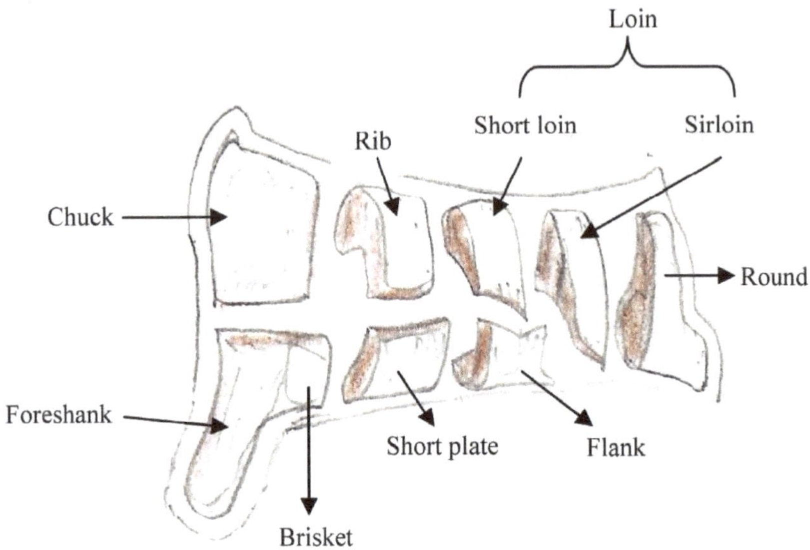

Wholesale cuts of beef/buffalo

Cutting and fabrication of goat and lamb carcasses

Carcasses of goat and lamb are generally fabricated into different cuts following the procedure of United States Department of Agriculture (USDA) or Bureau of Indian Standards (BIS) specifications. In USDA pattern, carcasses are separated into fore saddle and hind saddle by making a cut in between the last two ribs. However, BIS specifications advocated that carcasses should be divided into right and left sides instead of fore and hind saddle.

USDA pattern of carcass fabrication

In USDA pattern carcasses are first separated into fore saddle and hind saddle by making a cut in between last two ribs. The thin meat is usually removed from natural seam present between flank and leg.

Name of cut	Percent share in respective saddle	Location and cut site
Foresaddle (53%)		
Neck	4.0	Cut at last cervical vertebrae where it blends with the shoulder.
Shoulder	25.0	Cut between 5th and 6th rib

(Contd.)

Rack	10.0	Cut between 6th to 12th ribs.
Breast	8.0	Cut is made forward to the last rib at a point midway of the last rib and continued forward to a point 1/2" above the elbow.
Shank	6.0	Cutting of foreshank bones.
Hind saddle (47%)		
Loin	10.0	Cut just in front of hipbone and the last two lumbar vertebrae.
Flanks	3.0	Flank is a specified area contains thin meat. It is boneless cut in which natural seam starting from breast.
Leg	32.0	Remaining portion of hind saddle is leg cut.
Suet and kidney	2.0	Kidney and adjacent fat makes the suet and kidney cut.

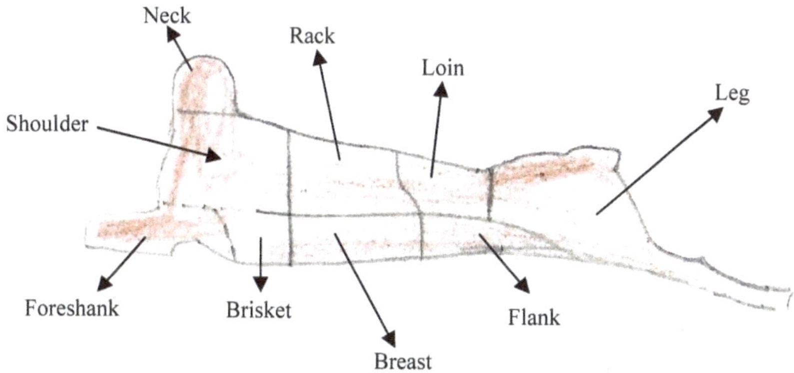

Wholesale cuts of goat and lamb -USDA

BIS pattern of carcass fabrication

BIS pattern of carcass fabrication is generally followed in India to make the cuts from goat and lamb carcasses. In this pattern consumers and traders are generally preferred to make only six cuts from the goat and lamb carcasses i.e. neck, shoulder, rack (rib), foreshank and breast, loin and leg.

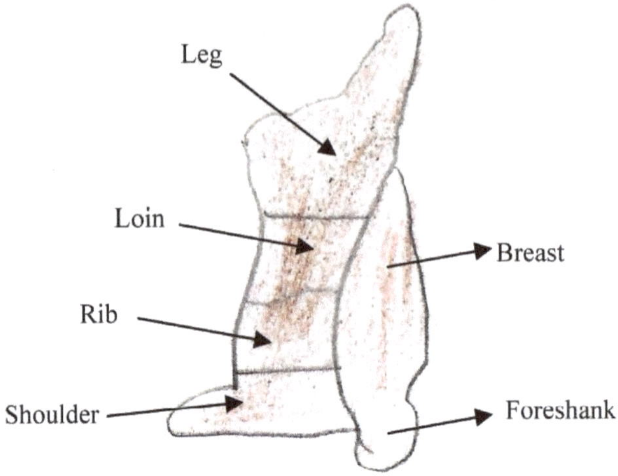

Wholesale cuts of lamb -BIS

Cutting and fabrication of pig's carcasses

Pig carcasses feet are firstly removed from fore and hind feet both. Fore feet is cut at 1 inch above the knee and hind feet at the lower of hock edge. The carcasses are then separated into right and left and again into six distinct cuts in each side.

1. The anterior part is called 'Rough Shoulder' is separated from the posterior 'Rough middle' and 'Rough Ham' portion by cutting between second and third ribs.
2. 'Rough shoulder' contains three distinct wholesale cuts i.e. Jowl, Boston Butt and Picnic Shoulder while 'Rough Middle' is made up of Upper Loin, Side or Spare Ribs or Bacon. 'Rough Ham' is the original ham portion of the pig carcass.
3. Jowl is obtained by making a cut close to the neckline.
4. Boston butt cut is fabricated as upper one third of the skinned shoulder. It is usually separated by making a cut parallel to back from a point just vertical to the exposed section of the shoulder blade.
5. Picnic shoulder is the lower two third portion of the shoulder region.
6. Rough middle as a whole is obtained by making a parallel cut to backbone at a point three fingers width below the vertebral column

at the shoulder end and extending it up to the leg end in a manner just to miss the tender lion muscle. Loin cut is upper portion of the section while lower portion of section is called Spare ribs and belly (bacon).

7. Rough ham is usually separated rough middle by a cut between second and third sacral vertebrae at right angles to the line of leg. The 'Regular Ham' is suitably obtained from rough ham by trimming the fat and lean on the exposed surface of the ham.
8. Thus wholesale cuts from each side of the pig carcasses can be categorized as Jowl, Boston Butt, Picnic Shoulder, Loin, Side and spare ribs and Ham.

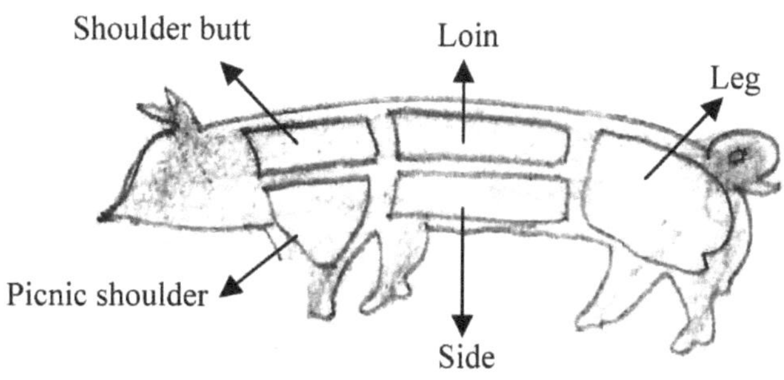

Wholesale cuts of pigs

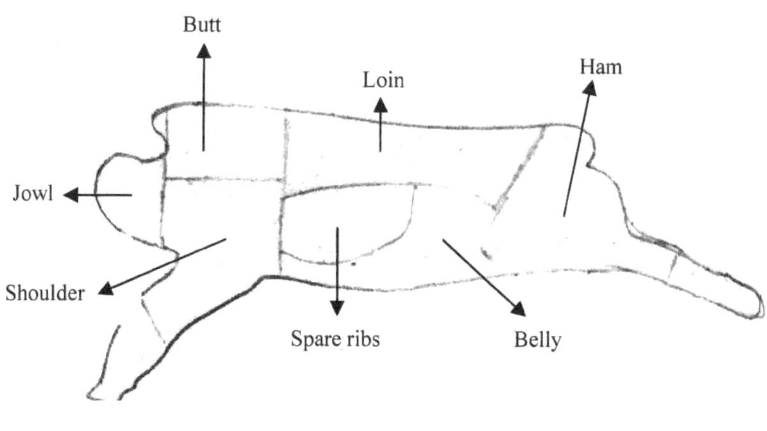

Wholesale cuts of pork

Cutting and fabrication of wholesale cuts of poultry

Food Safety Inspection Service (FSIS) of USDA specified the guidelines in 1986 for cuts of poultry. The salient features of guidelines can be summarized as:

i. There should be proper cutting of thighs, drumsticks and wings. These parts should be separated by making the clear cuts at connecting joints but care should be taken that medullary cavity (marrow) of bone shaft should not be exposed.

ii. Knee bone or patella should be included either in thigh or drumstick.

iii. Skin and fat is usually separated from parts of the poultry carcass.

iv. Leg and thigh contains pelvic meat but excludes pelvic bone. Leg and thigh also includes flank or abdominal meat but excludes rib bones.

v. The separation of carcass should be in such a way that there should be two equal halves-right and left. However, backbone should be the part of both right and left portion and cut should be one-fourth inch from breastbone or sternum.

vi. Leg quarter contains thigh and drumstick with one half of back portion. Abdominal fat and up to two ribs are also included in leg quarter.

vii. Breast portion should be free from abdominal fat, skin or fat and bone shaft should be unexposed but marrow of humerus may be exposed.

Whole sale cuts of poultry

Poultry carcass is usually separated into anterior (front) and posterior (rear) portion by making a cut between 6th and 7th ribs. Anterior quarter is generally separated by making a longitudinal cut at first thoracic vertebra and extending posteriorly through the sixth thoracic vertebra and cutting the keel in half. However, posterior cut separation is achieved by making a cut at seventh thoracic vertebra and extended posteriorly splitting the lumbar-sacral vertebra in half. The cuts of poultry carcass are basically depends on the choice of the consumers as well as on trade requirement. Basically there are six distinct cuts i.e. neck, breast, wing in anterior portion while leg, back and drumstick in posterior portion.

Carcass portion	Major cuts	Description
Anterior quarter	Neck	Cut at the end of cervical vertebrae and all cervical vertebrae are included in neck.
	Breast	A longitudinal cut started from first vertebra and extended posteriorly through the sixth thoracic vertebral column and sternum.
	Wings	By making a cut through shoulder joint at proximal end of humerus.
Posterior quarter	Leg	Each leg is cut at a point 2.5 cm above and 2.5 cm below the joint formed by the femur.
	Back	Cut begins at seventh vertebra and extended posteriorly on either side of lumber and sacral vertebra completely removing this portion of the back bone.
	Drumstick	Drumstick contains tibia and fibula bones and cut at 2.5 cm below the femur.

Extendable poultry cuts

Breast

i. *Breast with back cut*: breast with back cut can be obtained by making a longitudinal cut at first vertebra and extending posteriorly through the sixth thoracic vertebrae column and sternum.

ii. *Keel cut breast:* keel cut breast portion is produced by making a cut at distal end or at the tip of sternal crest and continued dorsally across the fifth and sixth vertebral ribs until the pectoralis muscles are separated from the whole breast.

iii. *Wishbone or clavicle cut*: it is obtained by putting a cut at anterior end of the sternum and extended dorsally along the coracoid. Thus a piece of cut is obtained from breast at the junction of clavicle and coracoid.

iv. *Quartered breast:* breast can be quartered into longitudinal cut and yield two halves as in breast with back cut and a cut through each half beginning at the point of sternal ribs and across the fifth and sixth vertebral ribs, severing the spine at approximately seventh lumber vertebra.

v. *Split breast:* split breast piece is obtained by making a cut on each side of vertebral column beginning at mid-point of sternal ribs and breast is completely separated from back.

vi. *Breast with ribs*: breast with rib cut can be splitted on each side of vertebral column. A cut is started at posterior to seventh rib and extended anteriorly to a point where breast with ribs and scapula were completely separated from back.

vii. *Stripped breast with scapula:* stripped breast with scapula is obtained by placing a knife in body cavity at anterior end of vertebral column and placed a cut in ventral posterior direction to split the breast through centre of sternum. The skin is loosen and separated in its full length and breast is split along with scapula from remaining ribs.

Wing

i. *Wings with breast:* wing with breast portion is obtained by making a cut approximately 2.5 cm of pectorals major with shoulder joint.

ii. *Wing segments:* Wing segment is produced by splitting the wing tip at distal end of forearm and forearm is cut at distal end of the humerus. The proximal wing portion is separated by cutting through shoulder joint.

Leg and thigh

i. *Three piece leg*: three leg pieces is usually contains femur, fibula and tibia and obtained from each leg by making a cut at a point 2.5 cm above the joint of femur.

ii. *Thigh with back portion:* thigh with back portion is obtained with the help of a longitudinal cut started at seventh vertebra and extending posteriorly on either side of the lumbar and sacral vertebra completely remove the back bone section.

iii. *Strip cut thigh:* strip cut thigh portion is obtained by cutting through the junction of thigh muscles with pelvic girdle to hip joints and disjointing the femur. The leg is separated from back by pulling the loin or 'oyster' muscle off with the thigh. The thigh and drumstick is separated at joints.

iv. *Square cut thigh:* the procedure is almost same as mentioned in stripe cut thigh but loin oyster muscle remains attached with back.

v. *Drumstick with thigh:* drumstick with thigh portion is obtained by making a cut at femur 2.5 cm above the joint formed by the femur, fibula and tibia.

vi. *Thigh back:* the thigh back portion is obtained by making a cut above 2.5 cm of femur joint and containing the portion of back.

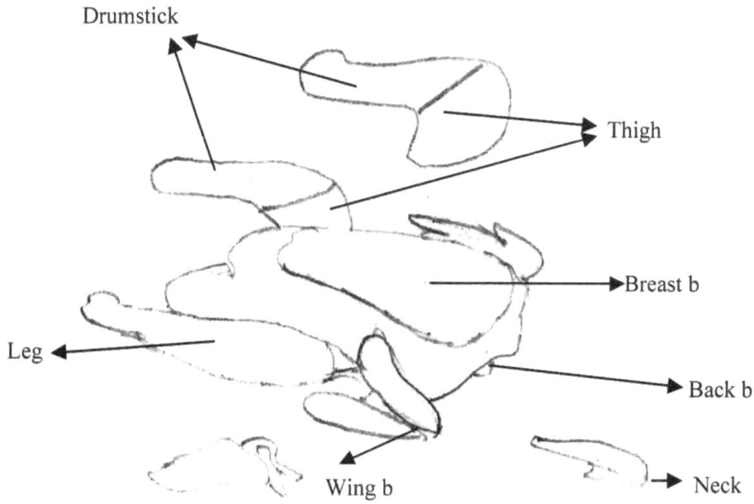

Wholesale cuts of poultry carcass

Cutting and fabrication of wholesale cuts of rabbit

The consumers and traders are now showing the interest in rabbit meat. Thus the knowledge of rabbit carcasses cutting and fabrication becomes important. In United States of America rabbit carcass weighing 800-900 g is referred as fryer. It is high in demand and inculcating the good prices. Normally rabbit carcass is splitted into seven distinct cuts i.e. two hind legs, two fore legs, two pieces of chest and back, one piece of loin. However, large rabbit carcasses can be splitted into 9-12 pieces depending on their requirement for example hind legs can be splitted into two portions if demanded. Loin and back portion can also be separated into five pieces and front portion of ribs and each foreleg can also be split into one piece. The medium size rabbit carcass can further be splitted as per the choice of consumers and traders. Sometimes whole small rabbit carcass is packed along with joints depending on demand of consumers and traders.

References

1. Barbut, S. (2002). Inspection, grading, cut up and composition. *In:* Poultry Products Processing: an industry guide, CRC Press, Florida. Pp 12-180.

2. Islam, M. A., Seeland, G., Bulbul, S. M. and Howlider, M. A. R. (2002). Meat yield and cooked meat taste of hybrids from different

genetic groups in a hot-humid climate. Indian Journal Animal Research, **36**: 35-38.

3. Namken, J. C., Farris, D. E. and Capps, Jr. O. (1994). The demand for wholesale beef cuts by season and trend. J. Food Dist. Res. 25: 47-61.

4. NAMP (2010). The Meat Buyer's Guide, (6th ed.). North American Meat Processors Association. Reston, VA.

5. Sams, A.R. (2001). Second processing: parts, deboning and portion control. *In:* Poultry Meat Processing, CRC Press, Florida. Pp 35-46.

❑❑❑

Chapter 11

Quality and Safety Management Systems in Abattoir

Hazard Analysis and Critical Control Points (HACCP)

Hazard Analysis and Critical Control Point is a comprehensive food safety system of food which starts from production to the ultimate consumption. HACCP monitors each and every step of production process, identify the specific hazards, implement the effective control programme and also verify the procedure. However, it is not a zero risk programme and there is possibility of risk of hazards in the process but the theme of programme is to minimize the risk of hazards upto a level which will be considered as safe. Thus HACCP programme is termed as risk management tool. It involves the management of all types of hazards like microbiological, chemical and physical.

The HACCP system came into existence in United States in 1971 by Bauman the Pillsbury Company in collaboration with the National Aeronautics and Space Administration (NASA) and the US Army Natick Research and Development Laboratories. These agencies had the initial responsibility for designing and manufacturing food products without contamination from pathogens, bacteria or viruses responsible for diseases and illnesses in human beings. Later, HACCP concept becomes reality at international level for management of food safety at all production, transformation, storage and distribution sites for foods to human consumption. In 1993, it was adopted by the European Union (EU) for all food processors and the Codex Alimentarius Commission as the principal food safety system. The HACCP concept involves in entire process of food production right from identification of specific hazards in raw materials, processing, operations, packaging, transportation, distribution or even at consumption point. It emphasizes on preventive measures rather than control measures in whole of the food production chain.

Pre-requisite programmes and bodies of Implementation

HACCP is a food safety management system and involves critical examination of raw materials, processes and products and maintains the hygienic conditions of products till it reaches to the consumers. There are certain prerequisite programmes which are mandatory to fulfill the necessary steps of HACP. Some of these prerequisites may be described as:

1. *Food certification*: In India, Bureau of Indian Standards (BIS) is officially recognized certification body. The certification mode may be Quality system certification against IS/ISO 9000; Environmental management systems certification as IS/ISO 14000 and HACCP with the integrated ISO 9000 system certification against IS/ISO 9000 and IS 15000:1998 Food Hygiene-HACCP system and guidelines for its implementation. The operation of BIS certification is conducted through its five regional offices and 24 branch offices situated all over the country. The team of certification includes trained auditors and HACCP experts. They are responsible for certification of those units which are having documented established and transparent quality and safety management system and assure the customers satisfaction through *inter-alia* complaint redress mechanisms.

   For food certification, HACCP system is recognized by the Codex Alimentarius Commission which is internationally recognized standard for world food trade under WTO Agreement. Sanitary and Phyto-sanitary (SPS) Agreement under the WTO Agreement makes it mandatory for all countries to maintain measures to ensure that food is to be safe for consumers and to prevent the spread of pests and disease among animals and plants. Thus the HACCP system which is called a preventive food safety management system emphasizes the strict control and inspection at all stages of raw material, product processing and ultimate use to achieve this goal. So to get certification from BIS all key elements like good product management, good hygiene conditions and good manufacturing practices must be followed. These goals can be achieved by critical examination of raw materials, processes and products; hygienic conditions from origin till it reach to the customer; identifying stages/processes where hazards could occur; instituting and maintaining controls at identified stages/processes; documenting HACCP process and keeping records; and ensuring that the system continues to work effectively.

To get certification the fresh and raw meat must have the total viable count in between 0.5 to 2 million per gram while the range in cooked product should be in between 200 to 10,000 million per gram. Similarly Coliform counts must have below 200 in a gram in fresh and raw meat and below 10 in cooked products. Salmonella, Shiegella must be absent in 25 gram fresh and 10 gram cooked meat respectively. The Staphylococcal count should be less than 100 in fresh and below 10 in cooked meat.

2. *Hygiene code:* In HACCP profile hygiene code is mainly meant for predetermined critical control points. The hygiene code is a basic requirement and predetermined the critical control points in small and medium sized food industries including abattoirs and meat shops. In this code of practice hazard analysis and risk assessments are done and preventive, corrective measures in form of standard protocol are adopted to minimize and control these risks and hazards. Infact hygiene code is an integral part of good manufacturing practices and guide the inspectors to judge certain points for efficacy assessment.
3. *Good manufacturing Practices (GMPs)*: GMP is an essential step to achieve standard quality final product. It must be followed at each and every step like personnel, plants, equipments, operations, cleaning and sanitation, transportation and distribution etc.
4. *Standards operating procedures (SOP)*: SOP assures the implementation of standards procedures for a particular product processing and must have standard protocol as per standard agency recommendations. So that essential safety and quality of products can be assured.
5. *Sanitation standard operating procedures (SSOP)*: SSOP have the essential step to be followed by the production agency to achieve the greater quality hygiene and sanitation in the product processing unit.

Objectives of HACCP

HACCP is a science-based analytical tool applied on microbiological, chemical and physical hazards affecting product safety. However, it also assures the products quality along with the safety and enables the management to introduce and maintain a cost-effective ongoing food safety program. It is so by preventing the spoilage and entry of pathogenic organisms in the food chain. Thus HACCP food safety system is considered satisfactory and its implementation in the food chain boosts the confidence of the consumers about the safety of particular product. The beneficial effects of HACCP in food chain may be summarized as:

1. It enables food manufacturing or catering companies of all sizes to move away from a philosophy of control, based primarily on end-

product testing (i.e., testing for product failure), to a preventive approach whereby potential hazards are identified and controlled in the food processing environment (i.e., prevention of product failure).

2. It is a logical and cost-effective base for better decision-making with respect to product safety.
3. It provides greater security of control over product safety which is not possible with traditional end-product testing and when correctly implemented may be used as part of a defense of 'Due Diligence'.
4. It has both National and International recognition as the most cost-effective means of controlling food-borne disease and is promoted as such by the FAO/WHO Codex Alimentarius Commission.
5. The HACCP system, which is science-based and systematic, identifies specific hazards and measures for their control to ensure the safety of food.
6. This system is capable of accommodating change, such as advances in equipment design, processing procedures or technological developments.
7. HACCP can be applied throughout the food chain, from primary production to final consumption, and its implementation should be guided by scientific evidence of risks to human health. It helps in enhancing food safety and implementation of HACCP can provide other significant benefits. In addition, the application of HACCP systems can aid inspection by regulatory.
8. It helps in improvement of business and built confidence of the consumers about a particular food product.
9. It enables the producers to meet the regulatory and commercial trade for a particular food items with the little efforts.

Limitations of HACCP

Besides all good things of HACCP it also has some limitations which can also effectively tackled during HACCP implementation programme. In countries like India these points are more realistic than western countries. Some of these points are as under:

1. HACCP requires the education of non-professional food handlers, especially in food service industry.

2. The concept of HACCP must be accepted by food processors, food inspectors and public. The failure of which may produces detrimental effects on food production.
3. The adoption of HACCP gives the false impressions if procedures are not full proof.

Terminology

1. **Control Point (CP):** any point in a specific food system where loss of control does not lead to an unacceptable health risk.
2. **Critical Control Point (CCP):** any point or procedure in a food system where control can be exercised and a hazard can be minimized or prevented.
3. **Critical limit:** one or more prescribed tolerance that must be met to ensure that CCP effectively controls microbiological health hazard.
4. **Hazard:** any biological, chemical or physical property that may cause an unacceptable consumer health risk.
5. **Monitoring:** a planned sequence of observations or measurements of critical limits designed to produce an accurate record and intended to ensure that the critical limit maintains product safety.

Principles of HACCP: there are seven principles of the HACCP system.

Principle 1: Assessment of hazards and risks associated with raw materials, ingredients, processing, packaging, distribution and consumption of meat products on the basis of flow chart.

Principle 2: Identification of critical control points to control and minimize hazards.

Principle 3: Establishment of critical limits or tolerance levels (standards) at each control points.

Principle 4: Outlining the procedures to monitor the critical control points.

Principle 5: Defining the corrective action if deviation is noticed during monitoring.

Principle 6: Maintenance of proper record or documents of HACCP plan.

Principle 7: Verification of methods, procedures and tests to oversee the compliance of plan.

Implementation steps of HACCP

1. Formation of HACCP team - Team members should represent from the entire quality food chain.
2. Description of the product - Nature of the product, brand name if any, specifications, microbiological, biochemical and organoleptic standards and storage temperature etc are to be clearly described and documented.
3. Identifying the indented use by customer - Intended use and the general public are to be clearly documented and allergens if any are to be specified and printed on the pack. For example chicken can be declared fit for consumption for all age groups from infants to geriatrics.
4. Developing the process flow diagram - A diagram involving all the process steps to be drawn and the process flow in progressive order is to be mentioned.
5. On site verification of the process flow - A declaration to the effect that process flow is true and correct representation of the actual production activities and process in terms of description and sequence is to be signed by team leader of the HACCP team.
6. Hazard analysis and identifying the preventive measures - Each step of the process flow is to be analyzed for the possible hazards which may be of biological, chemical, physical or quality by using hazard analysis work sheet.
7. Identifying the critical control points (CCPs) - By using the CCP decision tree each step of the process flow is to be analyzed for identifying the CCPs.
8. Establishing critical limits - Critical limits for each CCP shall be identified and established where the expected food safety hazards shall be eliminated or controlled to permissible limit based on the limits prescribed by the regulatory bodies or government agencies.
9. Monitoring the critical limits - A dedicated person is engaged online to monitor the established critical limits for each CCP.
10. Corrective action procedures - During monitoring if any deviations are noticed, deviation shall be recorded and reported to the person responsible for the corrective action. The person-concerned in-turn shall record the corrective action taken. These procedures are to be documented and made available to the certifying bodies during their surveillance audits.

11. Verification procedures - Verification of the records are to be done daily by the person responsible for the quality of product.
12. Record keeping procedures - Each record shall be given separate code for identification and traceability and documented regularly. These documents are audited periodically and used for system review.

CP and CCP's in the slaughter procedures of different animals:

Species of animals	CCP	CP
Cattle	AM Examination PM Examination Dispatch	Sticking Skinning Electrical stimulation Evisceration Washing of carcass Deboning Fresh packaging
Pigs	AM Examination Scalding PM Examination Chilling Freezing Dispatch and storage	Dehairing Evisceration Washing of carcass
Sheep & Goats	AM Examination PM Examination Chilling Freezing Dispatch and storage	Sticking Skinning Evisceration Packaging& weighing

Process Flow Chart

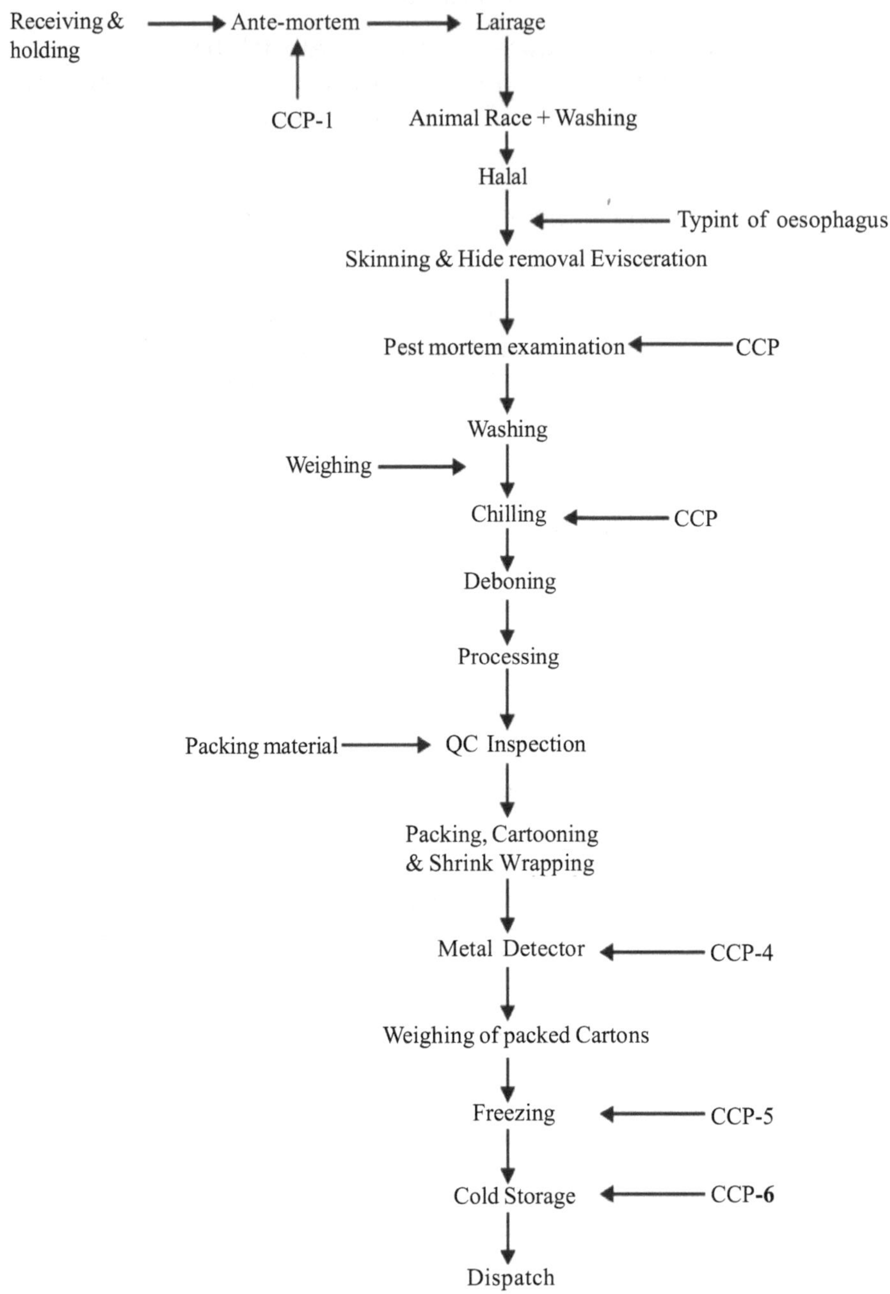

HACCP is a unique system of food industry which assures the consumers about the safety of food products if implemented in food processing industry. It monitors the processing steps right from raw materials to the ultimate product. Thus it enhances the quality of product and its shelf life. In the world of today HACCP becomes reality and most of the importers now require mandatory implementation of this food safety system.

Good Manufacturing Practices (GMP)

Good Manufacturing Practices (GMPs) are minimum sanitary and processing requirements for food companies to ensure the safety and suitability of food at all stages of the food chain. These requirements are defined by the Food and Drug Administration in 21 CFR, part 110. Good Manufacturing Practices must be adapted from point of production (farm) to point of consumption (fork). GMP measures are not a day operation but they should be adopted in routine practice.

Raw material

All the animals and materials supplied to the meat plant must be maintained hygienically and also adjudged for sanitary requirements. To ensure quality meat production trucks, containers and carriers of raw materials should be evaluated upon receipt. Raw material should be segregated depending upon its status and due attention is required for further handling and processing's.

Plant vicinity

The ground outside the meat plant must be maintained in such a way that there should not be the water logging, too much muddy surface, and plants, weeds and debris should be properly trimmed and maintained. Roads should be maintained properly and there should be separate passage for raw material and final product. There should be proper maintenance state of gate and sewage lines. So that wild birds and animal's particularly street dogs, crows and vulture can be avoided.

Plant design and equipments

Plant building and equipments must be in good maintenance condition. Exterior doors of plant must remain closed at all times and if possible they must be self-closing and tight fitting. The proper hygienic and sanitary status must be achieved all time. Building grounds must be free from dust, dirt and litter as well as dirty operations in plant must be taken care of all time. The meat plant building should be insect and bird proof with tight fittings. Building should be free from cracks or holes to avoid breeding ground and shelter of pests. Door and other openings should be narrow enough so that rodents could not get entry into building. Building openings must be covered with proper meshes. Containers and equipments made up of glass, including glass thermometers, should not be permitted in the production area.

Equipments should always be checked before assembling. All attachments and equipments must be thoroughly cleaned after each use and at least once each day after use. Clean, sterilized gaskets, screens, platforms etc. should always be used. Use of low quality and excessive lubricants on equipments should always be avoided. All cleaning equipments and chemicals should always be stored in a separate section in meat plant. Floor drains should be free from all debris with no evidence of any offensive odours. There should be regular cleaning and sanitization of drains and always prefer only black bristle brushes for cleaning of floor drains.

Pest control measures

There should be a routine pest control system particularly in areas where food is stored and passed for utilization. The accumulation of waste material and filth must be avoided. Continuous monitoring and residual precautions must also be adopted.

Personnel management

Persons working in meat plant must follow the sanitary and hygienic measures while working in the plant. Some of the important steps necessary in personnel hygiene are:

i. There should be a proper uniform for all employees in production areas. Uniform must be clean and good in house keeping condition. The uniforms should be changed daily or sooner if soiled for any reason. Shirts are required to be buttoned and tucked into trousers.

ii. Persons engaged in various meat production and handling operations required to wash their hands with a sanitizing soap prior and after completion of their work.

iii. Hairs are good source of contamination and required proper authorized head covering to avoid contact of loose hair with food product.

iv. Mouth and nose should also be covered with suitable proper mask to avoid contamination to the product. Hands should be preferably covered with disposable gloves.

v. Good hygienic measures must be practiced at all time. Chewing tobacco, smoking, trimming fingernails, spitting, use of snuff, chewing gum and open blowing of the nose in the production area or any area exposed to products or packaging materials are always avoided.

vi. Sanitary precautions are always required to be taken by employees when sneezing or coughing.

vii. Employees with infectious skin eruption, cuts and open sores on fingers unless they are covered by a band-aid with a finger are always avoided.

viii. Holding of toothpicks, matchsticks, or similar objects in the mouth of employs during working are not allowed. Pencils or other objects held behind the ears are forbidden.

ix. Persons suffering with communicable diseases or other infectious conditions should always be avoided in production and product handling areas.

x. The wearing of jewellery i.e. earrings, watches, rings, neck chains, etc. should be prohibited in working areas. Nail polish and/or perfume are not allowed in production or storage areas of meat processing plant.

xi. Consumption of beverage or food is allowed exclusively in the designated area and proper washing of hands and thorough drying is required prior and after meal.

xii. Safety glasses, goggles, or shields must be worn when handling hazardous materials such as cleaning chemicals, petroleum products, etc. Emergency arrangements must be there for mishappenings.

Sanitary measures

There should be sufficient and efficient hot and cold water supply. The maintenance of boilers and chillers should always be in good condition. Proper and potable water supply should always be ensured. All the building and parts, platform and instruments should always be sterilized. Proper and regular cleaning, washing and sanitization in meat plant should always be ensured. Clean and unclean operations must always be done in properly separated areas.

Process control

All the slaughter operations such as animal management in lairage, ante-mortem examination, stunning, sticking, bleeding, dehiding, dressing and carcass cutting must be performed in full proof system. Proper watering and feed withdrawal to the animals should be proper. All clean and unclean operations must be done in proper hygienic manners. Water used in washing and cleaning of carcass must be of potable quality. There should be proper temperature maintenance during cuts fabrication and storage.

Product handling

The product dressing and cutting should always be done on rails and floor contact should always be avoided. The handler and packaging materials must be sound in hygienic and sanitary manner. The cutting saws, knife and cleavers must be maintained in good condition. Wash, dry and sanitize hands thoroughly before starting work and after each absence from the work area is essential. Manual handling of meat should always be avoided and trolley or gambrel should be in good hygienic conditions. The equipment with wooden handles should always be avoided. Material handling equipments such as scoops, carts, lifts, etc. must be kept clean, covered and well maintained. There should not be direct exposure of meat to sun and adverse climatic conditions. Cutting and storage rooms and vans must be maintained on proper temperature.

Waste material and by-products utilization

The organic and inorganic wastes generated in meat plant must be handled properly. The meat plant waste must be treated in proper way by primary as well as secondary treatment as and when required. There should be a waste disposal and treatment plant near the meat processing unit. The edible and inedible by-products must be separated and utilized properly. Edible by-products may be collected and stored for sale and further utilization while inedible by-products may be utilized in sanitary way. Rendering plant and autoclaving as well as cooking and disposal facilities may also be added near the plant.

Record keeping

Process, maintenance, product storage and delivery pattern should always be maintained and continually monitored. The temperature maintenance and variation chart should be recorded and abnormality found should clearly be emphasized. Today traceability is utmost important aspect of quality meat production. So source of raw material and its previous history should always be recorded carefully. Identification of all raw materials must be recorded on batch sheets to enable tracing of finished goods from receiving to production, packaging and distribution. The permanent record on hard and soft copy should always be maintained in administrative office.

Visitors rule

Meat plant visitors as well as regulatory personnel must adhere to all plant rules and comply with sanitation and safety regulations. Authorized personnel admitted to processing areas shall confer all safety, hygienic and sanitary rules and/or regulations as applicable to personnel working in meat plant. All contractors and maintenance staff should always follow the GMP measures.

Good Hygienic Practices (GHP)

Good Hygiene Practices are the set of requirements to prevent contamination of food in order to provide safe food to the consumers. The major cause of food contaminations which are responsible for food borne illnesses are poor sanitation and lack of environmental hygiene, improper and inappropriate transportation, poor storage facilities, poor personal hygiene, unsafe source of food etc. There are different types of contaminants responsible for food illnesses which may be broadly classified as:

i. **Biological**: biological includes bacteria, viruses or parasites that are present in air, food, water, soil, animals or humans. They are most common contaminants and produces serious hazards to the consumers.

ii. **Physical:** physical contaminants are mainly foreign bodies and get entry into foods by accidental contamination and/or poor handling practices. These are mainly visible particles and can be avoided by very little efforts examples are pebbles, stones, metal, glass, wood, insects, soil, dirt, jewellery, hair, fingernails etc.

iii. **Chemical:** different types of chemicals are in use in various meat production operations. These are mainly cleaning and sanitizing chemicals generally used for food contact surfaces, pest control, paints and water treatment etc. Pesticides, fertilizers, fungicides and naturally occurring harmful chemicals like mycotoxins are also included in this group. The residual problem of these chemicals if not properly handled and continuously used may create a great danger to the health of human beings.

GHP is a comprehensive efforts of which includes hygienic and sanitary management in meat production and includes proper food safety at animal handling and transportation, management at lairage and abattoir, slaughter and dressing, cutting and washing of carcass, storage and distribution etc. All the measures of Good Hygiene Practices as per Schedule 4 of Food Safety & Standards (Licensing & Registration of Food Businesses) Regulations, 2011 must be taken care during production of meat food. Some of the essential steps of GHP in meat food production can be summarized as:

General requirements

i. Animal production for meat purpose must be done in good environmental and hygienic conditions. To achieve the objective, meat food contamination through air, soil, water, feed-stock, pesticides, veterinary drugs or any other agent used in primary production must always be avoided and managed properly. To protect food sources from faecal and other contaminants, washing, cleaning and sanitatization rules must be followed.

ii. Handling and transportation of animals from source of production to abattoir must follow the code of practices.

iii. Equipments and containers used in handling of animal foods during fabrication, storage, processing, packaging and serving shall be made of corrosion free materials. These materials should also be free from toxicity to the food and should be easy to clean and disinfect.

iv. Special care should be taken to minimize the contamination by pests, chemicals, microbiological or physical or other objectionable substances during handling and transportation.

Plant design and establishment

Establishment design and facilities of abattoir and meat processing plant must be such that it minimizes risk to ensure food safety. Premises and equipments to be used in various operations should be maintained in such a way that risk of contamination is eliminated. Nature of operations to be conducted and associated risks must be identified. Abattoir and meat processing plant location must be free from potential source of contamination such as obnoxious odour, fumes, excessive soot, dust, smoke, chemical or biological emissions and pollutants etc. Internal design, structures and layout of plant should be in such a way that they prevent contamination to the food. Following requirements should be considered important in GHP achievements:

i. Premises and equipments should be easy to maintain, clean, disinfect and monitor for day to day operations.

ii. Material of equipments should be durable, movable and capable of being disassembled for cleaning, disinfection and sanitization.

iii. Water requires for various operations in abattoir and meat plant must be of potable grade and should be free from contaminations.

iv. Ventilation systems should be supported with natural as well as mechanical facilities like air filters, exhaust fans etc. So that quality air can be maintained in plant and flow of contaminated areas to clean areas can be prevented.

v. Drainage and waste disposal system in abattoir and meat processing plant should be constructed in such a manner that risk of contamination to food or water can be avoided.

vi. There should be proper temperature control facility particularly in areas where carcass is to be fabricated and cuts are to be stored.

vii. Undistorted proper intensity natural and artificial light should be provided. So that employees/workers can operate in a hygienic manner. Sanitary measures must be adopted in installation of electricity fittings. So that it could not contaminate the food articles.

viii. There should be suitable and well thermocontrolled storage facilities separately for raw material, processed, reject and offal's. The provision of proper disposal of condemned and discarded parts and animals should be maintained.

Operational control

i. To control the hazards in food chain, Hazard Analysis and Critical Control Point's concept is acceptable worldwide. It is a systematic and preventive approach for food safety and helps in prevention of biological, chemical, and physical hazards in production processes. To develop a full proof system of operation in a food chain, monitoring and control of raw material, process of processing, storage, packaging, dispatch and transportation all should be taken care of in proper way.

ii. Standard Operating Procedure (SOP) must be developed to pinpoint problem and control damage faster as well as specific process steps must be set up to prevent microbial cross contamination, physical and chemical contamination.

iii. Always use the potable water for washing, development of steam and ice as well as other operations in the abattoir and meat processing plant.

iv. Packaging requirements must fulfill the Food Safety & Standards (Packaging & Labeling) Regulations, 2011. All the operations must be well designed and performed in well manner.

v. There should always be the sufficient trained and skilled workers in the plant. The knowledge of food hygiene principles and practices to ensure food safety and quality of products must always be set on priority.

vi. The judgments on food hazards, appropriate preventive and corrective action and effective monitoring and supervision must be the part of routine operational process.

vii. All the records pertaining to food production, processing, handling, storage, distribution, food quality, laboratory tests, cleaning and sanitation, pest control and disposal of materials must be maintained.

viii. A standard cleaning and sanitation protocol must be developed which can be monitored and judged for each operations and corrective measures must be adopted if required. Cleaning programmes must design keeping in view of the regulations of FSSAI.

ix. Pest control systems must be effective and always follow the principles of monitoring, detection and eradication.

x. Waste management system must be carried out systematically and a definite as well routine programme must be implemented. All the waste management system must be located away from food processing area and should be in covered plan as described in FBO regulations.

xi. There should be an effective monitoring system to ensure that all methods in place are effective. There should always be the provision of periodic audit of whole system according to the SOP. So that gaps in GMP / GHP system can be effectively filled up. There should be laboratory facilities for monitor the microbial and other quality standards in pant or food chain as prescribed by FSSAI.

Personal Hygiene

i. All the employees and workers of meat plant should be sound in health status. They should be necessarily free from communicable diseases as well as cuts and injuries in hands.

ii. Personal cleanliness of employees is utmost important aspect of GHP. To achieve this objective personal must wear clean clothes, coverings of head, face, hands and footwear. Hairs and nails should be clipped and trimmed in at a regular interval.

iii. Workers must have good habits and bad habits like smoking, spitting, chewing, sneezing, coughing, and eating near food preparation areas must be discouraged and never overlooked.

iv. Visitors in plant must be allowed only with protective clothing with full adherence to personal hygiene.

Transportation

i. There should be separate vehicles for raw material and finished products. All the sanitary and hygienic steps must be followed in washing and cleaning of vehicles after and before completion of each consignment.

ii. There should also be the proper separation in between different types of finished products to prevent cross contamination. At the time of storage and transportation, proper control and monitoring over time, temperature and humidity must be mentioned.

iii. There should be the proper packaging of finished products to avoid spillage, shrinkage and losses during transportation and preservation. Packaging must be of food grade and astringent to the regulations.

iv. Transportation rules and regulations for raw materials and finished products must always be followed.

Product information display

There should be proper packaging of finished products as per the guidelines issued by Codex standard and FSSAI and labeling should adhere with provisions given by Food Safety and Standards Regulations, 2011. The proper labeling over products enables the persons regarding handling, storage, preparations and to use the product safely and correctly. The nutritional parameters, safety measurements and quality issues must be declared clearly and necessary steps for their conservation must be passed in form of instructions.

Trainings

The provision of regular trainings to the employees and workers is an important aspect of GHP. The trainings aspect must be emphasizes on food safety hazards and incidents. The other issues of trainings may be about nature of food and its ability to sustain growth of harmful micro-organisms, handling procedures, further processing, storage conditions etc. The exposure visits and site demonstration of various activities related to product development and maintenance must be conducted to enable the employees and workers about food quality, safety and hazard management.

Total Quality Management (TQM)

Total Quality Management (TQM) is the optimization and integration of all the functions and processes of a business in order to provide satisfaction and quality product to the consumers through the process of continuous improvement. The concept of total quality management came into existence in 1990's with the generation of Globalization concept in business. It's a reality in today world because consumers are more conscious on quality of product and process rather than end product assessment. The world is now seeking the product of their choice with special products of health benefits. So to achieve the objective and sustain in the throat cutting business all the measures to develop a quality product with certain nutrients is reality of today business. The principles of total quality management can be achieved by the following steps which may call as objectives of TQM:

i. Process improvement.

ii. Defect prevention.

iii. Priority of effort.

iv. Developing cause -effect relationships.

v. Measuring system capacity.

vi. Developing improvement checklist and check forms.

vii. Helping teams make better decisions.

viii. Developing operational definitions.

ix. Separating trivial from significant needs.

x. Observing behaviour changes over a period of time.

Principles of Total Quality Management

To achieve the best quality product with highest consumer satisfaction, it is utmost important to have the full proof system of management practices in the plant. Best quality efforts are also required to monitor, regulate and verify the system and corrective measure adoption as required time to time and as per the demand of consumers. To get highest quality products following principles are required to be adopted:

Principle 1: Customer-focused organization

There should always keep in mind the ultimate use of product. The ultimate consumer satisfaction and their requirement for particular type of product must be fulfilled. The future need of consumers should also be considered. The plan and implementation of operational work must be focused on the customer expectations. So that a well planned operations and quality as well as quantity of products can be obtained with minimum wastage. The economic sustainability also depends on the consumer demands and supply.

Principle 2: Leadership

The leading instinct of company administrative makes them unique in particular food product. There should be a clear cut objective to the employees and workers. So that they can concentrate on a particular direction and desired lead can be obtained. The internal environment must be created to achieve a common goal. The specialty product or uniqueness of product provides recognition to organization in little efforts. However, quality maintenance is a key of success to any organization.

Principle 3: Involvement of people

The self realization and motivation about the ownness and belonginess to all workers of an organization decides the success of organization. So they will participate and work in an organization with their full involvement. It enables their abilities to be used for the organization's benefit. But the welfare of employees and workers must always be protected to develop credibility and faith in organization.

Principle 4: Process approach

The definite plan of product development and their proper implementation is a key to achieve the goal of TQM in any organization. The management of resources and activities in rational way opens the avenue of success. The defined plan and its proper implementation not only help in quality product development but also assist in development of faith and confidence towards organization.

Principle 5: Systemic approach of management

The understanding of management and site operators must be based on common goal to be achieved. Management should always think positive towards the workers and workers should be loyal to the organization. Effectiveness and efficiency of organization can be enhanced by developing a system of each and every work.

Principle 6: Continual improvement

The change in system and continual improvement in current plan as per the present and future demand of consumers and market always help in upgradation of organization. The theme of success and step forward of achieving the glory of organization is behind the continual improvement in system and processes.

Principle 7: Factual approach to decision making

The decisions should always be based on facts and findings must be verified on these facts. The record keeping of data generated at various steps must be analyzed for certain findings. The modifications and improvements in process must be done accordingly but consumer satisfaction must always be kept in mind.

Principle 8: Mutually beneficial supplier relationships

There should be the independent and a mutually beneficial relationship between organization and its suppliers. But consumer satisfaction should always be in the centre of understanding. The faith and satisfaction of organization, suppliers and consumers are key cycling wheels of healthy and wealthy business.

References

1. ftp://ftp.fao.org/docrep/fao/010/ai407e12.
2. GMP Association, 2001. Compilation of Food GMP Certification System from http:// www.gmp.org.tw/en/index2.asp.
3. National Advisory Committee on Microbiological Criteria for Foods (1992). Hazard Analysis and Critical Control Point System. Intl. J. Food Microbiol., 16:1-23.
4. Snyder, O. P. (1991). "HACCP in the Retail Food Industry", Dairy, Food Environ. Sanitat. 11(2):73.

□□□

Chapter 12

Abattoir By-products

By-products or offal's are basically every part or particle which is not included in dressed carcass. It can also be explained as everything produced from the animals except dressed meat is considered as by-products. Meat industry now demands the full utilization of by-products to make the industry profitable and economically sustainable. It is also important for environmental management and to enhance the social image of the meat industry. The yield of animal by-products ranges between 50-60% of the live weight. However, it depends on the age, sex, breed, growth, disease status etc. for example healthy animals yield less by-products in comparison to emaciated animals. As per the FAO (2004) report 106.75 million livestock and more than 650 million poultry birds were slaughtered annually in leading to the production of 5.76 million tonnes meat. It leaves huge loads of by-products. As per the estimate animal by-products fetch 10-15% of the value of the animal in advanced countries but in India and other developing countries it contributes very less to the abattoir business. It is also suggested by some agencies that if by-products are processed properly then the return will be almost equal to the value of the meat derived from an animal.

The term variety meat is used for wholesome edible by-products segregated, chilled and processed under sanitary conditions. Variety meat normally includes liver, heart, tongue, oxtail, kidney, brain, sweetbreads (thymus and/or pancrease depending on animals age), stomach or tripe, intestines, fries (lamb or calf testicles) etc. Term edible fat is generally used to the fat obtained during slaughter i.e 'caul fat' means the fat surrounding rumen and/or stomach, 'cutting fat' means back fat of pork, 'leaf fat' means kidney fat etc.

Need of by-products utilization

1. *For the industrial development and revenue generation*: By-products utilization units may be developed as cottage industries. The production of sterilized feed stock and various valuable by-products

may open the avenue for newer industry development. The conversion of by-products into valuable products further generates the revenues. Thus we can enhance the economic status of the people concerned and valuable things may be available to the common mans.

2. *Employment generation through by-products utilisation and value addition*: By-products collection, storage, processing and its conversion into valuable products opens the doors of employment. In this field illiterate and literate both youths, women and unemployed persons may get employment. Thus the social as well as economic status of the poor and rural peoples can easily be upgraded.
3. *Environmental management by reducing the environmental pollution*: Utilization of by-products prevents the breeding ground for bacteria and other organisms and avoids the attraction of flies, rats, jackals, stray dogs, vultures, crow and other vermin. Thus sanitary and hygienic status of meat plant improves. As a result high quality meat can be produced in these plants with good working conditions.
4. *To enhance the social image of meat industry*: Meat industry is not easily acceptable by the persons residing near the slaughter house or meat processing plant because they have a tendency that it will create a great pollution to the environment and bad air may harm the health of dwellers. By the utilization of by-products and animal slaughter house waste the thinking of the society about the bad image of meat industry can easily be changed. It is very important in countries like India where slaughter practices are taboos.
5. *To utilize valuable animal protein for human foods and animal feeds*: The utilization of by-products in value added foods, sources of feed may be a good alternative to fulfil the demand of animal protein to the population and animals for present and future with increasing population pressure. Organs and some other edible by-products may be the good source of animal proteins to the humans and other animal by-products may easily be converted into animal and poultry feed as a source of various nutrients and proteins.
6. *For the better return to the farmers*: The proper utilization of animal by-products may be helpful to gain more profit from the meat business. Thus the demand of animals may further enhance and the prices of livestock and other requirements may be helpful for better returns to the farmers concern.
7. By-products and animal slaughter house waste may be the source of various nutrients for soil thus may be helpful in crop production. The waste material from slaughter house, condemned meat, parts

of animal's body, detained meat, beddings, droppings etc. can easily be converted into the fertilizers. These fertilizers may be helpful in enhancement of the fertility of soil and may be used as a supplement for soil nutrients.

8. *To help in prevention and control of spread of various diseases and conditions in both humans and animals*: By the proper utilization of animal by-products and slaughter house waste as well as the animal's parts and bodies died after disease or in natural deaths if utilized properly may help in control of animal as well as the spread of diseases in human beings. By this way material obtained can be sterilized and sewage gets treated water thus the breeding ground for disease causing organisms can be prevented. It also helps in destroying of spores and pathogenic bacteria, virus etc. Thus it provides healthy environment to the humans and animals to live healthy.

9. *Increase in export revenue and tax*: by the utilization of by-products like intestines, bones, hairs, hooves, horns, glandular by-products etc. several types of valuable products may be exported in global market. By this way country may get huge revenue which will be helpful in up gradation of social and economic standards of the concerns and in general of the countryman's. The taxes on various products sale and export may further be helpful in revenue generation for developmental activities.

Classification of By-products of an abattoir

A. **On the basis of it edibility:** Edibility is a main criterion to differentiate various by-products. It is determined by customs, religion, consumer acceptance, availability of the product, economics and hygiene. Some of the by-products are totally prohibited in certain areas and same are very much popular in other areas like blood which is forbidden in Islam while it is being utilised extensively for preparing sausages in many western countries and as a curried fried product in Nepal. In general, edible by-products accounts almost 67 percent among all by-products obtained from animal slaughter. However, general classification of by-product is as follows:

1. *Edible by-products*: Edible by-products are those which are utilized as food for human consumption. A number of by-products are eligible for this category like glandular by-products (viz. liver, heart, brain, lungs, thymus, pancreas, testicles, tongue and gizzard), intestines, skin, stomach, bile etc. In US meat trimmings from the head are also included in edible by-products.

By-products	Approximate recovery % by weight	Principle uses
Blood	3.50	Pharmaceuticals, blood protein isolates, food, feed etc.
Liver	1.20	Liver meal, variety meat, liver tones
Heart	0.30	Food, variety meat, huggis
Tongue	0.25	Food, variety meat
Kidney	0.17	Pharmaceuticals
Sweetbreads	0.10	Variety meat
Brain	0.10	Variety meat
Lungs	1.10	Heparin, meal
Pancreas	0.01	Hormones, enzymes
Oxtail	0.15	Variety meat
Spleen	0.25	Meat sausages
Tripe	1.25	Variety meat, enzyme
Intestine	-	Casings, food, surgical sutures
Poultry giblets	-	Variety meat
Pig tail and pig fat	-	Tid-bits
Trimmings	-	Variety meat, fat
Poultry gizzards and proventriculus	3.5-4.2	Edible as a source of chitinolytic enzyme

2. *Inedible by-products*: Inedible by-products are those which are not used for edible purpose but have several uses in other forms and provide valuable products. They account around 33 percent among the whole by-products of animal slaughter. The major inedible by-products includes wool, hair, hide, fibre, skin, bones, horns, bristle, hooves, manure, litter, hatchery by-products, snout, teeth, trimming etc.

By-products	Approximate recovery % by weight	Principle uses
Blood	<1.0 as drip	Leather finishing agents, animal feed, blood meal
Bone	18-30	Glue and gelatin
Hide	6-8	Leather, gelatin
Intestines	-	Casings, suturing material
Horn/hoof	0.5	Neats foot oil, protein hydrolysate

Bile	0.06	Detergent
Fat	-	Soap, grease
Feathers	7-8	Feathers meal, protein hydrolysate, bedding material, decorative purpose, sporting equipments, manure, fertilizers
Ruminal contents	-	Biogas
Poultry litter and manure	-	Recycled feed, organic fertilizer
Hatchery by products i.e. egg shell, infertile eggs, unhatched eggs, dead and culled chicks	-	Hatchery by-products meal, egg shell meal
Poultry heads	2.5-3.0	Poultry meal
Poultry feet	3.5-4.0	Soap, technical fat/poultry grease
Poultry intestines and glands	8.5-9.0	Sportgats, meat meal, poultry grease and active principles as hormones and enzymes

3. *Borderline by-products*: these by-products may be edible and/or inedible depending upon the food customs and the purchasing capacity of the consumer. Among these are organs such as the uterus, spleen, testicles, lungs and blood. However, for use as edible by-products they must be collected and processed in sound hygienic condition.

B. **On the basis of ultimate use**: By-product may also be classified on the basis of their ultimate use. They may be processed as industrial level for various uses. Some common uses may be as:

1. *Agricultural by-products*: animal by-products may be processed in such a way that they can be utilized in various purposes in agriculture. They may be used as a source of certain nutrients for soil and their uses enhances the productivity of lands. Some common agricultural by-products are meat meal, bone meal, fertilizer etc.

2. *Industrial by-products*: industrial by-products include the by-products which can be converted into the commercial products. Great revenue can be generated by this way and these products can be utilized in various food items and industry purposes. Some common examples are gelatine, glue, casings etc.

3. *Pharmaceutical by-products*: Pharmaceutical by-products are mainly the glandular by-products which can be converted in life saving

drugs and also in form of production of certain medicines. Some common animal glands and their valuable uses are listed below:

Tissues and glands	Products/ drugs/ medicines
Adrenal cortex	Cortisone
Adrenal medulla	Adrenaline, noradrenaline
Gall bladder	Bile, bile salt, pigments
Duodenum	Enterogastrone, secretin
Brain	Steroid, cholesterol, lecithin, cephalin
Intestines	Heparin
Lungs	Heparin
Liver	Vitamin- B_{12}, heparin, catalase
Ovaries	Progesterone, relaxin
Pancrease	Insulin, glucagon, lipase, LPH
Parathyroid	Parathormone
Thyroid	Thyroxin
Pituitary	GH, TSH, ACTH, lactogenic hormones
Seminal vesicles	Prostaglandins
Testes	Hyaluronidase
Stomach	Pepsin, rennin

C. **On the basis of origin**

1. *Principle by-products*: these by-products are directly harvested from the animals. These are usually raw materials and perishable in nature. They need proper preservation and storage for further use. The major principle by-products are hides and skins, hair, bristle, wool, bones, blood, hoofs, horns, feet, intestines, condemned meat, inedible offal, trimmings, major glands etc.

2. *Secondary by-products*: these are derived from principle by-products and are quite stable and can be directly utilized in various forms. Some of the examples are leather, glue and gelatine, fertilizer, tallow, grease, stock feed from hide and skin, pelt, brushes, fabrics, yarns, lanolin, fertilizer etc from hair, bristle and wool, blood meal, haemoglobin, fibrin, plasma, albumin, dye setting, serum, liquid blood products etc. from blood, meal, fat, gelatine, glue, cutlery, buttons, bone articles etc from bones, combs, hairpins, novelties, toys, meal, fertilizer, glue and gelatine from horns and hoof, casings, catgut, suture material, musical instrument strings, stock feed etc from intestines, tallow, leather, meal and candles from condemned

meat, inedible offals, trimmings etc. and life saving drugs, enzymes and hormones from glandular by-products.

D. **As per English commercial slaughter practices**:

1. *Red offals*: they are highly perishable offals and needs immediate cooling treatment after collection. The storage of these by-products is requires refrigeration temperature till its disposal. The examples of red offals are liver, kidneys, heart etc.

2. *White offals*: fats, manyplies (IIIrd stomach), gut and bladder, weasand, rectum are included in white offals.

3. *Grey offals*: grey offals include stomach, intestines, lungs, spleen etc. They should be collected and stored in separate chamber maintained at cooling temperature.

4. *Dark offals*: head, feet, shanks etc are some of the offal falls in this category. These offals required cooling and separate storage chamber.

E. **Classification of offals as per Food Standards Committee of the Ministry of Agriculture, Fisheries and Food,1972 of U.K.**

1. *List -A offals:* these includes mammalian tissues and offals which can be utilized as cooked or uncooked. Examples are diaphragm, skirt of cattle only, head meat, ox cheeks, pig bath chip, heart, kidney, liver, pancrease, oxtail meat, thymus of cattle and sheep only, tongue. It also includes heart, liver etc of poultry birds.

2. *List-B offals:* Those offals of mammalian tissues which can not be utilized uncooked. They are brains, blood, blood plasma, cow heel, sheep and pig trotters, pig chitlings, small intestines, lungs (lites), oesophagus meat, rectum, spinal cord, non-ruminant stomach, tripe, first and second stomach after cooking, fourth stomach, lamb fries (testicles), udder. Gizzard and neck of poultry is also included in this category.

F. **As per Bureau of Indian Standards (BIS) classification**: BIS classified the animal by-products in three categories on the basis of its hazard to the human health.

1. *Category 1* : The highest hazardous material from animal body are grouped in this category i.e animal parts may harbour the avian influenza, BSE diseases, pet animals, zoo and circus animals and experimental animals etc. Later animals are classified in this group due to the level of veterinary drugs and residues.

2. *Category 2*: The high risk materials are classified in this group like fallen stock, manure and digestive content. By default, the materials which are not classified in category 1 and 3 are also included in this group.
3. *Category 3*: Category 3 includes low risk materials from slaughter houses such as animal parts not indeed for human consumption like hides, hair, feathers, bones etc.

Slaughter house by-products and their gainful utilization

By-product	Raw by-products	Processed by-product	Process	Uses
Blood	Edible raw blood	Serum, plasma and red blood corpuscles	High speed centrifuge/ separator	Adhesive for sausages, pharmaceutical products, blood sausages or puddings.
	Inedible raw blood	Blood meal, poultry feed, blood albumen	Drying	Additives for livestock feed; leather finishing agent, plywood adhesive, fertilizer, mordant. Albumin in weatherproof glue
Bones	Bones	Manufactured bones	Processing	Buttons, cutlery, handles, bone articles
	Bones	Ossein	Processing	Glue, gelatine
	Bones	Raw bones	Processing	Stock feed, mineral supplement, bone block
	Raw bone classified as edible	Edible fat pieces	Rendering	Shortening, bone gelatine, bone meal, livestock and poultry feed.
	Raw bone classified as inedible	Inedible fat pieces	Rendering	*Lubricant gelatine:* in photography, pharmaceutical, printing. *Tallow:* soap, cosmetics, food, bone ash, ceramic. *Glue:* adhesive, abrasive.
Hide	Hides	Preserved hide, hair and wool	Salt pack curing and air drying	Leather products, falls, upholstery, shoes, gloves, belts, luggage, handbags.

	Hide and pelt	Trimming for inedible rendering	Rendering	Fertilizers and textiles. *Collagen:* cosmetics face creams, shampoo, detergents.
	Pig skin	Edible	Processing	Used in various comminuted product up to 7-10 %.
		Tanned skin	Tanning	Leather products.
	Trimmings	Preserved	Processing	Glue, tallow, fertilizer and feed stock
Intestine	Intestines	Casings	Running and stripping	Edible sausage
		Intestines	Processing	Surgical sutures, sports racket, strings for musical instruments (from sheep), prosthetic materials, collagen sheets, burn dressing, dialyzing membrane, animal feed, heparin and protein meal.
Stomach	Stomach	- Calf stomach - Pig stomach	Processing Processing	*Rennin* which helps in digestion of milk in infants.*Pepsin:* It assists in breakdown of protein into proteases and peptones.
Horns, feet and hooves	Cattle feet	Neats foot oil	Cooking	Fine lubricant
	Animal feet	Tendons	Processing	Glue and gelatine
	Horns and hooves	Gelatine extracted protein	Hydrolysis	Gelled food products, foaming in fire extinguishers, felt, upholstery, brushes.
		Bony structures	Processing	Buttons, comb, hairpins and washers
	Toe nails	Meal	Rendering	Mixed with livestock feed or fertilizer.
	Horns, feet and hooves wastes	Meal	Rendering	Meat foot stock and fertilizers
Lungs	Lungs	Edible products	Processing	Direct consumption, variety meat, sausage ingredient.

Brain	Brain	Pharmaceuticals	Processing	*Cholesterol:* used in synthesis of vitamin-D_3 in case of rickets and as an emulsifier in cosmetics. *Thromboplastin:* used as a blood coagulant in surgery.*Cephalin:* assists in clotting of blood.*Lecithin:* as an emulsifier, antioxidant and in treating snack bites.
Bile/gall stone	Bile/ gallstone	Pharmaceuticals	Processing	Bile paste in detergents, cholic acid, deoxy cholic acid, chenodoxycholic acid used in pharmaceuticals.
Pancreas	Pancreas	Pharmaceuticals	Processing	Trypsin, bate, insulin pharmaceuticals.
Liver	Liver	Edible	Processing	Direct consumption, variety meat, sausage ingredients.
Fat	Edible raw fat	Edible fat oleostarein cracklings	Rendering	Fatty acids, frying purpose, margarine, shortening, candy chewing gum, pet foods or meat meal.
	Inedible raw and condemned materials	Inedible fat, meat and bone meal	Rendering	Lubricants, soap, candles, glycerine additives for livestock and poultry feed.
	Inedible raw fat	Inedible (rendered) fat	Rendering	Lubricants, soap, candles, glycerine, additives for livestock and poultry feed.
Hair and bristles	Hair and bristles	-	Processing	Brushes.
Condem-ned meat and parts	Condemned parts, meat and offals	Condemned parts, meat and offals	Rendering	Tallow: Soap, machine oil, leather dressing, stearin, candles Others: Poultry and livestock feed.

Ruminal and intestinal contents	Ruminal and intestinal content	Paunch and intestinal contents	Composting and methanization	Compost, fertilizers and methane.
Bezoars	In stomach and intestines	Phytobezoars Pilobezoars	Vegetable matter and salt of calcium and phosphorus Hair and other keratinous material	Reported as antidote of poisons.No commercial value.

General composition of various meals

Meal	Value in percent					
	Protein	Moisture	Crude fat	Minerals	Calcium	Phosphorus
Meat meal	>55.0	7.0	8.0	30	-	4.5
Meat cum bone meal (carcass meal)	<55.0	7.0	8.0	-	-	>4.5
Bone meal	26.0	-	1.0	-	23.0	11.0
Raw steamed	7.0	-	1.0	-	32.5	15.1
Blood meal	>80.0	-	-	-	Less	Less

Salient points of by-products industry

1. Blood meal usually contains 80 percent protein. Among all the proteins lysine accounts seven percent. Others predominant proteins in blood meal are tryptophane and methionine.
2. Meat and bone meal are not only the source of proteins but also act as the source of phosphorus, calcium and Vitamin-B_{12}.
3. Meat, blood, liver meal contains practically no fibre. So they are extremely important in pig, poultry and fish feed because they allows to higher intake of protein.
4. Lean or emaciated carcasses have higher moisture content than fat animal carcasses. They also yields lower amount of non fatty solids because some of the proteins are replaced with moisture during starvation and fever.

5. Rendered dry products made from by-products generally accounts one third raw material by weight. The conversion ratio from raw material to final meal in dry rendering is 3:1, in wet rendering 4:1, blood to blood meal is 5:1 and bone to bone meal is 3:1.
6. During by-products processing yield per beast is higher from naturally died animals than slaughtered animals due to presence of higher amount of blood in previous one.
7. Meat and fat trimmings collected from meat plant can be utilized to make pet foods while bones can be utilized in form of bone meal.
8. *Pluck* constitutes larynx, trachea, lungs, heart and liver in calf while spleen is also included in pluck of sheep and oesophagus in pigs.

Variety meat

Variety meat products contribute good proportion in animal slaughter products. Major variety meats are lungs, liver, spleen, heart, brain, ears, feet, stomach, tripe, kidneys, tongues etc. In opinion of meat industry these variety meats are less valuable and commonly not utilized in direct consumption. It is because of their unpalatability and presence of typical fatty acids and higher cholesterol. In general variety meat products are considered food of low income populations as a source of high quality protein and nutrition. But in real sense they are quite nutritious and posses good proportion of vitamins as well as other nutrients. They can be processed into value added products. Many countries particularly in Asian countries variety meats are considered as delicious food and are the basis for many traditional dishes.

Nutritional value of variety meat

Variety meat	Nutritional constitutes	Utility
Livers	High in vitamin A, B, C and D, iron, zinc, copper, and fatty acids.	Direct consumption and value added products.
Hearts	Large amounts of iron and are a good source of selenium, zinc, phosphorous, niacin, and riboflavin.	Direct consumption and value added products.
Brains	Rich in niacin, phosphorus, vitamin B_{12} and C.	Direct consumption and value added products.
Ears, feet, lungs, stomach and tripe	High in proline, hydroxyproline and glycine.	Value added products.
Kidneys	Good source of vitamin B_6, B_{12}, and folacin.	Value added products.

Utility of variety meat in different countries

Country	Variety meat product
China	In various recipes as blend in form of sharp tasting variety meats.
Japan	Cow tongues are considered expensive delicacies.
South Korea	Sliced beef feet in soup preparation.
Mexico	In preparation of different dishes like tripe and liver with tomatoes in *putzaze*, tongue with green chilies in *lengua*, and tripe as soup in menudo norteña.
Russia and Egypt	World's leading importers of edible offal as variety meats to supplement high quality protein and nutrition in values added products.

General utility of variety meat

i. Meat protein concentrate and meat extract derived from internal organs such as liver, lung, spleen, stomach, duodenum, kidney, heart, brain can be utilized for making soups, stews, sauces, canned meat and gravies.

ii. Variety meat protein concentrates and extracts can be utilized as an excellent flavouring ingredient for noodle soup mix, onion soup mix and dips.

iii. Variety meat products can be utilized in form of emulsion based meat products like sausages, patties, nuggets, meat balls, kababs and restructured meat products like steaks, cutlets, chops, roasts, rolls as well as in enrobed meat products.

Poultry industry by-products

Poultry industry by-products are everything's comes from poultry farm, hatchery and processing units. These by-products may be utilized as edible for man and animals and some of them may be considered as inedible. Major by-products obtained from poultry industry can be classified into three major groups as:

i. Poultry by-products recovered from production phase such as litter and manure from the farm.

ii. Poultry by-products emanating from hatchery include infertile eggs, shells of hatched eggs, dead embryos and dead chicks.

iii. By-products obtained from poultry processing plant i.e. blood, feathers, offals (feet, head and intestinal tract), condemned birds etc.

By-products from poultry industry

Group of poultry birds	By-products as per the live weight of bird			
	Total by-products	Offal	Blood	Feathers
Broilers	25-32 (29.0)	18.5	3.5	7.0
Fowl	25-30 (28.0)	18.0	3.0	7.0
Turkey	20-25 (23.0)	12.5	3.5	7.0

Poultry industry by-products and their utilization

By-product	Process	Product	Utilization
A. Poultry by-products recovered from production phase			
Manure and litter	Dehydration & sterilization	Feed Manure & litter	Livestock and poultry feed Surface dressing of agriculture fields. Fertilizer as a source of minerals and elements.
B. Hatchery by-products			
Infertile eggs, shells of hatched eggs, dead embryos and dead chicks	Rendering	Mixed meal	Feed of poultry and livestock. 3-5 percent meal can be added in layer feed.
C. By-products of poultry dressing plant			
Feather	Processing & sterilization	Feather stock	Bedding material, decorative items, sporting equipment, manure or fertilizer, feather meal etc.
Feathers, blood heads, feet, intestines, lungs, pancreas and spleen	Rendering	Poultry by products meal, hydrolyzed feather meal, mixed poultry byproducts meal as well as technical fat or poultry grease.	Feed and food.

Salient features in utilization of poultry by-products

i. Sterilized and dehydrated poultry manure contains about 27-29 % protein and can be used up to 20 and 25 % in the total diet of broilers and layers respectively.

ii. Poultry manure is not only a good fertilizer but it also improves the physical structure of soil.

iii. The hatchery by-products are cooked, dried and ground with or without removal of fat. It is a good source of protein and also contains about 18.10 % calcium and 413 mg per 100 g phosphorus.

iv. Poultry by-products industry involves feathers 6-7%, blood 3.5%, heads 3.0%, feet 3.9%, intestines, lungs, pancreas and spleen 8-9% of the live weight. The natural proportion of different byproducts viz. feathers, blood and offals is 4: 1: 6.

v. Commercial mixed poultry by-products processing industry meal should contain not more than 16 % ash and 4 % acid insoluble ash. Permissible incorporated level in ration is 5-7%. It can also be satisfactorily substitute the meat meal or fish meal.

vi. *Giblet* includes heart without pericardium, liver without gallbladder and gizzard without mucosal layer. It is a part of routine carcass weight of poultry.

Composition of one ton deep litter

Component	Contribution in kg	Comments
Nitrogen	29.48 kg	Equivalent 136.08 - 147. 42 kg ammonium sulphate
Phosphorus	20.41 kg	Equivalent to about 113.40 - 136.08 kg ordinary super phosphate
Potash potassium	20.41 kg	Equivalent to about 45.34 kg
Magnesium	6.80 kg	-
Sodium	6.8 kg	-
Calcium	27.21 kg	-
Trace elements like boron, copper, iron, sulphur and zinc	Traces	-

These by-products are valuable items and must be utilized in proper way. The utmost care is required during handling, collection, transportation, storage and processing. These steps entirely depend on the ultimate use and edibility of these by-products. In general edible by-products requires sound preservation and storage facilities whereas, inedible by-products and wastes can be handled and stored in separate unit till further use. In all way the by-products and slaughter house wastes must be utilized.

References

1. Kondaiah, N., Anjaneyulu, A.S.R., Lakshmanan, V. (1993). Incorporation of chicken by-products in mutton nuggets. J Food Sci. Technol., 30(2):143–144.
2. Liu, D.C. (2002). Better utilization of by-products from the meat industry 2002-10-01. Extension Bulletins. Food and fertilizer Technology Center for the Asian and Pacific region (FFTC publication database)
3. Mann, I. (1978). Preparation of stock feed and fertilizers on commercial scale. *In:* Animal By-products: Processing and Utilization, 3rd edition, FAO, Italy. Pp 1-25.
4. Ockerman, H.W. and Hansen,C.L. (2000). Rendering. *In:* Animal By-products Processing and Utilization, by CRC Press. Pp 1-83.
5. Ranganayaki, M.D. and Srinivasan, T.S. (1999). Hygienic processing and utilization of animal by-products. *In:* Souvenir cum Proceedings of National Seminar on Processing of Meat, Poultry and By-products for Value Addition at CFTRI, Mysore from 24-26 Feb. Pp 187-196.
6. Sharma , B.D. (2003). Plan and layout of by-products utilization plant. *In:* Modern Abattoir Practices and Animal By-products Technology, First Edition, Jaypee Brothers Medical Publishers,New Delhi. Pp 97-106.

❑❑❑

Chapter 13

Plan and Layout of By-products Utilization Plant

The vast livestock population requires proper harvesting of animal by-products to generate income to the farmers and to provide the employment to marginally educated masses. The density of livestock in our country demands atleast one animal by-product processing plant in each fifty kilometer range. Proper utilization of animal by-products will also serve in reduction of environmental pollution through slaughter house. Ultimately image of the meat industry can be enhanced by proper utilization of animal by-products. The proper disposal of animal slaughter house and by-products waste is further necessary to reduce the environmental pollution and to enhancement the livelihood of neighourers.

Animal by-products are entire bodies or parts of animals, products of animal origin or other products obtained from animals that are not intended for human consumption. The materials included in animal by-products are butcher and slaughterhouse waste, blood, feathers, wool, hides and skins, fallen stock, pet animals, zoo and circus animals, hunt trophies, manure, ova, embryos and semen not intended for breeding purposes. They are valuable and perishable items and requires due attention as soon as their collection.

Collection and transportation of animal by-products

The animal by-products must be collected, identified and disposed of without undue delay. It is essential to prevent risk of diseases and health hazard to human and animals. Animal by-products must be transported in sealed new packaging or covered leak-proof containers or vehicles from abattoir to the by-products processing plants. The containers and vehicles used for transportations must be specific in use for a particular animal by-product and if not possible they must be cleaned and disinfected after every use to avoid cross contamination.

Important considerations during establishment of a by-products utilization plant

Basic requirements

1. In India, by-product plant should be established adjacent to the slaughter house or it may be a part of the same building connected through chutes or gravity pipes. In earlier case, the passage between slaughter house and by-product plant must be constructed with concrete, stones or bricks and the slope should be towards by-product plant.
2. The establishment should preferably be away from inhabited area.
3. There should be the availability of labours, electricity and ample amount of water supply.
4. As far as possible, there should be provision of overhead rails from slaughter house to the by-product plant.
5. A by-product plant should have its own screened drainage with a gully fitted with individual grease traps.
6. The by-product plant should have clear clean and unclean sections. Charging platform or raw materials inlet from a part of unclean sections whereas processed and sterilized by-products are prepared, stored and disposed of from clean sections having separate exit points.
7. The floor, walls and ceiling should be made up of smooth and concrete material so that these can be easily and frequently washed. A floor slope of ½ inch per ft. is generally recommended.
8. A by-product plant should invariably have a hide/skin salting room, renderers, tripery, boiler, manure bunker, store besides common amneties.
9. The plant building should be open and ventilated to prevent humidity build up leading to corrosion of equipment and building. It will also check the growth of moulds and bacteria in the building. The roofing material may preferably be corrugated asbestos sheeting. There should be provision of exhaust fans from each partition.
10. The equipments to be installed should cope up with the by-product or offal accumulation expected each day. Renderer, fat settling tank, fat expeller, blood press, grind mill etc. are essentially required. A boiler of suitable capacity is inevitable for processing as well as cleaning operations.

11. The sections for inedible animal parts i.e. tripery, hide room, boiler, lavatories, laundry, store etc. should have separate entrance and exit.
12. The animals condemned at antemortem and received dead in slaughter house should be destroyed and cut into pieces and passed into by-products processing plant through chute.
13. Proper ventilation is a prime requirement of the plant. For this purpose steel structures with wall built up of six feet height or prefabricated steel structures with ventilators of top may be installed.
14. Roof of the plant may preferably be of corrugated asbestos sheets.
15. At initial stage, processing of one or two by-products can be taken up. The operations can be further extended in stages.

Hygienic requirements

1. To maintain the sound hygienic condition in plant, there should be the clear cut demarcation in clean (processed products) and unclean (raw materials) areas.
2. The by-product plant worker must have their own amenities.
3. The walls and floors of plant must be hard, smooth and easily washable with the floor slope not less than half inch in a foot.
4. There should be the provision of hot water and steam all time during plant operations.
5. There should not be any connectivity between slaughter house and by-product processing plant except chutes.
6. There should be proper packaging availability for the processed meal and other products. The metal containers or polyethylene bags lined with standard jute or sisal bag can be used for the purpose.

Provision of nuisance prevention

The nuisance production is a great problem of by-product processing plant. So the attempts must be done to minimize production and excretion of off odours from the plant. The following steps may be helpful in this work:

1. The proper construction, early processing of raw material and proper provision of off odour control measures must be taken care.
2. The provision of condenser in the way of renderer (where hot vapoures are produced) to boiler stack (where these vapoures dispersed in cooling water) must be installed.

3. The provision of chlorination and use of activated carbon for absorption of nuisance material greatly reduces the pollution in plant.

Requirement of equipments

The equipment and its capacity requirements for animal by-products processing are solely dependent on the type of by-products available and final products produced. However, some common equipment required for plant can be enlisted as:

1. Renderer
2. Renderer melter
3. Bone digester
4. Fat expeller/extractor/press
5. Mill (grinder/disintegrator/swing beater)
6. Autoclave
7. Fat settling tank
8. Blood press
9. Boiler

Boilers used in production of steam must have the working steam pressure not less than 80 lb. The requirement of steam for processing of one kilogram of by-products will be around 1.25 kilogram.

Sections of by-product processing plant

To obtain optimum return and to reduce the environmental pollution following basic facilities must be there in animal by-products processing plant:

1. Hides and skins section with salt store.
2. Tripery/gut processing section with cleaning tables, water taps etc.
3. Carcass utilization plant with renderer, bone digester, fat settling tank, fat expeller and adjoining milling room and store.

Besides, boiler, worker lockers, amenities and adjacent manure pit are other important requirements. The boiler should be of suitable capacity keeping in view the availability of raw material and consumption of renderer. The requirement of steam has been worked out to be 1.25 lb per lb of raw material to be processed.

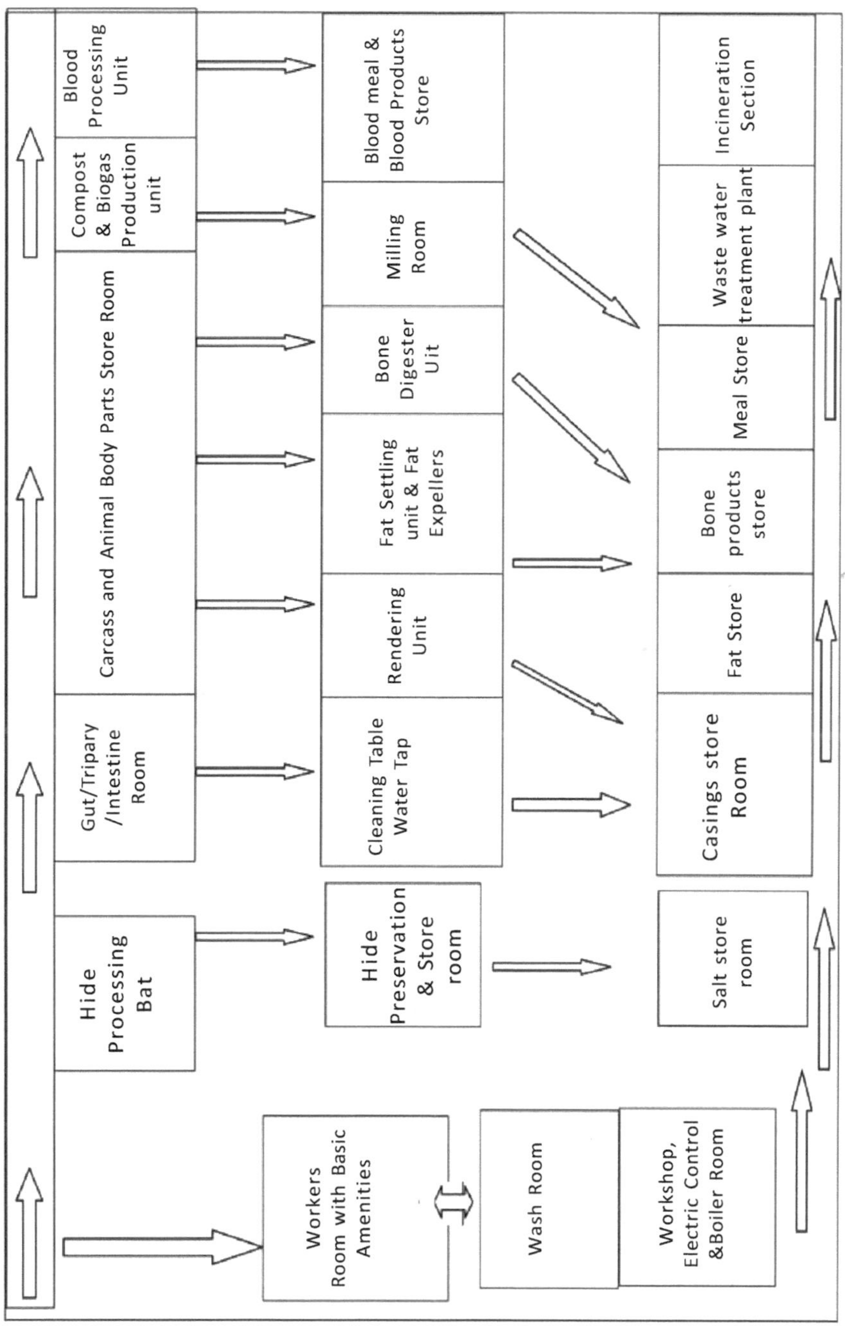

Figure 13.1: Layout of animal by-products processing plant

(a) **Rendering section:** Rendering plant is a basic need of animal by-product utilization plant. It must be according to the requirement of the capacity of by-products utilization unit. All the general hygiene requirements and processing standards must be fulfilled. The provision of type of renderer (dry, wet or continuous) in plant is depending on the product yield and material available for rendering.

(b) **Fat handling section:** To handle the fat comes after rendering requires fat extractor, expeller and press. Then there should be a suitable storage facility for technical fat and other types of fat.

(c) **Milling section**: Milling section is required to handle the material used for production of different types of meal. It must have the sufficient electricity supply and alternatives of the electricity to carry out the smooth functioning of the section. There must be a storage section to hold the raw materials and final products separately.

(d) **Hide and skin section:** Hide and skin section of the plant must have the facility of salt storage. It should have sufficient aeration, dryness and appropriate humidity to avoid dry ness as well as yeast and mould growth over the hide and skins.

(e) **Tripery and gut section:** There should be sufficient space for a table to handle the intestines and other parts of it. It must have the supply of sufficient quantity of potable water.

(f) **Blood processing room:** Blood is an important by-product of the slaughter house and having higher biological oxygen demand. It means it is capable to create greater pollution than all other by-products produced during slaughter of animal. There must be a facility of autoclaving and press to handle the blood.

(g) **Incinerators:** For incineration of waste material and parts of carcasses etc. requires incineration facility. These incinerators must have the provisions prescribed by environment agency and local authority like hygiene conditions, temperature requirements, water discharge requirements, human and animal health guidance etc.

(h) **Composting and biogas section:** They are the type of anaerobic digestion systems in which waste materials, intestinal contents and rendered material are utilized to produce biogas and compost.

(i) **Pet food section:** The animal parts used for pet foods must have the good hygienic and quality standards. All the measures related to sanitary and hygienic requirements must be followed. The provisions of nutritional and biosecurity must be taken care.

(j) **Intermediate plant section:** The plant section dealing with animal by-products after their collection must also meet the general hygiene requirements.

(k) **Storage section:** Storage section receiving raw products must comply with the general requirements and receiving derived products must comply with special requirements like sanitary, hygienic and quality standards.

(l) **Alternative sections**: Alternative section is required to process animal by-products by technologies or methods of disposing of animal by-products such as biodiesel and alkaline hydrolysis.

(m) **Workers amenity section**: Workers amenity section must have the separate entity to maintain the sanitary and hygienic requirement of the plant. The section must have the changing room, lavatory and supply of hot and cold water.

Now the time is to produce value added by-products but very few units are available in India in this field. The value added by-products having great export potential are dicalcium phosphate, ossein, gelatin, bone meal, bone grit etc. The potential products can also be obtained from blood, liver, glands for pharmaceutical purposes and intestines can be processed for casings. The organs like liver, heart, lungs, kidneys may be suitable alternative for pet food industry. Skin and hides can be properly utilized by little interventions of technology to high quality leather and leather products. The need is to optimize the plant and generate the vision to gain more profit from industry.

References

1. Kondaiah, N., Anjaneyulu, A.S.R., Lakshmanan, V. (1993). Incorporation of chicken by-products in mutton nuggets. J Food Sci. Technol., 30(2):143–144.

2. Liu, D.C. (2002). Better utilization of by-products from the meat industry 2002-10-01. Extension Bulletins. Food and fertilizer Technology Center for the Asian and Pacific region (FFTC publication database)

3. Mann, I. (1978). Preparation of stock feed and fertilizers on commercial scale. *In:* Animal By-products: Processing and Utilization, 3rd edition, FAO, Italy. Pp 1-25.

4. Ockerman, H.W. and Hansen,C.L. (2000). Rendering. *In:* Animal By-products Processing and Utilization, by CRC Press. Pp 1-83.

5. Ranganayaki, M.D. and Srinivasan, T.S. (1999). Hygienic processing and utilization of animal by-products. In: Souvenir cum Proceedings of National Seminar on Processing of Meat, Poultry and By-products for Value Addition at CFTRI, Mysore from 24-26 Feb. Pp 187-196.

6. Sharma, B.D. (2003). Plan and layout of by-products utilization plant. In: Modern Abattoir Practices and Animal By-products Technology, First Edition, Jaypee Brothers Medical Publishers, New Delhi. Pp 97-106.

Chapter **14**

Rendering Methods-Preparation of Meat, Bone and Fish Meal

Term rendering is generally used to recover the fat from animal material by heating. However, today rendering word is applied in broad sense in by-products industry to recover stock feed, fertilizers and fats from slaughter house offals, parts and condemned material from animal body. Today many products are recovered by rendering process and can be utilized in different ways. Some of them may be categorized as edible and inedible. The major examples are lard and tallow which may be edible and inedible depending on the processing. Other valuable products include chemicals, meat meals and bone meals. To get these valuable products, various animal by-products are processed like viscera, bones, trimmings, dead stock, feather and other poultry materials.

Rendering systems

Now a day number of rendering systems are used to produce various types of valuable products. Broadly they may be classified as *dry rendering, wet rendering and continuous low temperature rendering.*

i. *Dry rendering system*: dry rendering system is generally utilize horizontal steam jacket renderer in which steam is circulated in double walled jacket and material remains in inner part of the equipment. The material never comes in contact of steam and it is cooked by the pressure (75 Psi for 3-4 hrs) generated from moisture of material itself. The stirring process maintains the material in continuous motion and ensures uniform cooking of material. All the processes like sterilization, digestion and drying takes place in same vessel and in a single operation. So nutrient loss in this method is minimal. The fat released from cells but remains in dispersed in material called *cracklings*. It is a gritty, fibrous and non slippery material having moisture as low as 5 percent. The bones are separated and sent to bone digester for bone meal preparation. The fat content of cracklings can be reduced by hydraulic press and fat expeller based on continuous screw principle. The material is then subjected to turbine (centrifugal fat extractor) of 700 rpm speed to melt the fat and centrifugal force drives the material into storage tank. Fat is then extracted by solvent extraction method using petrol, ether, heptanes or perchlor ethylene etc. Sometimes antioxidants like butylated hydroxyanisole (BHA) are mixed to enhance the keeping quality. The crackling is converted into meat meal by using grinders, disintegrator and swine beaters and directly collected into packaging bags through cyclone. Dry rendering process saves energy, labour and yields 20% more meat meal than wet rendering process. Dry rendering process can be classified as batch dry rendering and continuous dry rendering systems.

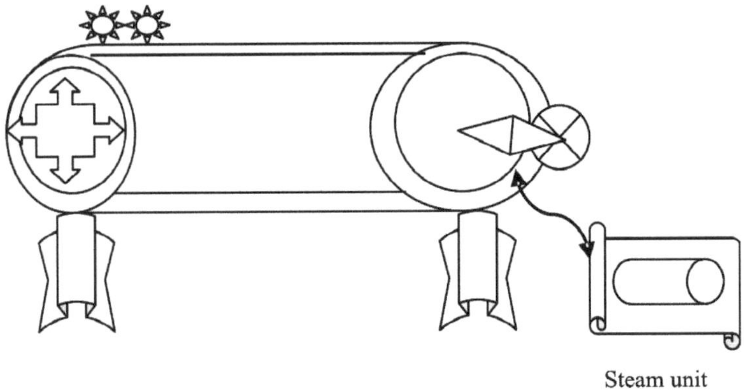

Horizontal dry renderer

a. *Batch dry rendering system*: in batch dry rendering system material is filled and discharged from cooker in batches. Steam jacketed cooker is used to sterilize the material and cooking temperature is 100-130^{0}C for 1.5 to 2 hrs. After cooking and digestion solid material is pressed to remove residual fat and free fat is drained. Solid is then grinded, disintegrated and milled to get meat meal while fat is purified by extraction procedure.

b. *Continuous dry rendering system*: it is a continuous dry rendering system in which flow is continuous and raw material is treated at atmospheric temperature. The process is completed in horizontal vessel consisting of two separate openenings, one for raw material and another for final product. Material is then discharged to percolator (tank with strainer screw and drainer screw) at bottom.

The material is then subjected to screw press and separated into solid and liquid fractions. Solid mass is grinded and converted into meat meal while liquid is centrifuged in bucket or pusher centrifuge for further use.

ii. *Wet rendering system*: wet rendering is generally performed in vertical wet renderer which is almost same as domestic pressure cooker. It is consisting of steam pressure regulator, manhole for feeding of raw material and three 8-12 inches diameter outlets for fat, water and tankage or slush. In wet rendering system material is fed to the cooker and steam of 40 Psi is generally passed through perforated plates at bottom of digester and material is allowed to cook for 5-8 hrs. Then material is allowed to settle for at least 2 hrs and pressure is released. Settling of material separates fat on top, water in middle and slush or tankage at bottom due to the hierarchy of specific gravity and heaviness. They can be discharged from the respective outlets. Fat is purified by distillation and bones from slush are passed to bone digester for bone meal preparation. Remaining slush is processed as meal. Wet rendering system produces good quality fat but 25% meal is lost in gravy. Wet rendering system based on processing can be classified as batch wet rendering and continuous low temperature rendering systems.

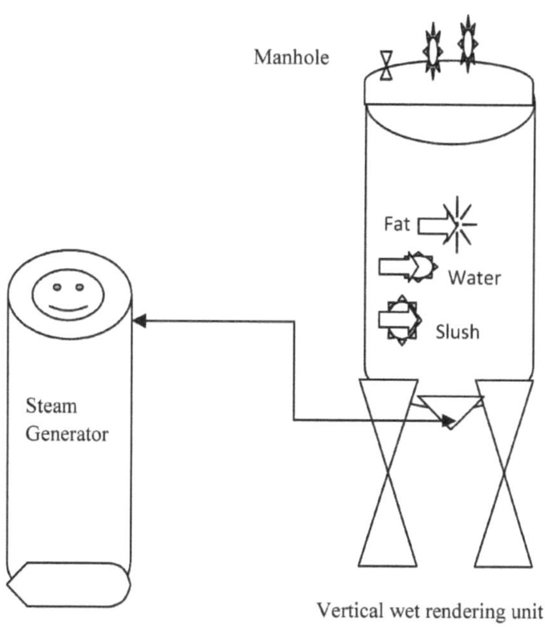

Vertical wet rendering unit

a. *Batch wet rendering or autoclave rendering*: in batch rendering system material is fed and discharges in batches. In the system pre-ground raw material is subjected to steam injection of 140°C at 40 Psi for 5-8 hrs. The high temperature of this system produces dark colour fat due to boiling of material and mixing of paunch colour.

b. *Continuous low temperature rendering (CLTR)*: continuous low temperature rendering is basically mechanical dewatering system in which fat, water and solids are separated by passing the steam injections. In the process, material is heated at 60-90°C for 10-30 minutes. The cell breakage releases tallow, liquid and solids. Tallow is purified by screw press in almost equal proportion with water. The water part is evaporated and fat is recovered by distillation. Solid masses are portioned, cooked and dried while liquid part is centrifuged by a tricanter and sent to evaporator after passing with vibrating screen. This system recovers higher percentage of tallow and only 7-10 percent solid part is converted into meat and bone meal.

Salient features

- This process produces high quality tallow because at low temperature colour of paunch and dirt is not mixed with tallow.
- Energy efficient process and require only 0.5 kg steam per kg of raw material in comparison to 1 kg steam per 1 kg of material in traditional rendering system.
- Fat and fat free solids recovery is better due to avoidance of washing step. Fat recovery is 99.5 % in comparison to traditional rendering system while fat free solids recovered 94 % than 96% in later system. Both fat and moisture content in meal is 8% in CLTR system while traditionally produced meal contains 12 % fat and 3 % moisture.

Products obtained during rendering

i. *Rendered fat:* rendered fats may be edible and inedible depending on its processing condition and raw material used for rendering. Basically two types of fats are obtained: tallow and lard. Tallow is a rendered fat obtained from fatty tissues of cattle or sheep while lard is a fat rendered from clean tissues of healthy pigs. The quality of fat is generally assessed on the basis of titre and free fatty acid contents. Titre is a temperature at which fatty acids of a fat solidify. It may vary with the animal species or even with the location of fat in animal body as loin fat has lower titre than kidney fat. Similarly corn fed pig shows higher titre than peanut fed pigs. Good quality lard and tallow must have following qualities:

a. Titre of lard should be 36-40^{0}C, tallow from cattle 42-45^{0}C and sheep 44-48^{0}C.

b. Good quality fat should not have free fatty acids (FFA) above 2.0 because higher FFA indicates the spoilage.

c. Colour of fat should be respective to species and it should be free from off odour, colour etc. As green colour in fat indicates gut and red blood contamination in fats.

d. Moisture in fat should be minimal (0.2%).

e. Bleach value of tallow should be <0.5 R.

f. Iodine value should be minimal as it indicates the degree of unsaturation.

g. Peroxide value of fresh fat should be in the range of 1-2 as it is a determination of rancidity.

The fats and fatty acids obtained from the meat processing industry can be utilized in various forms. As edible tallow and lard find use in margarine, shortenings and cooking fats while inedible tallow and lard can be utilized as explosive, paint, soap, solvent, industrial oil, lubricant, chemical, rubber, insecticide, floor wax, cosmetic, ceramic, medicine, tanning industries and many more.

ii. *Meat meal:* tankage obtained in wet rendering system is finally ground to a fine powder using grinder and if necessary digest the material using steam injection similar to dry rendering system. But care should be taken that material should be free from horns, hoof, manure and stomach contents. Digested tankage if contains phosphorus greater than 4.4% may be designated as meat and bone meal. Good quality meat meal must have cooked meat and tallow flavour, free from pathogenic organisms and must be stored in a room below 10^{0}C. On digestion with 0.2% pepsin, 87 % crude protein from meal should be digested with in 16 hrs at 45^{0}C.

iii. *Bone meal*: the long bones obtained in rendering process are separated and sent to bone digester. The long bones are first crushed into smaller size and feed to bone digester. The digestion of bones is achieved under steam at 60 psi for 2 hrs and fat as well as protein is separated. Material is then extracted the fat and gelatin using solvent extractors like petrol, ether, heptanes or perchlor ethylene etc. The remaining bony material becomes soft and chalky and can easily be converted into bone meal after grinding.

iv. *Carcass meal:* carcass meal can be obtained from condemned animals, parts, fallen and dead animals. It may also include the parts of animals like bones, heads, feets, trimmings, genitalia, fetus, udder, tripes and empty intestines, trachea, lungs, stomach and other condemned parts. To get a proper carcass meal a separate carcass utilization unit is required. The unit must have a renderer, bone digester, fat settling tank, fat expeller, grinder or mill etc. The processing steps may be almost same as discussed in rendering part.

Composition of various meals obtained from animal and poultry slaughter

Constituent	**Meat and bone meal**	**Poultry by-products meal**	**Blood meal**	**Feather meal**
Moisture	7	7	7	7
Crude protein	50	58	80	86.4
Fat	8.6	13.0	1.0	3.3
Calcium	10.1	3.0	0.3	0.33
Phosphorus	5.0	1.7	0.25	0.55
ME (kcal)	2740	3300	3420	3073
Pepsin digestibility	91.8	90.0	95.6	87.0
Amino acids				
Arginine	3.6	4.0	3.8	5.4
Lysine	2.6	2.7	8.9	1.7
Methionine	0.7	1.0	1.5	0.4
Cystine	0.3	0.7	1.5	0.4
Tryptophan	0.3	0.5	1.1	0.5

Source: Mann (1978); Ockerman and Hansen (2000)

Fish meal

Fish meal is a popular animal feed due to high nutritional value particularly rich in good quality protein. Fish meal is popular because it is rich in fibre and easy to produce. It can be added in feed of swine, cattle and poultry at the rate of 3% of animal diet. Good quality fish meal contains about 60% protein. Fish meal is also high in essential amino acids especially lysine, B-complex vitamins (Vitamin-B_{12}, choline, niacin, pantothenic acid and riboflavin) and minerals including calcium, copper, iron, phosphorus and other trace minerals. About 90% fish meal is produced using oily fishes of species Anchovy, Cepelin and Manhaden etc. and only 10% fish meals from white fish offal such as Cod and Haddock. The major problem of fish meal addition in animal feed is transfer of is fishy odour in eggs and milk. So to avoid off odour in animal products following quantity of fish meal in animals feed is recommended: cattle 907/day/454 kg, pig 113-227 g/day, not more than 5% of ration for chicks, 10% of ration for hens and 45-91 g/day for sheep according to weight.

Composition of fish meal

Nutritional component		Percentage
Digestibility		92
Moisture		6-12
Protein		50-77
Fat		5-15
Ash		8-33
Salt		3-4
Crude fibre		<1
Vitamins	Vitamin-B_{12}	0.1-0.33 mg/lb
	Choline	1500 mg/lb
	Niacin	30 mg/lb
	Riboflavin	3 mg/lb

Source: US Fish and Wildlife Science (1996)

Fish meal processing

Fish meal can be processed generally be rendering process. Generally by wet and/or dry rendering procedures.

i. *Wet rendering system*: wet rendering system is a continuous system of fish rendering and adopted to handle large number of fish. It is most suitable method for rendering of fatty fishes like menhaden, red fish, sea herring, pilchard/California sardine and salmon cannery waste.

Processing steps	Detail
Material collection	Fish and material is collected.
Cooking	It is done in continuous cooker and product moved through screw conveyor. Steam is then injected which coagulate protein and releases oil. Cooking rate is dependent on steam pressure which is normally in the range of 5-10 psi.
Pressing	Cooked mass is passed into continuous screw press encased in a cylindrical screen fitted with two meshes of

	1.2 mm diameter at inlet and 0.8 mm diameter at outlet. Pressing of mass causes cellular rupture.
Drying	Drying of mass is done over direct flame or in steam jacketed drier or in a steam tube drier.
	Liquid part is screened through vibrating screen and heated to 90^{0}C. After centrifugation water is evaporated and rest material is collected.
Storage	Dried fish meal cake can be stored in alcohol which is subsequently removed by azeotropic distillation.

ii. *Dry rendering*: dry rendering system is a batch method of fish meal production. It is generally adopted in non oily fish offals like codd, haddock, canning waste and carcasses of shark and grey fish etc.

Processing steps	Detail
Material collection	Fish and other material are collected.
Grinding	Large parts of fish and material is grinded to reduce their size.
Cooking	Cooking is done in steam jacketed cooker with stirring at 10-80 psi.
Drying	Drying is done under vacuum or atmospheric pressure.
Pressing	Mass is then pressed using hydraulic press to separate solid and liquid.
Storage	Solid fish meal cake is dried further and stored after cooling in polyethylene bags or air tight containers.
	Liquid part is heated and passes to settling tank where oil and water is screened. Resultant products are then stored accordingly.

Feather meal

Feather meal production is a largest market of feather industry. Feathers are rich in keratin protein which is broken down by hydrolysis to make it palatable. After complete rendering feather meal becomes digestible and provides good quantity of high value protein (80%). Feather meal is good source of cystine, threonine and arginine but lacks some essential amino acids such as lysine, methionine, histidine and tryptophane. The moisture content in feather meal is about 10%, fibre 4% and fat in some extent. Generally rendering system is adopted to obtain the feather meal which is a good supplement for poultry and pig feeds but can better utilize in ruminant feed. It can be added in feed @ 0.5-1.5 percent.

Processing technique

Step	Processing changes
Collection of feathers	Feathers are collected from poultry birds
Washing	Washing with water.
Dewatering	Dewatering with mechanical pressure instruments.
Cooking	Steam cooking at 138-149°C with 40 to 50 psi for 1-2 hrs.
Cooling	Cool the material to make meal.
Drying	Drying in tube dryer or air dryer.
Milling	To make the feather meal in fine particles.
Packaging and storage	Package the meal in air tight container and store at room temperature.

Rendering is a process of conversion of perishable by-products into stable and valuable products. However, product quality and its shelf life is mainly depends on raw material quality and safety. The main aim should always be in rendering is to obtain maximum yield and best possible product quality.

References

1. Mann, I. (1978). Preparation of stock feed and fertilizers on commercial scale. *In:* Animal By-products: Processing and Utilization, 3rd edition, FAO, Italy. Pp 31-40.

2. Ockerman, H.W. and Hansen,C.L. (2000). Rendering. In: Animal By-products Processing and Utilization, by CRC Press. Pp 85-126.

3. Prokop W. (1985). Rendering systems for processing animal by-product materials. Papers from the Symposium on Animal Fats presented at the 74th AOCS Annual Meeting held in Chicago, Illinois, May 8–12, 1983. J Am Oil Chem Soc. 1985;62(4):804–811.

4. Sharma , B.D. (2003). Plan and layout of by-products utilization plant. *In:* Modern Abattoir Practices and Animal By-products Technology, First Edition, Jaypee Brothers Medical Publishers,New Delhi. Pp 97-106.

❑❑❑

Chapter **15**

Blood

Blood is a first by-product of animal slaughter house. It accounts about 5-7 percent of animals live weight. It is highly nutritious material particularly rich in protein (17-18%) and essential nutrients. Blood is a rich source of amino acids like leucine, lysine, valine, phenylalanine, histidine etc. It is also rich in haem iron which is biologically most available form of iron. Protein efficiency ratio of plasma is 2.5 while 1.0 for globin. It contains about 80 percent water and responsible for effluent problems. It is a great source of pollution because BOD_5 of whole blood is 250000 mg/litre. It should be collected and processed as soon as possible because whole blood clots easily and is capable to clogs the drainage system, grease traps and septic tank of meat plant or abattoir. Blood rapidly decomposes, spreading bad odors and forming an excellent medium for bacteria growth within the abattoir itself, or its vicinity. It attracts flies and rodents and easily contaminates the carcass, organs or meat parts and seriously reduces the keeping quality. So proper utilization of blood not only enhances the aesthetic look of meat with longer shelf life but greatly reduce the pollution. It can create very substantial income to the butchers and abattoir owners and may be helpful in upgradtion of economic status of meat industry. Blood if properly utilized may serve as the base for industries like leather, textile, plywood, feed, fertilizer, ceramics, cosmetics, pharmaceutical and Scientifics etc. It can also be used to process blood into different foods.

Collection of blood

The utilization of blood is mainly dependant on its mode of collection. So it should be collected according to its ultimate use as given below:

i. For edible purpose blood should be collected hygienically as fresh and sound from healthy and well inspected animals. Blood collection can be done in Trocar knife with hollow handle and canula for hygienic recovery. The collection and storage vessel should be preferably of stainless steel and standard size should be 45 cm in diameter and 15 cm deep. The container must be sterilized before collection of blood using steam or hypochlorite solution.

ii. To preserve the blood in original liquid state for food or industrial use particularly to obtain plasma, serum and blood albumin, it should be maintained in liquid state by using one of the method described below:

a. *Defibrination*: In defibrination process blood is stirred by wooden ladle or by whipping with a wire whip. In this process fibrin is gradually set on ladle or whip in form of dark red coloured different lengths of threads. The developed fibrin can be utilized as valuable food for man or poultry and can be utilized in manufacture of peptone or lecithin. Mechanical stirring produces dark-colored serum due to the destruction of red cells which can be washed several times to get light colour.

b. *Chemical method*: chemical method is basically includes the *calcium removal* which can be achieved by using oxalates and citrates. Blood can also be preserved using one part citric acid, sodium citrate, sodium or potassium oxalate in two parts water.

c. *Use of anticoagulants*: It should be collected with anticoagulant like trisodium citrate, oxalate, EDTA or heparin at the rate of maximum 0.2% to prevent clotting.

iii. Conservation of blood for industrial use can be preserved under cold storage or alternatively with 3% salt, 2% ammonia, 0.3-0.5% of 40% formalin or 2% Lysol. However, such blood cannot be used for edible purpose. Most preferably this form of blood is used in tanneries.

iv. For meal and feed purpose blood should be collected in undiluted form, as early as possible before decomposition because decomposed blood with evil smell cannot produce palatable meal and feed. For meal, blood must be free from floor washing, detergents, insecticides and extraneous matter.

v. Special care is required when an animal is killed with Mohammedan method and contamination of blood with undigested food from the stomach can be prevented by grasping the esophagus firmly in one hand at the moment of killing. Alternatively in higher slaughter rate abattoirs a light metal clamp may be used instead of the hand. The blood should be collected in blood pans preferably of galvanized containers measuring 20 inches in diameter, 6 inches in depth containing two handles. In modern abattoirs where hoists or bleeding rails system is adopted, a blood-collecting tank or with blood gutters of two outlets, one at blood tank and another to sewer. In most modern way blood from abattoir to blood processing unit can be blown through a pipeline operating with steam or air pressure and device is called blood-blow tank.

Categorization of blood based on utility

Utility category		Use
Human food	i.	Blood sausages.
	ii.	Blood puddings.
	iii.	Plasma as protein booster in food and binder or stabilizer in meat products.
	iv.	Blood albumin as a substitute of egg albumin in ice-cream and bakeries.
Animal feed	i.	Blood meal.
	ii.	Lysine supplement.
	iii.	Mixed blood meal.
	iv.	Stabilizer in feed mixture and pet food.
Blood based industries	i.	*Plywood industry*–plasma as a water proof adhesive.
	ii.	*Tanneries*–light coloured protein finisher and gloss enhancer.
	iii.	*Photography*-lithographic coating solution with albumin and ammonium dichromate.
	iv.	*Textile industry*-dyeing.
	v.	*Fire services*- blood protein foam compound as fire extinguishers.
	vi.	*Food industry*-blood albumin as substitute of egg albumin.
	vii.	*Cosmetic industry*-cosmetic base.
	viii.	*Ceramics for ceramic industry.*
	ix.	*Fertilizer industry*-source of nitrogen and super-phosphate, seed coating, soil pH stabilizer.
	x.	*Biochemical and pharmaceuticals industry*-it is a source of amino acids like lysine, leucine, histidine, phenylalanine etc, blood clotting agents like thrombin and prothrombin, immunoglobulins, serotonin, peptone, plasma extender etc.
	xi.	*Laboratory and bacteriological media*-blood agar, tissue culture media, albumin and globulin, sphingomyelin, catalase etc.
	xii.	*Medical Profession:* as fibrin foam in nerve and arterial surgery and prostate operations, fibrin powder to check the bleeding in skin injuries and fibrin bioplast in joints problems.

Blood processing

There are various procedures routinely adopted to utilize the blood of slaughter houses. These processes includes very basic to sophisticate based on the final utility of blood. Blood can be utilized alone or in combination of other by-products. Techniques and procedures generally adopted in blood processing may be discussed as under:

i. *Plasma:* Plasma is mainly consisting of cells like erythrocytes (red blood cells or RBC's), leucocytes (white blood cells or WBC's) and thrombocytes (platelets). Plasma is basically contains serum and fibrinogen. It is obtained by collecting the fresh blood in blood anticoagulants like 4 percent trisodium citrate (1 ml in each 10 ml blood) or EDTA or oxalates or heparin as soon as possible. Then unclotted blood is centrifuged which separates blood cells and plasma. The storage of plasma for further use requires packaging and freezing storage.

ii. *Serum:* Serum is a fibrinogen free fraction of blood and mainly contains albumen and globulin. To get serum blood is collected aseptically and allowed to clot under slanting position in cold condition. Blood clotting time in large animals is about 3-6 minutes but poultry blood is clotted quickly. Fresh serum up to 2-3 hrs is not generally accepted for serum isolation due to colour. Serum obtained after 12 hours is almost clear with the exception of some RBC's which can be separated by using bucket centrifuge at 1000 rpm for 30 minutes. The obtained serum is then deactivated by heating at 55^{0}C for 30 minutes followed by filtration through Seitz filter paper to make it clear. It can be stored under refrigeration for one month and under freeing (-20^{0}C) for six months.

iii. *Haemoglobin*: the separation of plasma from blood erythrocytes yields 60-70 percent protein fraction in haemoglobin. Its one percent addition in meat products gives dark coloure product and act as catalyst in oxidation of unsaturated fat. But when used in higher concentration has an inhibitory effect on fat oxidation in products like blood sausages, blood puddings, blood breads and blood cookies. The dark impression can be removed by bleaching with hydrogen peroxide (H_2O_2). In this reaction 3% H_2O_2 oxidizes the haemoglobin into colourless verdomethemoglobin. Alternatively, heme group of haemoglobin can be removed by adjusting pH 2.0 which opens the organic chain and heme group is released. However, heme removal greatly reduces stability of globins' protein molecule and denatured easily with heat and other agents.

iv. *Blood albumin*: dried blood serum is generally called blood albumin and is considered as cheapest substitute of dried egg albumin. Blood albumin can be obtained from clotted blood without lime after chilling and cutting to the size of 0.5-1 inch and draining of serum at 10^0C. Clear yellow serum is then added with 0.05 percent phenol on weight basis and subjected to spray or vacuum drying at < 60^0C to obtain soluble fine blood albumin without denaturation. Alternatively blood albumin can also be obtained from liquid blood containing anticoagulant after 10-12 hrs chilling, centrifugation at 250-300 rpm and addition of warm calcium chloride. Material is then added with phenol and drying is done in similar manner as mentioned earlier. Yield is about 20% of blood plasma weight and 1-2% on the basis of whole blood. Yield may be 4-5 % higher in later method. Straw coloured good quality blood albumin containing 80% protein can be stored in cool conditions for several months.

v. *Fibrinogen:* Blood plasma is usually contain fibrinogen. To get fibrinogen, blood plasma is treated with sodium citrate acetic acid buffer in presence of aqueous ethanol to pH 7.2 and 8 % ethanol concentration. Fibrinogen is now precipitated and centrifuged, filtered and freeze dried to get it purified.

vi. *Fibrin foam:* Fibrinogen is converted into fibrin with the action of thrombin. Fibrin foam is a white to cream coloured spongy material which can soak in liquid upto 30 times. It is very useful compound in nerve and arterial surgery and prostate operations. It is digested in body system and does not hamper the action of antibiotics. To get fibrin foam, plasma is treated with citrate buffer at pH 6.0 and purified by centrifugation. After that it is diluted to less than 2 percent fibrinogen level and adjusted pH 6.25. The material is then vigorously beaten to obtain fibrinogen foam which is treated with thrombin to get fibrin foam. Fibrin foam can be stored under freezing for further use.

vii. *Fibrin powder*: fibrin is a good compound for dressing and treatment of wounds like external injury, cut wounds, burn wounds and ulcers. Fibrin powder used in wound prevents infection and stop loss of electrolytes from wound by acting as a haemostatic agent. Fibrin automatically arrests the bleeding by natural process of blood clotting by conversion of fibrinogen into fibrous netlike fibrin in presence of thrombin, a proteolytic enzyme. Fibrin can be isolated from fibrinogen and be made in form of sponge, film or powder. Fibrinogen is basically obtained from blood by centrifigugation in combination with cryoprecipitation or by using precipitation agents like ethanol, ammonium sulfate or polyethylene glycol. It can be converted to fibrin suspension by using thrombin. The mixture is then dried and pulverized to produce natural fibrin powder. However, shelf life of this powder is low due to use of crude protein. It is also not capable to couple with the drugs for better functionality.

viii. *Fibrin bioplast*: fibrin bioplast is a modified form of fibrin powder resembling with plastic. Fibrin bioplast from animal blood fibrin can be produced by compression moulding of fibrin and glycerol. It adheres with the body lifelong and need not to remove fibrin bioplast from bone joints once moulded.

ix. *Blood foam compounds*: Protein foam of blood origin is considered as cheapest type of fire extinguishers. Particularly by reduction of vapour formation, cooling of foam forming water, and retardation of oxygen supply to fire. Blood foam compounds are very effective extinguishers against fire generated from petrol, paints, fat, naptha etc. However, it is not very effective in fire induced with spirit and alcohol. Blood foam compounds can be generated from coagulated blood stock by treating with 2 percent saturated sodium hydroxide followed by heating with constant stirring in steam jacketed vessels at 90-95^{0}C for 4-5 hrs. The pH of stock is then adjusted to 6.8 with hydrochloric acid. Further it is heated to 60 to 70^{0}C to get 1.2 specific gravity. It is then added with 2.5 percent (w/v) of ferrous sulphate as stabilizer and 0.2 to 0.5 percent (v/v) cresol as preservative. The foams are then generated by mixing water and air under pressure. Blood foam is then can be stored in container for use.

x. *Organic fertilizers*: Waste and improperly collected, soiled blood can be utilized as fertilizer by treating with 2 percent formalin or 2 percent Lysol followed by sun drying. It is good source of nitrogen, iron and copper but phosphorus can also be supplemented in traces. It can serve the purpose of compound fertilizer by addition of super phosphate.

xi. *Blood char:* blood char or blood charcoal is a source of carbon from blood and can be utilized in absorption of gases and as an industrial decolorant. It can also be utilized as an effective antidote for chemical poisonings. It can be obtained by addition of activating agents like zinc chloride, potassium sulphide, potassium thiocynate, phosphoric acid, sulphuric acid, hydroxide and carbonates of alkali metals etc. followed by kneading, extruding, heating in airtight oven at 650-750^{0}C for 6-8 hrs, wet grinding, centrifugation, steaming or Co_2 activation, drying and packaging.

xii. *Blood sausages or puddings*: hygienically collected and aesthetically maintained blood particularly red blood cells consisting of 34-38%

protein and 62% water can be utilized in formulations of black sausages and puddings.

xiii. *Blood and paunch meal*: blood and paunch meal may be a good source of feed for pigs and poultry because dried blood and paunch may supply 40% true protein. In mixed type meal, blood supply protein, amino acids particularly lysine while paunch manure is rich in vitamins, minerals and fibers. It can be utilized up to 10% level in poultry feed. It can be prepared by heat treatment at 100^{0}C for 30 minutes followed by pressing, cooling and fumigation. Storage can be done in suitable polyethylene bags or air tight containers.

xiv. *Blood meal*: blood meal is a dark brown coloured granular product rich in protein (80%) and amino acids particulary lysine (6-9%) and show characteristic iron smell. The yield of blood meal from raw whole blood is about 20%. It contains 5-10% moisture, 10-12% nitrogen and <5% ash. Blood meal can be utilized as pig and poultry feed and as a lysine supplement. It can also be used as a fertilizer due to presence of sufficient quantity of nitrogen.

Steps in blood meal preparations

Processing steps	Detailed procedure
Blood collection	Collection of blood should be in such as manner that it should be free from floor washing, insecticides, detergents and other extraneous matter.
Preservation	Blood can be preserved by adding equal quantity of absorbent like rice bran or cassava. It can also be preserved in 1% lime in form of rubbery consistency mass with calcium addition. Alternatively blood can be preserved by addition of 20% salt.
Heat treatment	In blood cookers on open fire till dry. It is not advisable now due to high fuel requirement, stickiness in vessel and lower food value. In double jacketed boiler at 100^{0}C for 30 minutes with continuous stirring. In can also be heated by passing direct steam injection into the blood mass to sterilize the material.
Pressing	Heat treated blood mass is stored in hessian bags or any other porous bag, hang in a stand and squeeze to reduce moisture up to 40-45% manually or mechanically. Pressing can also be done in screw press for better results.

Drying	*Sun drying*: on concrete platform or in a shallow tray to the moisture level of 10-12%. *Cabinet drawing*: at pilot level drying can done in cabinet dryer in which steam coils are fitted at bottom while exhaust fans at top. The chest of dryer may have six trays each of 2 feet wide, 3 feet long and 6 inches deep size. These trays remain stationary in position. The hot air generated from charcoal burner of 1400-1500 rpm is blown from bottom to the material. *Tunnel drier*: in tunnel drier, trays are moving from one end to another to make the operation continuous. Hot air blow is in counter direction to material or in parallel flow tunnel. *Rotary drier*: rotary driers are consisting of rotating drums of 2 feet 6 inches diameter and 6 feet long dimension fitted with two doors, one at top for feeding and another to discharge the material. The excess moisture in this drier is drawn by small fan and heat is generated through furnace to one side of the casing, using charcoal or wood as fuel.
Cooling	Dried material is cooled to ambient temperature.
Milling	Material is subjected to milling to get a fine powdered meal.
Fumigation	Fumigation of blood meal is commonly done with methyl bromide or ethylene oxide to disinfect the material.
Packaging	Packaging of blood meal can be done in polyethylene bags or air tight containers.

Blood management and utilization is an important aspect of by-product handling. It is utilized for gainful return and sustainability of meat and by-products industry. The prime need is to collect the blood in best manner. So that it can be utilized in edible as well as in industrial uses. However, all efforts should be made to collect and process even of single drop of blood comes from slaughterhouse.

References

1. Kondaiah, N., Anjaneyulu, A.S.R., Lakshmanan, V. (1993). Incorporation of chicken by-products in mutton nuggets. J Food Sci. Technol., 30(2):143–144.
2. Liu, D.C. (2002). Better utilization of by-products from the meat industry 2002-10-01. Extension Bulletins. Food and fertilizer Technology Center for the Asian and Pacific region (FFTC publication database)
3. Mann, I. (1978). Utilization of blood. *In:* Animal By-products: Processing and Utilization, 3rd edition, FAO, Italy. Pp 61-76.

4. Ockerman, H.W. and Hansen,C.L. (2000). Blood utilization. *In:* Animal By-products Processing and Utilization, by CRC Press. Pp 325-353.

5. Sharma, B.D. (2003). Utilization of blood. *In:* Modern Abattoir Practices and Animal By-products Technology, First Edition, Jaypee Brothers Medical Publishers, New Delhi. Pp 107-112.

Chapter **16**

Hides and Skins

Hides and skin are the important and widely used animal by-products of slaughter house industry. Human beings are utilizing animal skins since time immorial and nomadic people still depend upon them for shelter, clothing, weapons, food containers etc. In general on live weight basis yield of hide is 7 percent while skin is around 11 percent. Though it is also obtained from the fallen animals but the superior quality hide is always of slaughtered animals. Source wise slaughtered animals account 20-25 percent of hide and 80 percent of skin whereas fallen animals contributes around 75-80 percent of hide and 20 percent of skin. So the major sources for hide are fallen animals and skin is from slaughtered animals.

Hide	Skin
Skin of fully grown large animals such as cattle, buffalo is called hide	Integral body covering of small animals like sheep, goat, pig and very young calf is called skin
It is large, heavy and thick	It is small, thin and light in weight.
Generally it is of above 13.6 kg in weight.	It is generally lower than 13.6 kg in weight.
Major source is fallen animals.	Major source is slaughtered animals.

Classification and Nomenclature of Hides and skins

Nomenclature of hides and skin

- *Hide:* Skin from a fully grown large animal.
- *Skin:* Skin from small animals i.e. goat, sheep and pigs.
- *Slunk:* Skin from an unborn calf which is often used for prach ment, light suede or drum beats.
- *Kip:* Skin from an older calf which has still not reaches maturity.

- *Renderer/Murrain hide/Fallen hide:* Hide removed form an animal that died from some cause other than slaughter
- *Natives:* Hides which have not been branded.
- *Packers hide:* Hides originating in large meat-packing houses. These are usually of the finest quality because of excellent conditions under which they are flayed and preserved.
- *Frigorifico:* Hides originating in South-American meat-packing plants.
- *Green hide:* hide which has not been preserved but it is just as it comes from the animal.
- *Ordinaries:* Terminology denoted to hides in East-Pakistan which are baldy fleshed, improperly cured and heavily damaged.
- *Kurbanis:* Terminology denoted to hides of good quality in East-Pakistan

2. Classification of hides/skin

A. According to weight

Origin	Wt. of green hides		Designation	Uses
	lbs	kg		
Unborn calf	-	-	Slunk skin	Furniture, drums and gloves.
Immature calf	9-15	4.8-6.8	Calf skin	Book binding and shoe.
Calf	15-25	6.8-11.34	Kip skin	Gloves and apron.
Heifer	25-30	11.34-13.60	Heifer skin	Shoes, furniture and car seats.
Cow	> 30	> 13.60	Cow hide	Garments or upholstery.
	< 53	< 24.04	Light cow hide	Workboats and car seats.
	> 53	> 24.04	Heavy cow hide	Strong and durable leather products.
Steer	32-48	14.51-21.77	Extremely light hide	Clothing's.
	48-58	21.77-26.30	Light steer hide	Clothing's.
	> 58	> 26.30	Heavy steer hide	Jackets.
Bull	60-100	27.21-45.35	Bull hide	Country boots.

B. According to branding:

Texas or Colorado hides are hides branded on butt or side. However, native hides are unbranded hides.

C. According to time of flaying:

Flaying from slaughtered animals- Slaughtered hides

Flaying from fallen animals- Fallen hide or
Rendered hide or
Murrain hides

D. According to quality of flaying-

Flaying by highly skilled workers- Big packer hides

Flaying by less skilled workers- Small packer hides

Goat and sheep skin classification: Goat skins are more valuable than sheep skins. They are larger to produce better lasting leather. Sheep skins are mostly of medium size without much regional variation.

Class	Wt. (kg)	Length (cm)	Region	Uses
Big goat skin	1.3	96.5 (above)	Punjab, Kashmir, Punjab border, Orissa, U.P	Rugs and carpets bindings
Medium goat skin	0.91	96.4	Rajasthan, Maharashtra, A.P, Kerala, Karnatka	Parchment
Small goat skin	0.86	76.2	Eastern part of India	Gloves, shoes and accessories

In India: buffalo hides are generally classified as:

Buffalo (Buff) calf skin- used in back pack leather, vellium and parchment.

Buff heifer hide- utilized in form of clothes and moccasins.

Buff hide- used for beddings and parfleches.

Buff bull hide- utilized in making of saddle covers and water bags.

Grading of hide/skin: FAO expert, stew (1955) has suggested a useful system of grading hides on basis of faults-

1. First grade- A hide that is free from holes, cuts, deep scores or gouges, visible grain defects and broken grain (over 25mm or 1

inch long) and which has substantially correct pattern and is sufficiently cured. An exception is that the rear shanks may contain one hole below the hock which is less than 25mm or 1 inch long.

2. Second grade- A hide that is off pattern, or contains a hole, cut, deep score, or gouge less than 152 mm or 6 inch long, or visible grain defects or warts less than one square foot (located above the line through the break in the hair on the fore and hind flanks).
3. Third grade- A hide that contains hair slips, five or more holes, cuts, deep scores or gouges, any holes or cuts longer or equal to152mm or 6 inch, insufficient cure, a pepper box, warts or any defect covering 1ft^2 or more of the hide.
4. Reject grade- Irregular shape or pattern with extensive damage on back or butt.

Sheep pelt grades according to wool length:

Grade	Wool length (inches)
Number 4	Bare to 1/8
Number 3	1/8 to 1/4
Number 2	1/4 to 1/2
Number 1	1/2to 1
Fall clip	1-2
Wool pelts	1.5

Structure of hide

Hide is basically tri-layer structure in which epidermis, dermis or corium and subcutis are generally found.

1. *Epidermis*: it is an outer pigmented surface and tubular invaginations for hair follicles.
2. *Dermis or corium*: it is elastic, reticulum and collagenous fibres. The inner portion of corium is interwoven with bundles of collagen. It is a part which is used for preparation of leather.
3. *Subcutis*: it is a loose membrane network and contains fatty deposits.

Hide/skin operations during its processing

Flaying: refers to the skinning operation performed by skilled worker following a uniform pattern. In modern abattoirs skinning of buffalo and cattle is done on priteh plates. These are steel plates of 20 cm diameter having 120 cm length and 60 cm. width anchored to the floor with bolts. Wheras, flaying of fallen animals is carried out over wooden flaying cradle which can easily made by nailing two smooth wooden logs of 150 cm length and 15 cm diameter at a distance of 30 cm. Properly flayed hide has certain qualities i.e. rounded rumps, equal width from centre of the back to the belly edge on each side, medium length in the shanks, regular dewlap, square outline etc.

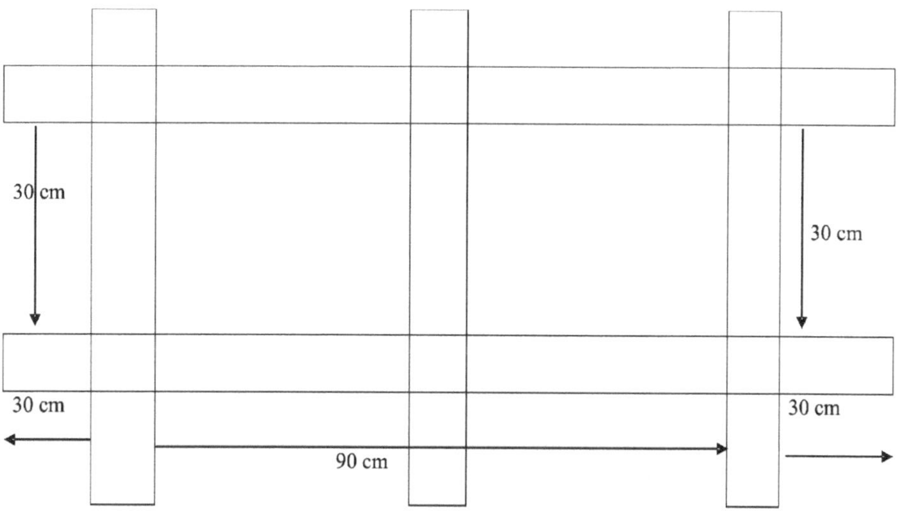

Wooden cradle for flaying fallen animals

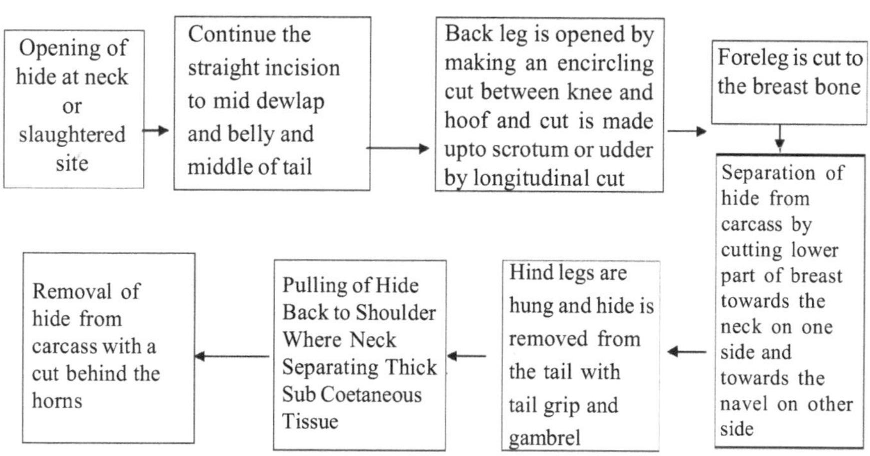

Flaying operations

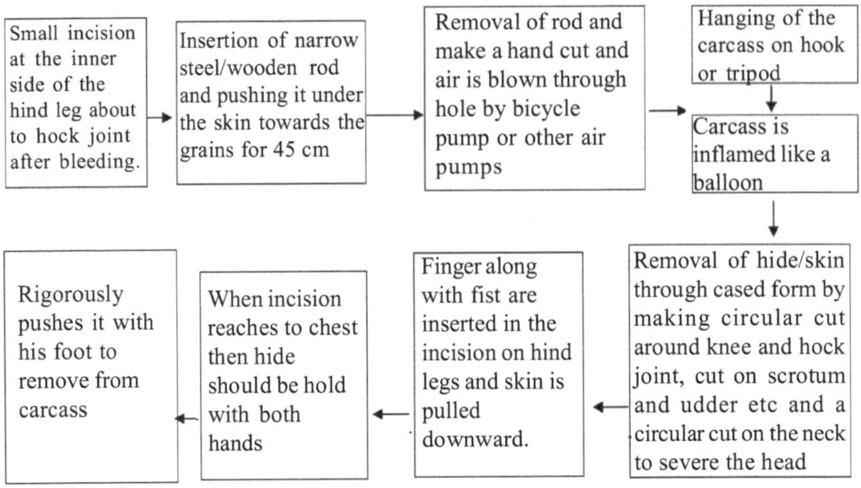

Case–on flaying technique for sheep and goat

1. **Preservation of hides and skins:** After flaying hides/skins should be cured quickly to arrest bacterial and enzymatic decomposition and spoilage. To achieve this goal hides/skins are washed just after flaying to remove blood, dirt etc. This is done with the half of scrubbing brushes under ramming cold water and putting them on draining racks. To get good quality hide/skin certain precautions are required:

   i. Provision of enough water and withdrawal of feed for at least 18 hrs facilitates flaying and avoids useless cuts on the skin.

   ii. Hoisting the animal improves bleeding and keeps the skin clean.

   iii. Skin of sheep and long haired goat are washed on the flesh side only.

Methods of preservation

Similar to other livestock products hide/skin is also very susceptible to the putrefaction due to certain micro-organisms or some other means. So the proper utilization of hide, its preservation is having paramount importance. Basically there are two major preservation techniques for hides/skin:

1. Air drying
2. Curing

1. *Air drying*: in air drying procedure water is removed from the hide

which is naturally present in it with the help of air. It is most suitable procedure for low relative humidity areas. It is time taking procedure and in any of the following cases minimum 7 days time is required to complete the drying operation. There are various air drying procedures in vogue to remove the water from hide/skin:

a. *Ground drying*- It is most popular technique of hide preservation since ancient time. In this procedure hide/skin is air dried by stretching out the hides with their flesh side up. In this technique hide is held on ground with the weight of stones or pegging the edges with sticks to the ground. It is cheapest and easily adoptable for rural people with talent hides. In this technique one side of hide remains in contact of ground without air circulation and putrefy easily leads to development of blemishes, hair slip and blisters. It produces uneven drying of hide because upper side gets over-dried and may have pocket of gelatinous material in the centre of corium invisible before tanning but resulting in holes afterwards. Greater exposure of heat on surface of hides leads to degradation of fat which penetrates deep in between fibres and greatly interferes in tanning. Over drying in this technique also produces denaturation of collagen and becomes hard and tend to crack on folding.

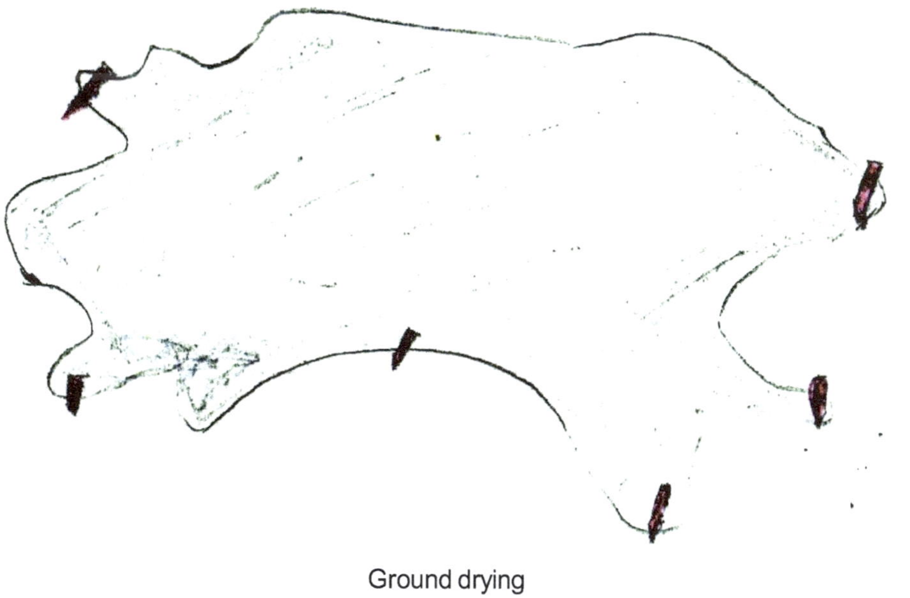

Ground drying

a. *Suspension drying*- in this procedure hides are suspended so the sun rays strikes obliquely and cooling of hides' takes place readily. Number of techniques is adopted for this purpose. Among all the most common techniques for this purpose is frame drying, line drying (drying on cords/wires/poles) and tent or parasol drying.

i. *Frame drying*- it is done on angled frame which is apron privately oriented to the sun. Frame drying facilitate free circulation of air on both sides of the hide or skin. It facilitates the draining of rain on surface away from the hide puddles. In this technique sun rays strikes obliquely instead of direct which prevents over-drying. Cooling is also rapid due to exposed surfaces from both sides.

Advantages: There are least chances of hair slip or putrefaction, less defects, longer keeping quality, easy transporation due to light weight of hides. The continuous pressure on hides/skin leads to constant equal tension thus hide remains completely flat and wrinkles free.

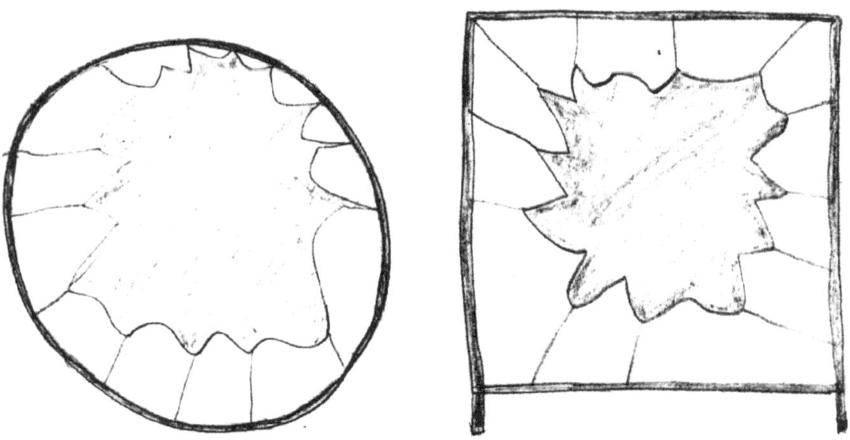

Frame Drying

ii. *Line drying (drying on cords/wires/poles)*: in this drying technique, hides are dried over thin cords or wires or poles etc with flesh side up. Though line drying leads to wrinkle formation and cracks on stretching such hide. Use of heavy poles, wires for drying damages skin along the line of contact due to impeded drying. So to avoid these conditions, the sides of the skins should be in sufficient distance and folds must be stretched on shanks with small sticks or straws.

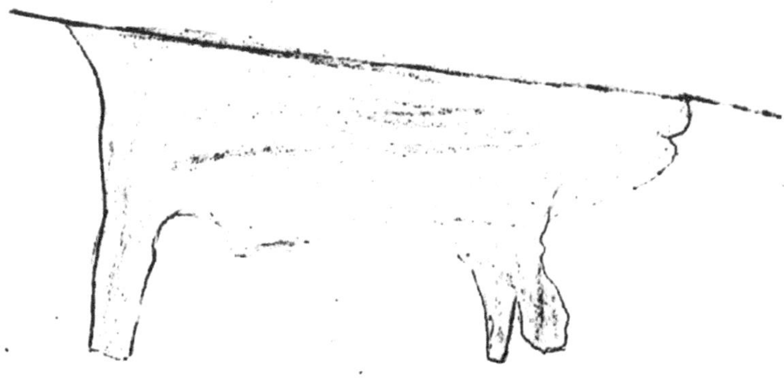

Line Drying

iii. *Tent or parasol drying*: in this technique hides are dried over the ground on tent or parasol wires, posts and cords. So the technique is also termed as umbrella drying.

2. *Hide curing*: in hide curing procedure drying of hide is performed with the help of uniform finally ground salt. The application of salt over hide is depends on moisture content and final use of the hide. However, some common salting procedures are as under:

   a. *Dry salting*: dry salting of hide or skin is generally adopted in tropical countries. It involves stacking the hides flesh side up and applying 2-3 mm fine salt evenly on that side. However, stacking should not be more than one meter in height because moisture drains onto the floor. Dry salting retains only 12% water in hide.

   b. *Salt pack system*: salt pack system helps in initial removal of moisture. Further water removal from hide is carried out by air exposure on hide. In Ideal condition for salt packing, it should be carried out at 15^0C with relative humidity of 85-90%. This procedure also requires good ventilation and salted plate form. It is not suitable for tropical countries because higher relative humidity and temperature leads to degradation of leather forming substance and the hides/skins tear and fall into pieces during tanning operation.

   c. *Wet salting*: it is done by preparing a curing solution consisting of 23 kg pure salt and 62 kg of water for 100 kg of hides. Hides are soaked in this solution in a pit of 1.25 meters for few days. Time involve in this procedure is 48 hrs for fleshed hides and 2 weeks for unfleshed hides. In wet salting of hides salted platform is required for draining the moisture upto 35% water of total retention in hide.

Defects that affect the quality of hides and skin

Ante-mortem defects

1. *Poor substance*: Poor substances are responsible for poor strength of hide/ skin which is due to genetic factors and species variation.
2. *Defects due to diseases*: Number of diseases is important for quality hide/skin production such as pox, mange, warble fly, dermatitis etc.
3. *Grain damage*: Good grain is a desirable characteristic for hide/skin but it can be adversely affect by thorn or wire fence scratches or branding, abscesses, abrasions, tick damage, bacterial action.

Post mortem defects

1. *Bad shape or pattern*: Bad shape or pattern is undesirable characteristic which are generally observed due to faulty ground drying, fallen hide etc.
2. *Bad flaying*: Flaying is a skilled operation and faulty flaying leads to bad quality hide/skin due to knife cut.
3. *Curing defects*: Curing is an important mean of hide preservation but faulty curing may lead to salt burn, improper application etc.
4. Smoke damage: Exposure of hide over smoke may give rise to colour and other defects in hides/skins.

Tannery

Tannery is an ultimate destination of hides and skin where hide or skin is converted into leather. Leather is a stable product of hide and can be utilized in making several goods and upholsteries. Some of the important quality characteristics of leather are:

1. Excellent flexibility due to high tensile strength over a wide range of temperature and moisture.
2. High tear and puncture resistance due to in-built fibrous network.
3. Ability to breathe which provides cooling in hot weather and insulation in cold weather.
4. It has excellent moulding ability.

Conditioning of hides and skin

The preserved hides and skins are first conditioned at tanneries before tanning under the following steps-

1. *Washing and soaking*: It is done for several hours in water containing zinc chloride and a mixture of soda ash and borex. During this process salt is removed alongwith proteins of blood and lymph. In the process hide absorbs water and restore their original shape and dimension.
2. *Fleshing*: It is done on a convex wooden beam by scrapping the flesh with serrated knife.
3. *Liming and dehairing*: The application of saturated solution of lime and 0.1% sodium sulfide removes and loosen hair and epidermal cells.
4. *Washing and dehairing*: The hides are now washed with weak acid to neutralize the lime. Mild heat can also be used if necessary.
5. *Bating*: Bating is a process of treating hides with proteolytic enzymes (pancreatic juice mixed saw dust) at pH 8.5. It results in soft and pliable pelt which can be tanned by vegetable tanning.
6. *Pickling*: It is done for chrome tanning wherein pelts are pickled in bath of 1% H_2SO_4 and 10% salt in water at pH 2 to 2.5 for 2-3 hrs.

Tanning

Conversion of hides and skins into insoluble and non putrescible leather without destruction of original structure is called tanning. There are two main methods most widely prevalent for tanning like vegetable tanning and chrome tanning.

1. *Vegetable tanning*: Vegetable tanning is a traditional tanning procedure practiced since time immoral. It's a time consuming process and involves immersion of hides and skins in infusion containing tannin bearing plants extract and barks. Some of the tannin bearing plants are avarum (*Casia auriculata*), babul (*Acacia arabia*), myrabalan (*Terminalia chebula*), konnan (*Cassia fistula*) etc. It is known that vegetable tanned leather is more suitable for sole, belts, harness, saddler and other heavy leathers. It is also the suitable leather for carving and stamping. Vegetable tanned leather is not stable in water and tend to discolour if left soaked and shrinks on drying and becomes supple and harder. In hot water it shrinks drastically and partly gelatinized and becomes rigid and eventually brittle. Boiled leather is a type of leather which hardened when

boiled in hot water or boiled wax or similar substances. It is generally used for book binding and occasionally as armor.

2. *Chrome tanning*: Chrome tanning technique was invented in year 1958. In this technique chromium sulfate and other salts of chromium are generally used. It is a modern technique for production of soft, supple and strong leather. It is less time consuming process and takes only 5 to 6 hours. It is more stable in water and do not discolour and misshapen on exposure to water. It is also termed as 'wet blue' and is more suitable for isoteric colors. There are two techniques in chrome tanning are most popular depending on bath processes adopted.

   a. *Single bath process*: In single bath process of chrome tanning chromium sulfate or chrome is directly applied in tanning solution which gradually enhances the strength of leather.

   b. *Double bath process*: In this process chromium salt is formed on the fibres by the interaction of chemicals. Sodium bichromate is reacted with a reducing sugar maltose and sulphuric acid to get chromic sulphate. It is applied in 1.5 to 3 percent range initially at pH 2.8 and later at 3.5 pH to enhance the affinity of collagen to chrome. Chrome tanning actually takes place due to formation of cross linkages between chrome ions and free carboxyl groups in the collagen side chains.

3. *Aldehyde tanned leather:* In this tanning procedure glutaraldehyde or oxazolidine compounds are used. The leather produced by this procedure is termed as wet white leather because it is pale cream or white in colour. It is the main group of chrome free leather and mainly utilized in automobiles and shoes for infants. Examples of aldehyde tanned leathers are formaldehyde tanned leather, brain tanned leather and chamois leather. *Formaldehyde leather* is now a day not practiced due to danger to the workers and sensitivity to the people. *Brain tanned leather* is produced by using emulsified oils, often those from animal brains. It is labour intensive process. The leather produced in this process is known for exceptional softness and ability to wash. Chamois leather is highly water absorbent leather alike to brain tanned leather. It is also produced by using oils traditionally with cod oil which is oxidized easily to produce aldehyde and can be used for tanning and in production of different colours.

4. *Synthetic tanned leather:* Synthetic tanned leather is produced using aromatic polymers like novolac or nerodols or syntons. Synthetic

leather was invented during Second World War when vegetable tannin was short. This type of leather is usually white in colour. Generally melamine, amino functional resins and urea formaldehyde resins are used for this purpose.

5. *Alum tanned leather:* Alum tanned leather is generally obtained using aluminium salt mixed with variety of binders and proteins such as flour, egg yolk. Purists argon that is not technically suitable for alum tanned leather and that material rot in water and produces very light shades leather.

Post tanning operation

To attain good quality finished leather there are certain post tanning operations are essential. Some of them may be listed as:

i. *Setting out or wringing*: Setting out or wringing are the processes generally applied to remove excess tan or moisture from the leather. To achieve this aim tanned hide is passed between two large rollers.

ii. *Splitting or shaving*: Splitting or shaving is a process of adjusting the desired thickness of leather for a particular use.

iii. *Dyeing*: To obtain a particular colour in leather dyeing process is generally adopted.

iv. *Fat liquoring*: It is a process of adjustment of softness and firmness of leather by lubricating the fibres with oil. Fat liquoring is also useful in enhancement of tensile strength of the fibre.

v. *Staking*: Staking is a process of softening the leather to make it more pliable.

vi. *Buffing*: Buffing is a process of leather production in which grain surfaces of leather are makes smooth. It also helps in diminishment of blemishes. Buffed leather is called corrected grain leather and leather without buffing is termed as full grain leather.

vii. *Glazing*: Glazing is generally applied in chromic leather after seasoning and drying. A glass cylinder clamped to the end of moving arm made to roll on the leather. Heat generated by frictions softens the wax in the finish and produces a continuous plastic coat of high lusture on the grain surface.

As the leather gets ready it is graded for temper, uniformity of thickness, colour etc. The graded leather is properly packed for convenience and to fetch a better price for this viable product.

References

1. Liu, D.C. (2002). Better utilization of by-products from the meat industry 2002-10-01. Extension Bulletins. Food and fertilizer Technology Center for the Asian and Pacific region (FFTC publication database)

2. Mann, I. (1978). Hides, skins and glue stock. In: Animal By-products: Processing and Utilization, 3rd edition, FAO, Italy. Pp 80-138.

3. Ockerman, H.W. and Hansen,C.L. (2000). Hide, skin by-products, glue and gelatine. In: Animal By-products Processing and Utilization, by CRC Press. Pp 127—216.

4. Ranganayaki, M.D. and Srinivasan, T.S. (1999). Hygienic processing and utilization of animal by-products. In: Souvenir cum Proceedings of National Seminar on Processing of Meat, Poultry and By-products for Value Addition at CFTRI, Mysore from 24-26 Feb. Pp 187-196.

5. Sharma, B.D. (2003). Plan and layout of by-products utilization plant. In: Modern Abattoir Practices and Animal By-products Technology, First Edition, Jaypee Brothers Medical Publishers,New Delhi. Pp 97-106.

Chapter **17**

Bones, Hoofs and Horns

Bones of the animal body makes a skeleton system and helps in locomotion and support soft tissues. The proportion of bones in animal body varies with the animal species as they contribute 12-28 percent in cattle and buffalo, 17-35 percent in sheep and lambs, 50percent in bobby calves, 25 percent in veal calves, 12-20 percent in pigs and 8-17 percent in poultry. As the age advances bones becomes rigid due to ossification of cartilages but in older age bones becomes brittle and fragile due to reduction in bone organic matter. Compositionally fresh bones contain 50 percent moisture, 15 percent red or yellow marrow, 12 percent organic matter and 23 percent inorganic matter while dried and defatted bones contains organic or inorganic matter in a ratio of 1:2. These bones contain 33.3 percent organic matter (ossein or bone collagen) and 66.7 percent inorganic matter (57.7% calcium phosphate, 3.5% calcium carbonate, 3.5% sodium carbonate and chloride, 2.0 % magnesium phosphate). Structure wise bones are composed of blood vessels, lymphatics and nerves and long bones also contain medullary cavity or marrow. Bone marrows are basically of two types red and white. In fetal stage or even in newborns marrow is red in colour due to blood farming activity while in adults marrow becomes white which is rich in fat (96%) and yellow in colour. In poultry bones are light in weight and contain air sacs.

Classification of bones

Type of bones	Description	Utility
According to overall function and shape		
i. Long bones	Femur, tibia-fibula, humorous, radius and ulna manufacturing.	In live animals they enlarged to extremities and act as lever and support the soft tissues. Preferred for glue and gelatin
ii. Flat bones	Scapula or shoulder blade	In live animals these bones provides large area for muscle attac-

		hment. Mostly used as source of calcium and phosphorus.
iii. Short bones	Tarsal and metatarsal, carpal and metacarpal	Helps in movement of fore limb and hind limbs. Can be used as glue stock, bone meal and fertilizer.
iv. Irregular bones	Vertebrae and axial skeleton	Helps in body movement and balance. Can be used in bone meal and fertilizers.
According to source		
i. Green bones	Bones obtained from freshly killed animals.	Contains high percentage of moisture, protein and fat and serves as a stock for feed and other commercial uses. Can be processed to glue and gelatin.
ii. Desert bones	Bones of fallen/dead animals which are exposed to bacterial, atmospheric and insect action for long time.	Bones are light in weight and contain only calcium, phosphorus and other minerals with dried ossein. Bone meal and fertilizers can be prepared.
According to commercial utility		
i. Bones as a source of glue and gelatin	Bones with intact collagen and ossein	Glue and gelatin
ii. Bones as a source of calcium and phosphorus	Decomposed bones	Bone meal and fertilizer

Nutritional value of bones obtained from different animals

Bones	**Nutritional components in percent**				
	Water	**Protein**	**Fat**	**Calcium**	**Ash**
Cattle bones	62.8	11.3	6.9	4.6	14.4
Pig bones	62.7	12.3	9.6	3.6	11.8
Sheep bones	65.1	11.7	8.8	3.2	11.2
Chicken bones	65.6	16.3	14	1	3.1

Major uses of bones

Bone product	Processing technique	Utilization
Edible uses		
Mechanically deboned meat	Mechanical deboning	Used in ground and comminuted meat products.
Technical grade fat	Rendering	In margarine, shortenings, cooking fat etc.
Glue	Controlled hydrolysis	As adhesive in plywood industry, gummed tape, sizing agents, manufacturing of wool, silk and other fabrics etc.
Gelatin	Controlled hydrolysis	In foods industry- ice-cream, mayonnaise dressing, emulsion flavours. In wine, beer and vinegar industry- clarifier. In pharmaceutical industry- capsules and pills coatings. In Scientifics- as bacterial culture medium. Others- in photography, adhesives, electroplating etc.
Ossein	Demineralization	As raw material for gelatin extraction.
Isinglass	Controlled hydrolysis	As source of gelatin.
Bone paste	Bone grinding and digesting	As raw material to make bone paste cookies, high-calcium rice noodles, meatballs, meat stuffing, sausage, rice dumplings and bone paste floss.
Bone powder	Bone grinding and digesting	The superfine bone powder is used for fast food, snack food, puffed food, catering food, health food and seasoning, etc.
Bone soup	Controlled heating	As a delicious food and drink.
Inedible uses		
Bone and meat meal	Rendering	Bones, adhering meat, tendons and other offals are processed under pressure to obtained meal. It can be utilized in livestock, poultry feed and pet food.
Bone meal	Rendering and bone digestion	Raw or steamed bones are milled after removal of adhering material and ossein

		to obtain meal as source of calcium and phosphorus.
Meat meal	Rendering	Adhering meat, tendons and other offals are processed under pressure to obtained meal and to free ossein. Meal can be utilized as livestock, poultry feed and pet food.
Calcified bone or bone ash	Bones are burned for 30 minutes to 1 hour and then powdered.	In fertilizers as source of calcium, phosphorus and other minerals.
Bone char	Controlled heating (500-700° C for 46 hours) and grinding of bones to 25 mm.	As energy source and bone oil is a byproduct of bone char.
Bone china	Controlled heating and burning but Pig bones are unsuitable.	In development of potteries and crockery's.

Mechanically deboned meat (MDM)

Mechanically deboned meat is termed as separated meat. It is generally recommended for use in ground or comminuted meat products. It is usually recovered by mechanical separation or mechanical deboning or bone pressing or extraction by water jets/ice wiping/ acid or alkali or proteolytic enzyme treatment. Mechanical deboning machine was initially invented in Japan for fishery industry in 1940s. Later it was adopted in poultry industry in 1950s followed by red meat industry in 1978. Mechanically deboned meat usually contains adhering meat, part of bone marrow, powdered bone and connective tissues.

Important facts on MDM

i. For better quality and safety bones should be processed within one hour for recovery of MDM. If not possible they should be stored at 4^0C and processed within four hours or frozen at -18^0C and processed within 72 hours.

ii. It is 25-35 percent of the total bone weight if recovered properly. Recovery is better in machine extraction than hand deboning.

iii. Composition varies with the age of animals, meat-bone ratio, cutting and separation methods etc.

iv. It normally contains sarcoplasmic and myofibrillar proteins, non protein nitrogen and stromal proteins.

v. Younger animal's bones provide higher hemoglobin than aged animals which enhances iron absorption in diet of human beings.

vi. Cold-boned meat provides higher minerals than hot or pre-rigor boned meat.

vii. The ash in mechanically separated tissue is primarily calcium which helps in people having lactase deficiency and cannot tolerate milk as calcium source.

viii. In deboning of poultry bones, kidneys should always be removed before deboning otherwise they may contribute unwanted cadmium to the product.

ix. It is rich in essential amino acids like lysine, leucine and histidine which are often limiting amino acid in many diets.

x. It is good in water binding capacity, emulsifying capability, cooking stability as well as in cooking yield when used in emulsion type products.

xi. In fish mechanical deboning, cellular disruption leads to breakdown of trimethylamine oxide (TMAO) which is responsible for typical fish flavour into trimethylamine (TMA) or dimethylamine (DMA).

xii. The increase in pH in MDM is mainly due to addition of red bone marrow. Increased pH improves water holding capacity, emulsification, meat processing, cooking and freezing properties.

Nutritional value of MDM (Ockerman, 1988)

Nutritional component	Percent of bones
Moisture	55-58
Protein	13-15
Fat	25-28
Ash	1-3
Calcium	0.029-1.39
Protein Efficiency Ratio (PER) (g gained/g protein eaten)	2.5

Uses of mechanically deboned meat

i. It can be utilized in least cost formulated products.

ii. Admixture of bone marrow and MDM improves palatability, texture, juiciness of meat products.

iii. The permitted level of MDM in comminuted meat products like meat patties, sausages, hamburger, ground meat products and fabricated steaks is 5-20 percent.

iv. For better products MDM is used along with soy proteins in meat products because mushy texture of MDM can be compensated with lighter colour, course and rubbery texture of soy.

Recovery of fat

Fresh and green bones are generally used to extract good quality fat by solvent or steam extraction methods. Dry bones can also be utilized for fat extraction but they give poor quality fat. Bone marrow fat is more unsaturated than subcutaneous or intramuscular fat and requires higher processing temperature. Usually the fat extracted from bones contains various impurities which can be clarified by heating at 85-90^{0}C followed by settling. For further purification recovered fat is washed with 70^{0}C hot water or 3.0 percent salt water heated at 100^{0}C followed by rewashing with water or 0.03-0.1 percent citric acid or with 10 percent tri-sodium phosphate. Finally purified fat is allowed to settle before use. There are various techniques for fat extraction from bones is in practice:

i. Rendering of bones with adhering material produces either cracklings (dry rendering) or tankage (wet rendering). Fat from cracklings can be separated by centrifugal expeller while in tankage fat floats on top and can be removed easily. Recovery in wet rendering is better than dry rendering. Further rendered long bones from cracklings and tankage are subjected to bone digester at a steam pressure of 60 psi for 2 hrs. Steam in bone digester separates fat and proteins.

ii. Boiling of bones in open kettle freeing the adhering materials and dissolve some portion of ossein and cooked bones are drained dried and pulverized to obtain bone meal. During the process, fat of either edible quality or technical grade is recovered depending on quality of raw material used.

iii. Boiling of bones under pressure can also be utilized to recover the bone meal and fat. Ossein recovered in process can be preserved for gelatin production but cooking should not be beyond 70^{0}C to obtain superior quality gelatin.

iv. The exposure of sun and weather to bones for longer time loose fat and such bones are termed as weathered bones. These bones can be used for recovery of little quantity of poor quality fat but ossein for gelatin or other material for raw bone meal can be utilized.

Utilization of fats

i. Inedible fat recovered during bones can be utilized in livestock and poultry feed as high energy additives. Fatty acids purified from animal fat can be utilized in preparations of soaps, detergents, candles, deodorants, synthetic rubbers, polishes, paints etc.

ii. Edible fat can be utilized as margarine, shortenings, cooking fats etc.

Gelatin and glue

Commercially glue and gelatin is most valuable uses of bones. Both are physically as well as chemically similar products but glue is considered as low grade gelatin with comparatively dark colour and has only inedible uses. Gelatin is a derived protein of albuminoid class and has both edible and inedible uses based on raw material origin and hygiene maintenance. Pure gelatin can be identified on the basis of its amorphous nature, transparency, colour, taste and smell. Gelatin becomes brittle on drying, soft on heating and decomposes on burning with hair like smell. Gelatin is hydrophilic and water soluble which absorbs 5-10 times cold water than their original weight and dissolves on warming at 30^{0}C.

Glue and gelatin is mainly produced by the controlled hydrolysis of water insoluble collagen. Collagen is actually composed of tropocollagen monomers arranged in overlapping fibrils made up of three non identical coils of peptide chains. In production of glue and gelatin from tropocollagen, hydrogen bonds are breaks and stabilize triple helix and transformed into random coil configuration of glue and gelatin. The quality characteristics of gelatin such as water solubility, viscosity, adhesiveness and gel strength are basically based on their molecular weight. Generally low molecular weight gelatin has lower viscosity and gel strength and vice versa. In general, molecular weight of collagen ranges from 3,45,000 to 3,60,000 while of gelatin is in the range of 10,000 to 65,000.

Raw materials for glue and gelatin

Collagen is basically a raw material for production of glue and gelatin. So the parts of animal body contains collagen can be utilized for the purpose. Collagen contributes about 30 percent of the animal body's total organic matter and 60 percent of the total animal body's protein. It means large parts of the animal body can be utilized as base for glue and gelatin production.

Raw materials for glue	Raw materials for gelatin
The parts of animal body used for glue production are generally termed as *glue stock*. They are mainly hide and skin trimmings, ear pieces, poultry skin, sinews, tendon, horn pith, coney (dry rabbit skin), tail, puzzles, casings etc.	The major source for gelatin production is long bones like femur, tibia, metatarsus, humorous, radius and ulna, metacarpus. However, pigskins, ossein (bone protein), sinews can also be used for gelatin production.

Production techniques

All the techniques adopted for glue and gelatin production are based on three basic principles. They are extracted from collagen by digestion and removal of other adherent material to bones, controlled hydrolysis for conversion of collagen into gelatin and drying of final gelatin.

Alkaline extraction technique

It is most common method of glue and gelatin extraction from collagen materials. Alkaline extraction method is generally adopted for production of type-B gelatin from collagen materials like hides, skins, ossein from bones, sinews etc.

Processing step	Material used	Reaction observed
Washing	Cold water using cone mill or tumbler of barrel mill.	Stock hydration and removal of extraneous materials.
Liming	Saturated solution of calcium hydroxide with lime in water. The quantity of lime should be @10 percent of the stock. Exposure time should be one week to 3 months	Dissolution of non-collagen materials such as keratin, globulins, mucopolysaccharides, elastin, mucins, albumins etc. Conversion of fat into polar products. Hydrolytic reaction in collagen to enhance solubility by cleavage of intermolecular cross link units.
Washing	Cold running water for 1-2 days.	To remove the lime.
Neutralization	Dilute Hydrochloric acid or Sulphuric acid @4-10%	To make the collagen deplumped or limp or flaccid.
Washing	Dilute Aluminium Sulphate or Zinc Sulphate	To harden the collagen and improvement in colour. Now

		collagen stock is ready for extraction.
Extraction or cooking	Controlled hydrolysis at 54-60^{0}C for 3-5 hrs and continue upto boiling	Super quality gelatin at 60^{0}C. Medium quality gelatin at 65-70^{0}C. Low quality gelatin at 80^{0}C. Glue at 100^{0}C.
Filtration	Pressure filtration through steam sterilized cellulose paper	To enhance clarity and remove small particles.
Deionization	Through cation exchange resin of 20-50 mesh or ultrafiltration with a membrane of 25000 molecular weight size.	For demineralization and necessary if ash content is <0.5%.
Evaporation	Vacuum evaporation in pan	For concentration of gelatin by 20-25%, hide glue liquor 11-17%, bone glue liquor 33-42% and low quality glue by 50%.
Drying	Steam heated drums are used for drying for less than 1 minute or spray drying.	Dried glue or gelatin is removed by knife but in spray drying vacuum suction can be used to collect the glue and gelatin.

Acid extraction technique

Acid extraction technique is suitable for the production of type-A gelatin from collagen stock material contains cartilage or bones but it is a best suited method for extraction of edible geletin from frozen pig skins.

Processing step	Material used	Reaction observed
Washing	Cold water	Removal of salt, extraneous material, blood etc.
Fat extraction	Heating the skin with 55-60^{0}C hot water twice or thrice	After stirring for 4-6 hrs fat skimmed from the top of the material.
Washing	Hot water maintained at 40-55^{0}C	Washing of material to remove residues.
Acid treatment	Hydrochloric acid or Sulphuric acid or Sulphurous or Phosphoric acid for 10-72 hrs	The pH reaches to 4.0 which cause the swelling of collagen and coagulation of non-collagen material.

Washing	Water or sometimes with 5-8% sodium hydroxide to raise the pH 6-6.5	To remove the acid residues, coagulated non-collagen material and to raise the pH.
Extraction or cooking	Controlled hydrolysis at 54-60^{0}C for 3-5 hrs and continue upto boiling	Super quality gelatin at 60^{0}C. Medium quality gelatin at 65-70^{0}C. Low quality gelatin at 80^{0}C. Glue at 100^{0}C.
Filtration	Pressure filtration through steam sterilized cellulose paper	To enhance clarity and remove small particles.
Evaporation	Vacuum evaporation in pan	For concentration of gelatin by 20-25%
Drying	Steam heated drums are used for drying upto less than 1 minute or spray drying.	Dried gelatin is removed by knife but in spray drying vacuum suction can be used to collect the glue and gelatin.

Glue and gelatin extraction from bones using ossein as raw material

Processing step	Material used	Reaction observed
Primary steps		
Selection of bones	Long bones of animal body	Long bones like femur, tibia, metatarsus, humorous, radius and ulna, metacarpus are selected as stock material.
Washing and degreasing	Washing with water and dilute Sulphuric acid and degreasing using benzene	To remove residues and fat adhered with bones.
Cutting	Cutting to remove knee cap and knuckles	To facilitate action of hot water by exposing marrow.
Cooking	Cooking in water at 80-95^{0}C for at least 6 hrs	To remove adhered meat, gristle and fat. Fat is skimmed off as it settled on top.
Washing	Using warm water in rotary washer or high pressure spray	To remove adhering material after fat extraction.
Drying	Sun drying in net wiring or slow drying on steam coil heated air	To make the material stable and bones are now called *packer bones*.

Processing steps

Milling	In stone crusher	Screening to a size ranging from 1-2 cm cubes used as stock while small pieces are converted to bone chip, grist or bone meal and sinews can separated and subjected to alkaline gelatin extraction.
Washing	Ethylene chloride for glue and food grade hexane for gelatin	To extract out the fat.
Drying	In hot air oven at 50-60^{0}C	To remove the solvent.
Deminera-lization	Counter-current demineralization with hydrochloric acid using six to eight cycles at 25^{0}C until waste water pH become 6-6.5 or exposure of acid from 1-6 days in continuous way.	Ossein production after removal of minerals. Ossein can be used fresh for extraction or can be stored after hot convection air drying oven to the moisture of 8-10%. Stored ossein can be utilized within 6 months and it is soaked for 12-14 hrs before liming or acid treatment.
Extraction or cooking	Controlled hydrolysis at 54-60^{0}C for 3-5 hrs and continue upto boiling	Super quality gelatin at 60^{0}C. Medium quality gelatin at 65-70^{0}C. Low quality gelatin at 80^{0}C. Glue at 100^{0}C.
Filtration	Pressure filtration through steam sterilized cellulose paper	To enhance clarity and remove small particles.
Evaporation	Vacuum evaporation in pan	For concentration of gelatin by 20-25%
Drying	Steam heated drums are used for drying upto less than 1 minute or spray drying.	Dried gelatin is removed by knife but in spray drying vacuum suction can be used to collect the glue and gelatin.

Facts in production of glue and gelatin

i. Liming time in alkaline extraction for ossein is 3 months, sinews >1 month, pig skin -half month.

ii. Tanned leather is first soaked in mild alkali like sodium carbonate and then extracted by alkaline procedure.

iii. During filtration glue and gelatin usually clogg the filter. So to avoid clogging during filtration diatomaceous earth or activated carbon is added at 55-60^{0}C. Alternatively clarification can also be achieved using aluminium sulphate or heat coagulable egg albumin followed by heating to dissolve protein.

iv. Zinc sulphate or sulphur dioxide is used in glue as preservative to enhance the shelf life.

v. Glue is available in form of sheets or coarse broken but gelatin is usually sold as flakes, pulverized powder or granulated gelatin.

vi. In gelatin production from pigskin fat can also extracted by the solvent extraction procedure using food grade hexane or ethylene dichloride. However, it is not a method of choice for commercial purpose because material becomes hard.

vii. Gelatin obtained after acid extraction has pH in the range of 8.5-9.4 and molecular weight in between 70,000 to 90,000. In collagen structure only physical rearrangement takes place without much alteration in hydrolytic changes.

viii. Geltain produced from pigskin using acid extraction technology has better gel strength, clarity and colour.

ix. Isinglass can be extracted from fish bladder with water at 55-60^{0}C for 4-6 hours.

x. Bone crushing on stone crusher yield fragments of bones of size 1-2 cm cubes is used for gelatin production while small pieces who passes through 0.2 cm mesh are used as bone meal.

xi. In demineralization of bones for ossein production requires equal amount of acid to that of bone weight.

Uses of glue and gelatin

Edible uses of gelatin

i. Gelatin can be added in ice cream and soft chocolates @ 0.3-0.5 percent and act as foaming or whipping agent and as modifying agent for body, texture, shelf life and retardation of ice or sugar crystal formation.

ii. In milk gelatin is used to lower the curd tension and to enhance digestibility.

iii. In cottage cheese and sour cream gelatin prevents watering and provides smooth texture.

iv. In frozen products like cream pies, gravies and sauces gelatin prevents crystal formation and curdling.

v. Gelatin can also be added in meat products like jellied meat products, meat loaves, scrapple, brown sauces, meat pies etc @ 1-5 percent. However, its permitted limit is 0.4-1.5 percent in canned meat, turkey, chicken rolls and sprinkled in bone cavities of ham. It is added to enhance water retention and binding thus provides more stable juicy product.

vi. In alcohol industry (beer, wine, and vinegar) as well as in fruit juices, gelatin is used as thickening and emulsifying agent while isinglass can be used as clarifying agent.

vii. In pharmaceutical industry gelatin is used in making of capsules, as binder in tablets and as plasma extender in blood transfusion.

viii. Gelatin can be used as therapeutic agent for infant feeding, patients having digestive problems, peptic ulcers, muscular disorders and encouragement of nails growth.

Inedible uses of gelatin

i. Gelatin type-A can be used in delay absorption of heparin, ACTH and epinephrine. Absorbable gelatin foam powder and sponges can be used in absorption of blood during surgery and dusting of gloves.

ii. Gelatin can be used as sizing agent in textile and leather industry, as foam in fire extinguishers, photography, micro-encapsulation of minerals and in manufacturing of smokeless gunpowder etc.

iii. In cosmetic industry as adhesive and emulsifying agent.

iv. Gelatin can also be utilized in scientific field as culture media and enzyme strengthening.

Uses of glue

i. Glue is an important adhesive in plywood, furniture, sand paper, gummed tape etc.

ii. It can also be used as sizing agent, printability enhancer, in creation of permanent waves in papers and fabrics etc.

Bone meal

Bones particularly green bones are normally utilized in form of glue or gelatin or some other way into valuable products. But desert bones are mostly stored and lost their adhered meat, connective tissue and bone marrow which cannot be utilized in production of other valuable products is usually converted into bone meal. These bones are generally poor in sanitary condition and contain only calcium, phosphorus and lesser minerals with dried ossein. During rendering process bones are usually subjected to bone digesters and during glue and gelatin production they are crushed by can crusher into small pieces. The bones below the size of 2 mm are generally not utilized for glue and gelatin production so they can be converted into valuable bone meal. These bones are sterilized either under bone digester under steam at 60 psi for 2 hrs and fat as well as protein is separated. The materials like extracted fat and gelatin is usually removed by petrol, ether, heptanes or perchlor ethylene etc. and remaining bony material becomes soft and chalky. This material is further utilized for the conversion of bone meal after grinding. Bone meal may be a good source of phosphate in live-stock and poultry feed. Bone meal is actually gives one third yield to the actual weight of raw bones used for its preparation. So the yield ratio is 3:1.

Nutritive value and composition of bone meal

i. Bone meal generally contains 30.5% calcium, 15.5% phosphorus, 15-27% protein, 1.0% fat and other minerals.

ii. Bone meal is usually added in livestock and poultry feed as a source of calcium and phosphorus. The ratio of calcium and phosphorus which is required for ideally in ration to absorb and utilization is 2:1 is exactly in bone meal.

iii. Bone meal can also be utilized in cattle licks. In cattle licks generally 66 parts of bone meal is added with 33 parts of red oxide salt contains iron and 1 part each of copper sulphate, potassium or sodium iodide, cobalt nitrite, sulphate or chloride or other trace elements.

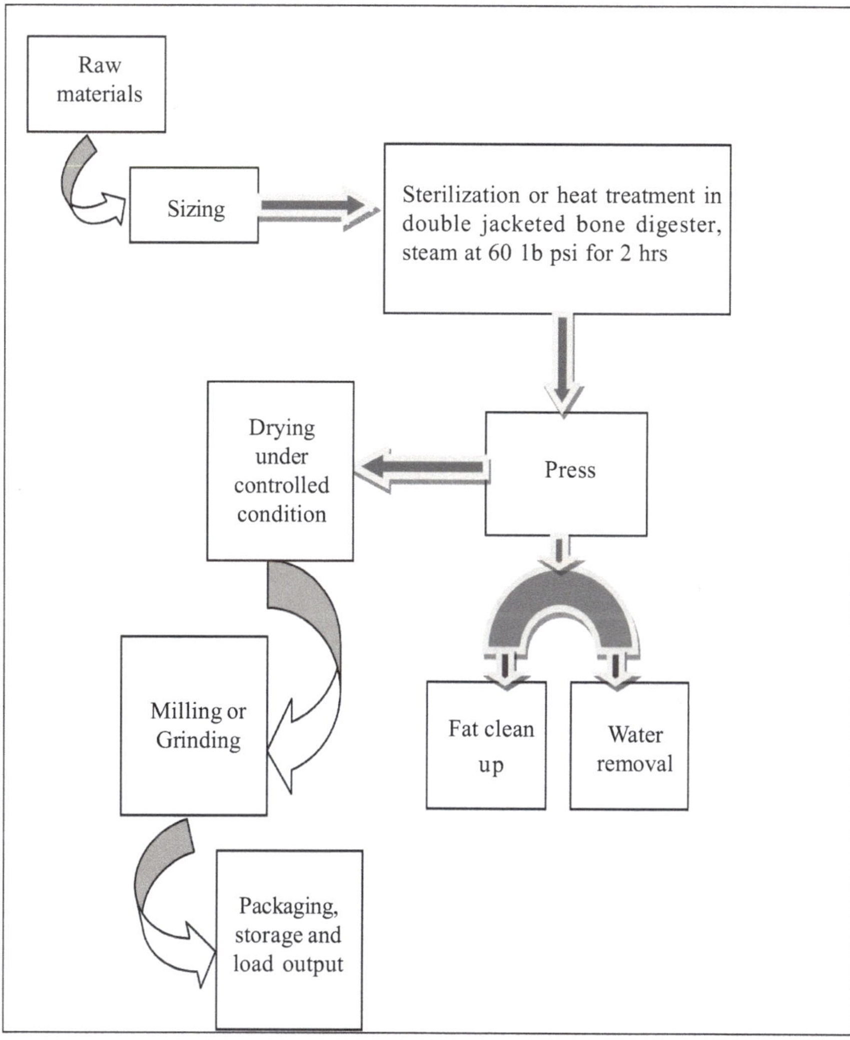
Raw materials
Sizing
Sterilization or heat treatment in double jacketed bone digester, steam at 60 1b psi for 2 hrs
Press
Drying under controlled condition
Fat clean up
Water removal
Milling or Grinding
Packaging, storage and load output

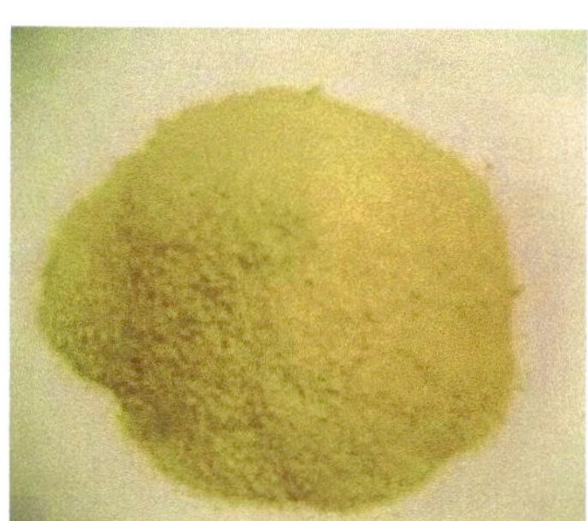

Bone meal

Bone ash or calcined bones $\{Ca_5(OH)(PO_4)_3\}$

The utilization of bones in form of bone ash is a good option. Actually bone ash is a white material produced by the calcination of bones because calcination retains their cellular structure. Bone ash can also be obtained by burning on grilling or by trench firing to yield spongy and brittle bones and pieces are then ground to ash. Typical bone ash consists of about 55.82% calcium oxide, 42.39% phosphorus pentoxide, and 1.79% water but its exact composition varies upon the type of bones being used. Physically bone ash has density around 3.10 g/ml and melting point of 1670 °C.

Utilization of bone ash

i. Bone ash can be utilized as fertilizer because of good source of phosphorus and it can enrich the soil with phosphorus for better crop production. It can be used alone as organic fertilizer and after treatment with sulphuric acid it is converted into single superphosphate which is good fertilizer and more water soluble. Bone ash when treated with phosphoric acid produces triple superphosphate which is more concentrated phosphorus fertilizer.

ii. Bone ash can be used as a baseline for development of bone china and may contribute upto 50% of raw material for bone china. Bone ash is good material for bone china because phosphate of bone ash generates beta tricalcium phosphate and creates a calcium crystal called anorthite. However, it is a fact that most of the bone china is produced with synthetic alternatives like dicalcium phosphate and tricalcium phosphate.

iii. Bone ash powder has good thermal stability as well as adhered well on metal, easy in cleaning. So it can be utilized in machines as polishing agent, protective coating, sealant etc.

Bone paste

Processing of bones into bone paste is a good alternative to utilize the bones. However, hygienic recovery of bones is an essential step in bone paste development. Bone paste development was initially started in Denmark in the year 1970s but now it is a common practice in Sweden, Japan, America etc. The bone paste tastes as good as meat and contains various nutrients like calcium, protein, fat, vitamin, collagen, chondroitin and micro-elements along with phospholipid and phosphoprotein for human brain as well as chondroitin, ossein for supplementing body energy and delaying senescence.

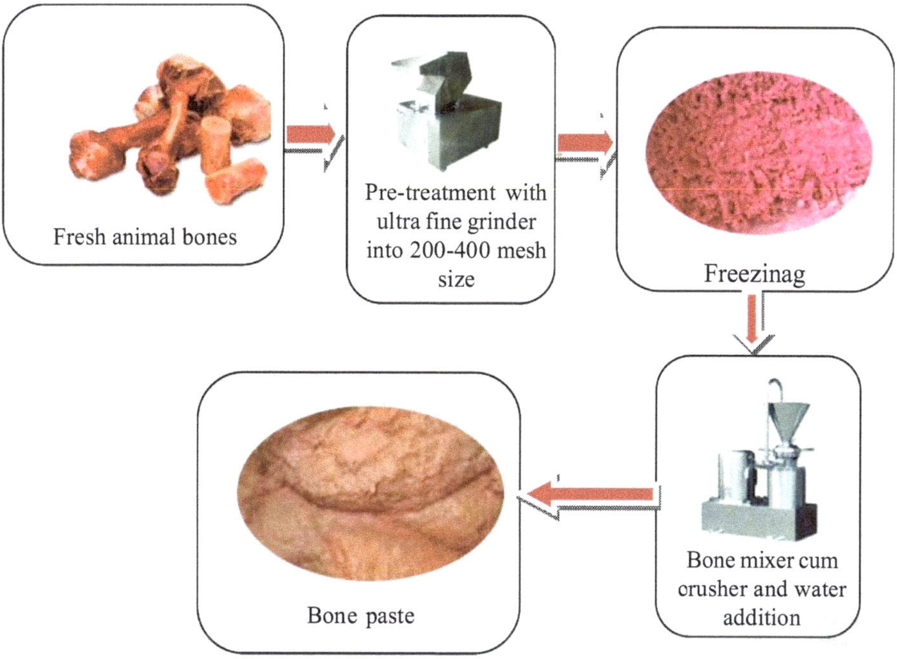

Process of bone paste development

Utilization of bone paste

There are number of products can be developed using bone paste like bone paste cookies, high-calcium rice noodles, meatballs, meat stuffing, sausage, rice dumplings and bone paste floss.

Bone Powder

Bone powder is a good source of kalium, calcium, phosphorus, iron, protein, micro-element, amino acid, etc. It could be a good calcium supplement because bone powder contains the ratio of calcium and phosphorus is 2:1 which is very near to the requirement of human body. Actually there are two forms of bone powder-*crude bone powder* and *superfine bone powder. Crude bone powder* is a good additive for animal feed and helps in animal growth. It can also be utilized as efficient organic fertilizer to improve acid soil and promote crop growth. While *edible superfine bone powder* is a good food nutritive fortifier and easily absorbed by human body. Generally super fine powder is utilized in form of fast food, snack food, puffed food, catering food, health food and seasoning etc.

Processing Technology

Crude bone powder	Edible superfine bone powder
Fresh animal bones	Fresh animal bones
Degreasing	Cleaning
Drying	Dehydration
Crushing	Crushing
Bone powder	Crude bone grinding
	Fine bone grinding
	Degreasing
	Superfine bone grinding
	Cooling
	Packaging

Bone china

Bone china is a great creation in field of potteries. The first incidence of development of bone china was recorded in 1748 by Thomas Frye in East London in which he used 45 percent bone ash and he gave the name of product as fine porcelain. However, first commercially widespread bone china was developed by the English potter Josiah Spode in the early 1790s. Now bone china is a precious product of countries like Bangladesh, India, Indonesia, Iran, Srilanka and Thailand. In India, Rajasthan has become a hub of bone china with the production of about 16-17 tonnes per day. Bone china is quite expensive and having status of luxury articles because of strongness, very high mechanical strength and chip resistance as well as its high levels of whiteness and translucency.

Bone china is soft paste porcelain but it has lower plasticity and a narrower vitrification range than porcelain. Traditionally bone china constitutes 25% kaolin, 25% cornish stone and 50% bone ash. The bone ash that is used in bone china development is preferably of cattle bones that have lower iron content. For production of bone china, bones are first crushed before being degelatinised and then calcined at up to 1250°C. Bone ash is then milled to a fine particle size and subjected to unfired body plasticity for definite shape using kaolin. The mixture is then fired at around 1200 °C to get a final body of bone china. The modern day bone china is basically consists of two crystalline phases, anorthite and β-tricalcium phosphate or whitlockite embedded in a substantial amount of glass.

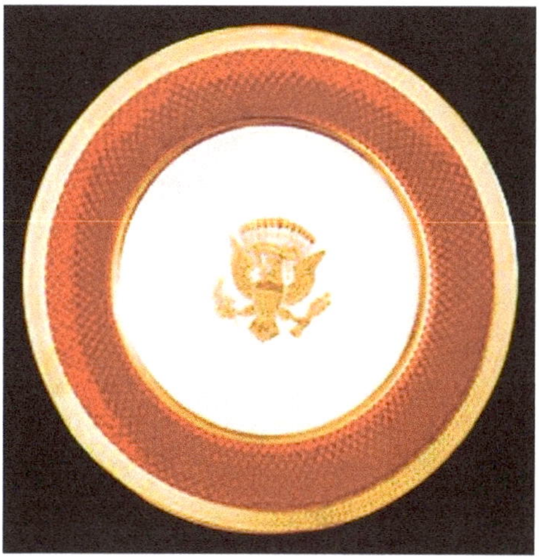

Utilization of hooves

Hooves are valuable by-products which can be separated from feet by steeping in hot water. After drying they can be further separated into white hooves and black hooves. White hooves are basically used for manufacturing of comb and buttons like articles while black hooves are processed by steam cooking and drying followed by grinding into meal and fertilizers. Hooves can also be utilized in form of foam type fire extinguishing fluids. Different types of dog chews can also be developed from hooves. The most valuable product obtained from hooves is 'Neatsfoot Oil'.

Neatsfoot oil

Neatsfoot oil is precious and valuable oil extracted from shin bones of hooves. It is actually pale yellow liquid possess unique quality characteristics like odourlessness and liquidity even at freezing temperature. Thus it can be utilized in machineries which are normally exposed to extremely lower temperature. It is a suitable lubricant for delicate machineries such as aeroplanes, ships, costly watches etc. However, its major use in manufacturing of leather. The production of Neat's foot oil is economical only in places which are adjacent to the large abattoirs. It is because only few milliliters of neatsfoot oil are produced from a pair of hooves and fresh stock is more suitable for its production. But it fetches very high price in market. Till date no single unit is working in India to process the neatsfoot oil.

Processing steps

Step	Purpose
Collection of hooves	Hooves are removed from feet in fresh condition
Washing	To separate adhering material like blood, dirt etc.
Scalding	Hooves are exposed in hot water (77^{0}C) for 15 minutes. Claws are separated and shells are loosened which can be separated with the help of hammer. Thus, shin bones are fully exposed.
Cooking or Extraction	Shin bones are immersed in water at 85^{0}C for about 8 hours in open tank or large kettle or wet rendered at 20psi for 4 hrs. Thus oil floats on top is skimmed off.
Purification	Raw neatsfoot oil is shifted to another kettle and heated at 85^{0}C for 8 hours and impurities are allowed to settle for 2 hours. Neatsfoot oil is then collected in separate vessel.
Filtration	Collected neatsfoot oil is filtered through sodium sulphate and silicon impregnated filter paper to remove traces of moisture.
Dehydration	Remaining moisture is then removed by heating at 100^{0}C for 2 hours.
Packaging and storage	Pure neatsfoot oil is usually packaged in coloured bottle and stored in dark room at room temperature.

Utilization of horns

Horns of animals particularly of indigenous animals are a typical structure present over head of the animal. They are different in different animals and varying in shape, size, colour and structure. The variations in horn are also dependant on species, breed, sex etc. However, almost all types of horns are basically made up of two structures like horn pith (inner core) and horn proper (outer cover). These both parts are generally separated by scalding in water at 60^{0}C followed by hitting with hammer. Outer cover of horn or horn proper is mostly contains keratin which can be converted into combs, buttons, hairpins, ornaments, knife handles and other decorative articles by controlled heating, pressing and cutting operations. Horn pith may be very good raw material for gelatin preparation or can be utilized for the production of bone meal and fertilizers.

Hooves and horns meal

Hooves and horns can be converted into meal by rendering. It may serve as very good fertilizer for enhancement of soil fertility because of rich nitrogen content. However, hooves and horns meal is not generally utilized as livestock and poultry feed because of poor digestibility and palatability. Hooves and horns meal may also be utilized in making of foam type fire extinguishing liquid. Meal is generally produced by rendering using steam under pressure to digest the hooves and horns for 8 hours. The resultant material is dried and milled to get fine hooves and horns meal.

References

1. Gracey, J.F. and Collins, D.S. (1994). Treatment and disposal of by-products. *In:* Reprint of 9th Edition, Meat Hygiene, ELBS, The Bath Press, Avon. pp 110-121.

2. Ockerman, H.W. and Hansen, C.L. (1988). Edible tissue from bone. *In:* Animal By-Products Processing, Jointly Published by Ellis Horwood Ltd., Chichester, England and VCH, Weinheim, New York (USA), Pp 158-175.

3. Ockerman, H.W. and Hansen, C.L. (1988). Glue and gelatin. In: Animal By-Products Processing, Jointly Published by Ellis Horwood Ltd., Chichester, England and VCH, Weinheim, New York (USA), Pp 132-157.

4. Ozgundogdu, F.K. (2005). Bone China from Turkey. Ceramics Technical, 20: 29-32.

5. Sharma, B.D. (2003). Utilzation of bones. *In:* Modern Abattoir Practices and Animal Byproducts Technology, first edition, Jaypee Brothers Medical Publishers (P) Ltd, New Delhi, Pp 122-128.

6. Whitewares (1987). Production, Testing and Quality Control. By W.Ryan & C. Radford. Pergamon Press, Pp 212-221.

Chapter 18

Processing of Animal Stomach and Intestines

Stomach and intestines are important part of animal body. Stomach mainly constitutes rumen, reticulum, omasum and abomasums. In which rumen, reticulum and omasum are utilized in form of edible uses, petfood and meat meal while abomasums can be converted into petfood and meat meal but abomasums of suckling calf can be utilized in extraction of rennet. Sheep rumen can also be utilized as haggis casings and pig stomach can be processed as petfood, pepsin, haggis casings and chitterlings. Organic content obtained from stomach and intestines can be utilized in form of compost, fertilizer and sometimes as feed. Intestine is also constitutes large intestine (colon, caecum and rectum), small intestine and oesophagus. In which large intestine and small intestine if not in condition to convert in casings can be utilized by rendering in form of meat meal. Serous membranes of caecum can be utilized in perfume industry to seal bottles. But major use of intestines is in casings preparation and small intestine as surgical sutures, collagen sheets, strings of musical instruments and tennis racket as well as in pepsin and heparin production. Oesophagus can also be utilized in form of casings and meat meal. The references of animals intestines use in making thread for sewing footwear and fur clothing are also available since long back. The use of animal intestine in valuable product is long back as 16th century in Russia.

Casings are generally used as container for various types of sausages. Some 55 percent of the sausage casings are made from animal intestines and rest of casings are made from polymeric materials. Natural casings that serve as containers or packaging materials for comminuted meat products like sausages, salami etc. can be obtained from various parts of digestive and excretory tracts like oesophagus, large and small intestines, caecum, rectum, bladders etc. India is capable to process animal casings of high quality with excellent calibration and shining colour. All these qualities make the India one of the major exporter of animal casing in world. The country has exported 352.21 MT of casing products to world for the worth of Rs. 28.45 crores during the year 2013-14 (APEDA, 2014). The major export destinations of Indian casings are Vietnam, Italy, South Africa, Portugal, Germany, Denmark, Spain, Albania, Romania, Japan, USA European union and Lebanon. The major export quality casings is salted sheep casings while dried cattle casings is exported to Gulf countries only.

Structure of intestine

Casings are soft cylindrical containers used to contain sausage or alimentary tract of sheep, goat, cattle and pigs, sometimes urinary bladder when used as food containers are called casings. Basically there are four distinct layers in intestine arranged from outer to inner as Tunica serosa or serous coat or outer coat, Tunica muscularis or muscular coat or longitudinal and circular layer, Tela submucosa or submucosal layer and Mucosal layer. Casings are mainly produced from strongest sub mucosal layer which is made up of dense connective tissues with elastic network having good quantity of collagen. It provides fine structure, good flexibility, strength and delicacy to the casings. Serosal and muscular layers may or may not be utilized for casings depending on the final utility of casings and strength of these layers at the time of extraction. But mucous membrane is always discarded during processing because it is weakest layer.

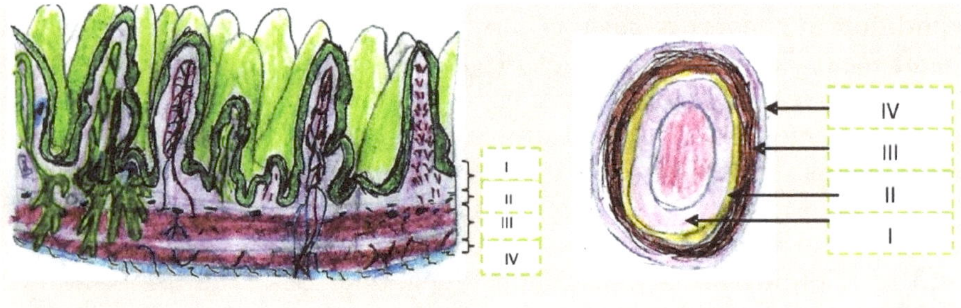

I. Mucous coat with finger like outgrowth for enlarged surface area.
II. Sub-mucosal layer or tela submucosa with firm elastic structure contains connective tissues.
III. Muscular layer or tunica muscularis, circular in structure.
IV. Serous layer or tunica serosa is a thin coating covering the abdominal cavity from inside and surrounding the organs.

Cross sectional view of intestine

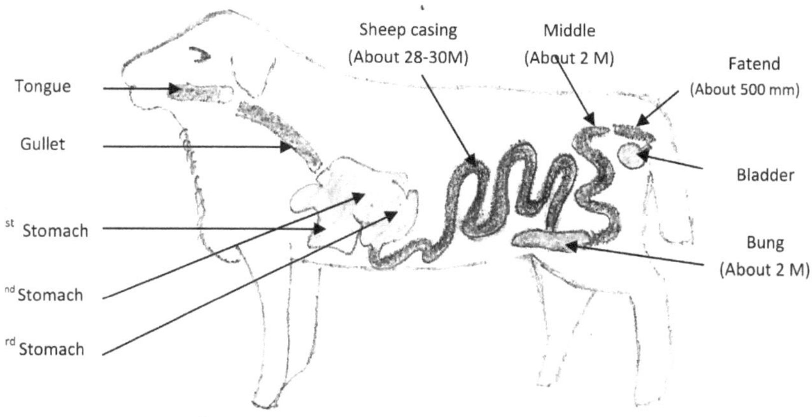

Parts of sheep and goat casings

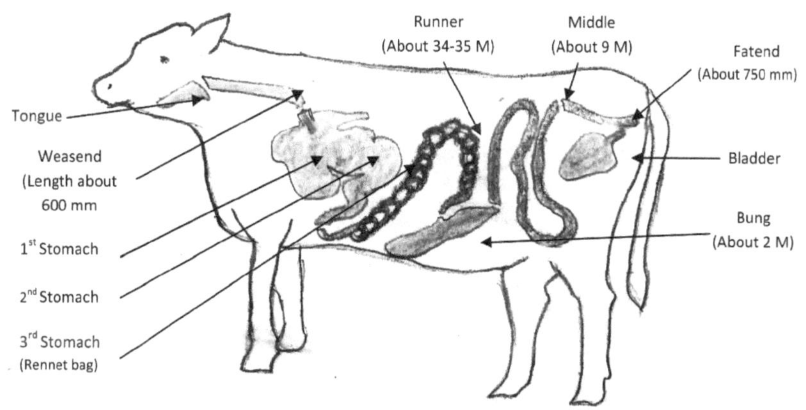

Parts of cattle and buffalo casing

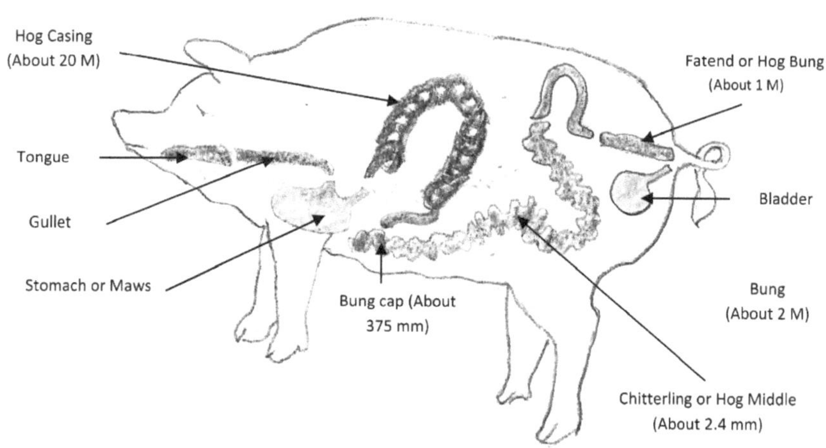

Parts of pig casings

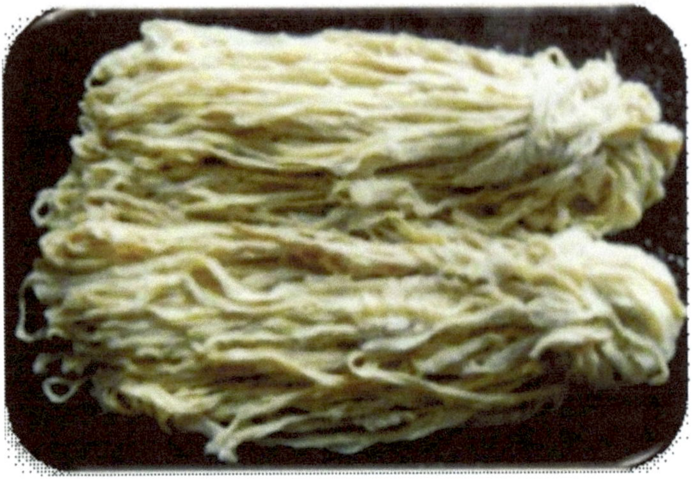

Terminology used for casings

Term	Description
Animal casings	Separation of sub-mucosal layer or tela submucosa after removal of tunica serosa (serous layer), tunica muscularis (muscular layer) and mucous coat.
Casing	Term generally applied for casings from small intestine of sheep and goats.
Small casing	Casing from small intestine of pigs.
Rounds	Casing from small intestine of sheep, goat or pigs.
Runner	Casing from small intestine of cattle and buffalo.
Middles	Casing from large intestine of cattle and buffalo and sometime pigs.
Bung	Casing from caecum or blind gut of cattle and buffalo.
Cap	Casing from caecum or blind gut of sheep and pigs.
Chitterling	Casing from black gut or part of large intestine of pigs.
Maws	Casings from cleaned pig stomach.
Weasand	Casings from oesophagus of cattle and buffalo.
Bladder	Casing from urinary bladder of cattle, buffalo or pigs.
Stump casing	Casing less than 6 ft in length.
Dry pack	Pack of overnight drained casings.
Slush pack	Pack of undrained casings.
Hank	Salted casing of sheep, goat or pigs measuring 100 yard or 91.4 meter in length.Dried casing of cattle and buffalo measuring 180 meters for runners and 90 meters for middles.

Classification of casings

Characteristics	Casing types with degree of characteristics		
	Natural animal casing	Collagen casing	Cellulose casing
Source	Submucosal layer of intestine and other casing stock.	Reconstituted collagen protein from hide of cattle and buffalo.	Cotton is regenerated into casings.
Presentation	Salted	Dried	Dried
Strength	More fragile	Less fragile	Least fragile
Edibility	Edible	Edible	Peeled before use
Mechanibility	Least degree	Less degree	Best degree
Printability	Not suitable	Limited suitability	Best suitable
Smoke penetration	Best	Very good	Good
Shelf life	Least	Less	Best
Diameter	Variable	Uniform	Uniform
Storage requirement	Refrigeration	Refrigeration	Room temperature
Cost	High	Less	Least

Quality characteristics of natural casings

Natural casings are generally obtained from healthy and well inspected animals after slaughter. For casing production animal intestine should be free from parasitic infestations and ulcers and must be handled hygienically. Casings should be permeable to water vapour, smoke and gases and can expand or shrink as per the requirement of product. They should also have the sealing property. For grading of natural casings Indian Standards (IS: 1981-1962) is generally followed. Natural casings must be inspected for following parameters before final dispatch:

i. Casings should be inspected for colour (transparent), flavour and defects. Common defect encountered due to faulty cleaning is dull/greyish/greenish colour of casings.

ii. Casing should be free from parasitic infestations. Common types of nodules of oesophagostomum are very common.

iii. Casings should also be inspected for cicatrices (scars of healed up intestinal wounds), domestics (small grease spots in casings), kink (twisted loop in the casting), rust (black spot caused by putrefaction due to bacterial of fungal action) etc. It is because they may be cause of lower price and even discard of casings.

iv. Casings should have enough strength to hold the weight of material during sausage preparation. It should also be free from holes, tears and lacerations.

v. There should be a desired diameter and length of the casings for a particular purpose.

vi. There should be the proper salting of sheep and goat casings and drying of cattle and buffalo casings. Prolong salting may lead to development of scars or patches in casings due to salt burn.

vii. Grading should be done calibre wise and accordingly they should be packaged in suitable containers.

Name of casing	Average length	Average diameter	Principle use
Round	75-90 ft	35 mm	Bologna, liver sausages, metwurst
Middles	20-25 ft	55 mm	Salami, Bologna
Runner	90-135 ft	>55 mm	Salami, Polish sausages, Bologna
Sheep casings	33-64 ft	14-25 mm	Sausages, Bologna, Salami
Bung	4-5 ft	-	Large Bologna, Salami
Bladder	-	7-14 inch	Mortadella and speciality products

Grading system as per Animal Casings Grading and Marking Rules, 1964

Parameters	Primary Quality (PQ) Grade	Grade-1	Grade-2	Grade-3
Dried Cattle and Buffalo Casings				
Colour	Natural colour and free from discolouration and spots	Slight variation	More variations	Short pieces of all grades
Defects	Free from defects like black nodes, cicatrices etc.	Few black nodes	Large black nodes	
Hank	Proper rolled values	Few folds	Defects in roll	
Others	Proper strength and free from laceration	-	Rough textured with some fat streaks	
Salted Sheep and Goat Casings (PQ & Grade-1 is same grade but for export AGMARK allows one more grade)				
Colour	Natural without discolouration		Slight variation	More variations

Defects	Free from all types of defects	Free	Some nodules
Hank	Proper hank and salted	Fit for sausages	Defects in salting
Others	Proper strength without any torn or laceration	Slight variation in strength	More variations

Processing of casings

Step	Processing detail
Viscera removal	i. Removal of viscera by opening the brisket. ii. Breaking of aitch bone but bung should remain intact. iii. Removal of pizzle cord and bladder. iv. Anal opening and bung dropping into carcass.
Separation of organs	i. Organs like stomach, heart, lung, liver should be separated from intestine. ii. Separate out the rounds, bungs, middles, bladders, weasands etc. based on the preference to dry and salting.
Pulling/Running	i. Removal of ruffle or mesentery fat from sheep, goat and pig intestines using hand or air operated knife is called pulling due to soft and delicacy. ii. Thick and strong intestines of cattle and buffalo are usually subjected to running in which knife is used to separate the mesenteric fat.
Chilling	Chilling of intestines at 10-15^{0}C is essential when 'green intestines' are not utilized in abattoir. It is done to reduce the bacterial and fermentative changes in intestines.
Stripping	i. Squeezing of intestinal contents of pig, sheep and goats by hand in between first and second fingers or instrument or machine. ii. Intestines of large animals like beef middles are stripped under fresh stream of running water.
Fatting	The fat in small diameter intestines of small animals is usually separated by scrapping while fat from beef casings requires pulling with knife.
Fermentation	i. Intestines of small animals are immersed in warm water with or without salt and soda (pigs' intestines at 21^{0}C for 1-2 days and sheep and goat intestines at 37^{0}C for half to one hour). It is done to loose different layers by enzymatic and bacterial action.

	ii. Intestines of large animals are not subjected to fermentation due to stronger muscular layer and cleaned manually.
Turning	Turning is performed only in intestines of large animals due to stronger muscular layer. Intestines are usually turned inside out using two fingers in a tank of warm water. Intestines of small animals are not required turning because they can easily cleaned by stripping and sliming.
Sliming	i. Sliming is the process of removal of mucous lining or slime with a wooden or plastic sliming stick at an angle of $30^{0.}$ ii. Sliming can also be achieved by crushing in crusher and soaking of intestines in water at $38-42^{0}C$ for 30-45 minutes. iii. So after removal of greyish coloured slime casing becomes transparent.
Inspection	Casings are inspected for proper strength, freeness from defects and cleanliness.
Measurement	Fresh ready casings are then measured for length and width. Width is usually calibrated with gauge in inflated or water filled condition.
Salting or drying	i. Casings of sheep and goat are generally salted while large animals are dried according to the demand of traders. ii. Curing is done with the help of fine salt for 5-7 days while large animal casings are controlled dried.
Packaging	Casings packaging is done in tierces, barrels or boxes. Salted casings preferably in wood barrels or in metal drums lined with cotton and plastics while dried casings in wooden boxes or barrels.
Storage	Salted casings can be stored for one to two years at $0-10^{0}C$ but dried casing at room temperature with less than 65% relative humidity for a year. However, casings should always be protected from direct sunlight.

Processing of collagen casings

Collagen casing is basically of two types-small casings or edible or chewable casings and inedible or large casings. Edible collagen casings are generally used in preparation of fresh pork sausages while large collagen casing are peeled before use because they are treated with aldehyde to provide the strength by cross linking the collagen. Edible collagen casing is soluble on cooking and primarily made from animal protein collagen extracted from beef hides. The essential steps in its extraction are soundness and kosher nature of hide from slaughter of sound and healthy animals. Collagen casings are available in natural colour or in red or smoke colours.

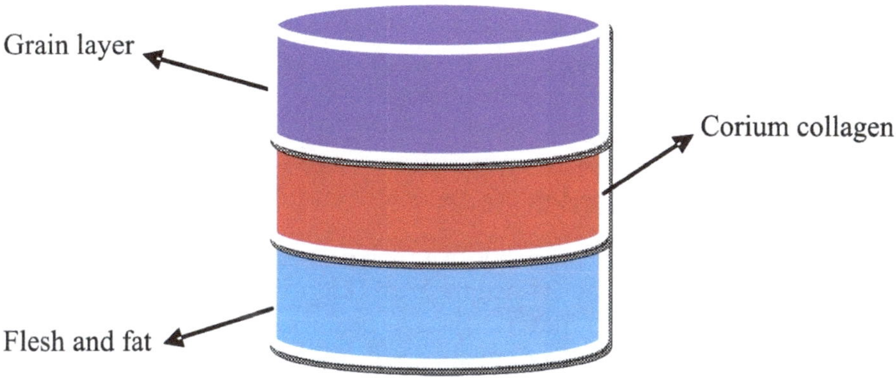

Layers in animal hide

Processing steps

Step	Processing detail
Removal of hide	Hide should be removed in kosher condition from slaughter of kosher animals.
Washing	Proper washing is required to remove all adhered materials.
De-fleshing	To remove the flesh and fat from hide with hand or knife or machine.
Removal of hair follicles	Hair follicles are removed by the treatment of hide with weak acid or alkali.
Splitting	Splitting of grain layer with corium (inner collagen layer).
	Neutralization and grinding Corium layer is neutralized by washing and coarsely ground.
Chopping	Production of shammy by chopping with ultrafine chopper.
Acidification	Shammy with 5 percent collagen is acidified with acetic acid to produce pasty gel.
Filtration and homogenization	To produce uniform stretch and burst strength fibres and arrangement of casing size, diameter and wall thickness upon extrusion.

Extrusion	Extruder's helps in alignment of collagen fibres through annular die to produce tube of uniform diameter, length, strength and wall thickness.
Neutralization and chemical treatment	Casing is neutralized by washing and treated with sugar to incorporate strength and glycerine for pliability.
Drying	Casings are controlled dried to remove the moisture to a desired level (13-18%). Now casings become ready to be 'shirred' or pleated into 'slugs'.
Sizing	Desired size of casings is obtained as per the demand and assures uniform size, weight and lengths.
Packaging	Packaging in hermetically sealed containers and put into outer cartons for storage.
Storage	Collagen casings are stored at 2-10^{0}C for further use.

Catgut suturing material

The word catgut is probably originated from 'cattlegut'. There are some references showing its origin from 'kitgut' in which 'kit' means fiddle. Catgut suturing material is a type of natural fibre originally developed from collagen present in small intestine of sheep and goats but it can also be obtained from intestines of cattle, pigs, horse, mules and donkeys. Catgut is a widely used material for surgical suturing. The prepared catgut can be sterilized before use in sterilizing fluid containing ethylene oxide, isopropyl alcohol and distilled water. Naturally it is commercially available in straw-colour with variable sizes as USP 6-0 (1 metric) to USP 3 (7 metric). Animal intestine based catgut can also be used as strings of harps, lutes, violins, violas and cellos, acoustic guitars and other stringed musical instruments, as well as older marching snare drums. The other uses of catgut are in strings of tennis rackets.

Step	Processing's
Collection of small intestine	Small intestines of sheep or goat are collected carefully. So that whole intact mass can be obtained without cut and tearing or lacerations.
Cleaning and steeping	Intestines are cleared from content, trimmed of fat and cleaning and steeping is done with water to remove the extraneous material.
Scrapping and steeping	External membranes of intestine are scaped off using blunt knife and steeped in potassium hydroxide for few minutes.
Drawing	Draw out the intestine to equalize and make them smooth.
Twisting	Twisting of strands of collagen in gut together to make the string.

Drying	Dry the string under controlled condition.
Polishing	Polishing of string is done to obtain desired diameter through centerless grinder.
Bleaching and disinfection	Bleaching and disinfection is done by using sulphur dioxide.
Dyeing and sizing	To achieve proper colour and size of catgut.
Treatment with chromium salt solution	It is done to provide the resistance to catgut against body enzymes and to slow the absorption process. Treated sutures are called catgut chromic sutures while untreated suture are termed as catgut plain sutures.

Biodegradable plastics

In present world there is a huge demand of biodegradable packaging materials. In particular environment friendly plastics manufactured from renewable resources may be a good source of such type of materials. Though some of the biodegradable plastics are available commercially but they are price competitive with traditional oil-derived plastics such as polyethylene and polystyrene. So to provide biodegradable packaging materials in affordable price animal intestine may serve as fruitful purpose. Biobased plastics can be developed from animal intestines by fermentation processes. These materials can be utilized in coating of food, pharmaceuticals, and industrial products. However, the packaging material obtained from animal intestine or protein films is quite brittle. So the use of plasticizers such as glycerol, propylene glycol, triethylene glycol, sorbitol, sucrose, and polyethylene glycol may help in reduction of brittleness of materials. The positive quality changes in protein films can also be achieved by modifying the cross linking of protein molecules. It can be achieved by using various physical and chemical processes such as heat, pressure, shear, irradiation, or acid or alkali treatment etc.

Miscellaneous products form stomach and intestines

Product	Processing technique	Uses
Bungs	Cleaning, trimming, turning, salting and chilling	Casings for sausage production.
Maws	Trimming, cleaning, turning, slimming and salting.	Casings for sausage production.
Bladder	Washing, turning, salting, inflation, trimming, chilling and drying.	Casings for sausage production.
Weasand	Washing, turning, inflation, drying	Casings for sausage production.

Chitterlings	Trimming, cleaning, turning, chilling, bleaching, salting,	Casings for sausage production.
Mucosa	Soaking, crushing, stripping, squeezing	In pharmaceutical industry as heparin and stock feed.
Intestinal content	Sterilization	Fertilizers and livestock feed.

Thus it can be concluded that intestines are very important by-product of slaughter house origin which can be utilized in various ways. The need is to exploit the technology and sound extraction of intestine. The products obtained from various parts of stomach and intestines are useful in day to day life of human beings. Some of them like catgut help in upgradation of human life by providing the game and entertainment instruments. It also protects and prolongs the human life through assistance in surgery.

References

1. Gracey, J.F. and Collins, D.S. (1994). Treatment and disposal of by-products. *In:* Reprint of 9th edition, Meat Hygiene, ELBS, The Bath Press, Avon. pp 110-121.

2. Ockerman, H.W. and Hansen, C.L. (1988). Sausage containers. *In:* Animal By-Products Processing, Jointly Published by Ellis Horwood Ltd., Chichester, England and VCH, Weinheim, New York (USA), Pp 285-321.

3. Roenigk, R.K. and Roenigk,H.H. (2010). Catgut sutures are made from sub-mucosal layer of the small intestine of sheep and the serosal layer of the small intestine of cattle. *In:* Roenigk and Roenigk's Dermatologic Surgery: Principles and Practices. Pp 93.

4. Rusakov, V. N. (2010). The Great Soviet Encyclopedia, 3rd edition (1970-1979). The Gale Group, Inc.

5. Wray, D. (2006). Suture and suture materials: Absorbable sutures: surgical gut. *In:* Remington: The Science and Practice of Pharmacy, 21st ed. Baltimore, Maryland; Philadelphia, Pennsylvania; Lippincott Williams and Wilkins, Pp 1974.

Chapter 19

Utilization of Animal Organs and Glands in Pharmaceutical, Cosmetic and Food Industry

India is bestowed by nature with a vast livestock resources comprising of 190 million cattle, 108 million buffalo, 135.17 million goats, 65.06 million sheep, 10.29 million pigs, 729.2 million poultry, 0.29 million mithun and 0.07 million yak (Department of Animal Husbandry, Dairying and Fisheries, 2014). The livestock sector is an important segment of agriculture and contributes nearly 25.6 percent of value in agriculture, fishing and forestry sector. The total share of livestock in GDP of India is 4.11 percent and meat is an important sector to generate foreign revenue by export. The share can further be extended by utilization of animal by-products because it is a sector of livestock neglected most. It is an old saying that 'each and everything comes from animals can be utilized except last cry of animals'. Among all by-products produced from animals, glandular by products constitute roughly 0.28% of the live weight of animal slaughtered. As per a estimate 9.13 thousand metric tons of glandular by-products are available for processing in the country. These ductless glands have vital role in human life because some of them can be utilized in production of life saving drugs. However, they are not fully utilized due to lack of modern abattoir facilities for proper collection, storage and transport of various byproducts, lack of awareness about the intrinsic value of the glandular byproducts and lack of scientific and technical competency for processing of these glandular byproducts.

The glandular products produced from animal body can be utilized in extraction of enzymes, hormones, pigments and vitamins. These are involved in the metabolic process in living cell and hence their availability in their natural form is very useful in pharmaceutical industries. Major glands serves the purpose are pituitary gland, intestinal mucus, adrenals, liver, lungs, thymus etc. The amount and extent of active ingredients in these glands depends on species, sex, and age of the animals. The major concern for extraction of active ingredients from these glands is solely dependent on collection, preservation and processing of glands.

Principles in glands utilization

i. Glands should always be collected from healthy animals and positively within 15-20 minutes.

ii. The adhering fat and connective tissue must be trimmed before preservation. So that effective preservation can be achieved.

iii. The glands should always be chilled as soon as possible in metal buckets containing ice but some of the glands like pituitary and suprarenal glands can also be preserved in dry ice. Care should be taken that ice or water should not come in direct contact of glands otherwise active ingredient of gland can leach to the ice or water.

iv. The best method to retard autolysis and destruction through bacterial growth of glands is quick freezing. Quick freezing is generally done within hour of collection in clean and pre-chilled trays on waxed papers and transferred to a sharp freezer at -18^{0}C or less, but never above -9^{0}C. So hard freeze glands after 48 hrs of freezing are shifted from trays or waxed papers to covered containers without leaving the air space. It is to avoid the direct contact of air to the glands and prevents freezer burn. In no case thawing is allowed until extraction of pharmaceutical products from glands.

v. Glands can also be preserved using chemicals like one part glands with one part acetone or phenol or two parts of 37 percent formalin.

vi. Some glands like pancreas, pituitary, thyroid, adrenal can be preserved by drying with acetone. These glands are initially defatted before drying. The dried powder of these glands can be developed by immersing in four part of acetone for three hours. After cutting the glands into pieces they are again immersed in three parts of chilled acetone for 2-3 hrs. After mincing these glands are again treated with three parts of chilled acetone and fine powder is achieved after grinding. Drying inactivates the enzyme of glands thus they can preserve for longer period of time.

vii. Special precautions are required for particular gland like hard frozen gland in water is suitable for liver extract, acidulated alcohol for insulin and dry state of gland for Adrenocorticotropic hormone (ACTH) because it losses potency in contact with water. Heat sensitive glands like anterior pituitary and suprarenal cortex are lyophilized (high vacuum freeze dried) to produce the extracts.

viii. Some glands like ovary and testes are not essentially defatted because their active ingredients are fat soluble. So these glands are converted into powder by milling with adhered fat.

ix. All the extracted products of glands must be tested for potency and suitability for most effective dispensing mode like powder, capsules, tablets, injections or liquid.

x. Vacuum drying of glands is generally performed at low temperature (24-32^{0}C) and 0.7 kg/cm^2.

Utility of various glandular byproducts

Glands are usually preserved by freezing and frozen glands appear bright pink in color except for suprarenal gland, which is light brown in appearance. These glands can be utilized for production of number of pharmaceutical preparations and drugs. Some of the major glands used for medicinal, pharmaceutical, food and cosmetic industries can be summarized as:

Utilization of animal organs

Organ	As food	As medicine or pharmaceuticals
Brain and spinal cord	Brain, nervous system and spinal cord are used for table purpose by cooking after blanching and removal of piamater and arachanoid meninges.	*Cholesterol* is used as emulsifier for cosmetics. *Cholesterol* helps in synthesis of male sex hormones. *Thromboplastin* and *cephaline* can be used in blood coagulation during surgery.
Heart	Heart is used as table meat in form of whole heart by roasting or braising or sliced heart by grilling or braising.	*Heart valves* of young pigs can be used for implantation of defective heart valves in human being.
Liver	Most widely used organ as food in form of processed meat like liver sausages and paste.	*Liver extract* in treatment of anaemia. *Desiccated liver* as nutritional supplement. *Catalase* an enzyme obtained from hog liver can be used in various catalase activities like splitting of hydrogen peroxide. *Dehydrocholic acid* from liver bile in treatment of indigestion and constipation. *Heparin* in blood clotting.

Lungs	As processed meat and sausages.	*Heparin* as anticoagulant and in treatment of emboli, gangrene, frostbite and burns. *Aprotinin* as trypsin inhibitor.
Spleen	As flavourings in meat pies and as ingredient in processed meat.	Spleen extract can be used in influencing the capillary permeability and blood clotting time. It can also be utilized in treatment of certain blood and lymphatic diseases.
Stomach	Rumen and reticulum in processed meat and sausages. Pig stomach after removal of mucosa lining by braising or in sausages. *Rennet or Rennin* is an enzyme obtained from 4th stomach or abomasums of milkfed calf or unweaned calf of cow or buffalo used in cheese industry.	*Pepsin* obtained from mucosal lining of hog stomach helps in digestion of protein. *Peptone* from hog stomach and used in laboratory work. *Glycoprotein* obtained from pyloric lining of stomach enhances utilization of vitamin-B_{12} in case of pernicious anaemia. *Gastrin*- a polypeptide hormone stimulates gastric juice production. *Mucin*-a hog stomach product treats peptic and duodenal ulcers.
Kidneys	As food by broiling or grilling or braising after removal of fat capsules, ureter and blood vessels.	-
Tongue	As food by salting, boiling and braising.	-
Udder	Bovine udder as food after slicing, frying or boiling.	-
Uterus	As food after poaching or boiling.	-

Utilization of animal glands

Gland	Location	Active ingredient	Utility
Adrenal or Suprarenal	Reddish brown in colour near pelvis and kidney	Adrenal cortex secret adrenocortico steroids Adrenal medulla secret epinephrine / adrenaline or nor-epinephrine/ adrenaline	In treating the deficiency diseases like Addison's disease, anti-neoplastic, anti-inflammatory conditions and treatment of surgical shock. Stimulate food utilization, arrest the haemorrhage, prolong local anesthetics, stimulate heart action and overcome shock. Reduce symptoms of hay fever, allergies of nasal mucous membrane, control bronchial asthma and reduce inner eye pressure during glaucoma treatment.
Pancreas (Gut sweet-bread)	Reddish brown shape of oak leaf attached with back of liver	Islet cells of Langerhans (β-cells) secret Insulin Islet cells of Langerhans (Alpha-cells) secret Glucagons LPH or lipase Chymotrypsin & trypsin Proteolytic enzymes Pancreatin Pancrelipase	Treatment of diabetes. Increase blood sugar; treat insulin overdose or low blood sugar due to alcoholism. Used as a digestive aid and absorption of fats and oils. Used as digestive aid, speedy healing of wounds. Trypsin can also be used in tanneries. Used in cataract surgery. Treatment of faulty digestion. Pork source enzyme act as digestive aid in pancreatic insufficiency and gelatin digestion in x-ray films.

Parathyroid	Little larger than wheat grain near thyroid	Parathormone Thyrocalcitonin	Treatment of human parathyroid deficiency, abnormal tooth development, muscular spasms, paralysis and stimulate the loss of calcium from bones. Used in prevention of tetany. Stimulate the calcium deposition in bones.
Pineal	Cone shaped reddish colour in brain cavity near third ventricle	Melatonin hormone	In treatment of schizophrenia, insomnia and mental retardation. Control the formation and release of gonadotrophic hormone.
Pituitary	Grayish or pinkish yellow at base of brain	*Anterior lobe* Growth promoting hormone (G.H.) Thyroid stimulating hormone (TSH) Prolactin Adrenocortrico-trophic hormone (ACTH). Follicle stimulating hormone (FSH), Luteinizing hormone (LH) *Posterior lobe* Oxytocin Vasopressin	Control growth (giantism and dwarfism) Regulate metabolism and activity of other endocrine glands. Mammary stimulating or lactogenic hormone Treat rheumatism, arthritis, eye inflammation and multiple myeloma. Control of gonads and their reproductive functions. Oxytocin initiates uterine contraction and also used as milk ejecting factor. Vasopressin is an antidiuretic hormone (ADH) and used as vasoconstrictor.
Thymus(True sweetbread)	Pinkish white in thoracic cavity but grayish yellow in pigs	Thyroid extracts	Assists in improving the resistance of body to infection and prevention of rickets.

Thyroid	Maroon colour at either side of trachea	Thyroxin Calcitonin or thyrocalcitonin Thyroid as substance	In treatment of hypothyroidism and diseases due to thyroid deficiency like creatinism in infants and myxoedema in adults. Lower calcium and phosphorus in blood and regulate heart beat and treat paget's disease. In lowering calcium level in blood and regulate heart beat.
Ovaries	Abdominal cavity above uterine horn	Oestrogen Progesterone Relaxin from corpora lutea of pregnant sow ovaries.	In treatment of reproductive problems and as contraceptics. Oestrogen is used in treatment of breast and prostate cancers and menopausal syndrome. Progesterone prevents abortion by preventing the ovulation and inhibiting the secretion of luteinizing hormone. Helps in normal parturitions by relaxes the pelvic ligaments.
Testes	Scrotum	Hyaluronidase or invasion enzyme Androgen or testosterone	Enzyme used as a spreading factor for drugs and androgen. Testosterone as male sex hormone and responsible for sexual behaviour.
Gall	Gall bladder	Cholic acid, deoxycholic acid, chenodeoxycholic acid and dehydro-cholic acid	Can be utilized as steroid precursor, precursor to dissolve gallstones etc.
Bile	Gall bladder and bile duct	Cortisones like prednisone or prednisolone Bile extract	Treatment of arthritis as an anti inflammatory agent. Increase secretary activity of liver.

Insulin production

Insulin is a hormone produced from pancreatic cells called islets of Langerhans. It is responsible for regulation of amount of glucose in the blood and smooth functioning of human body. The generation of insulin from cells is a continuous process as a result blood glucose level enhances. Then insulin allows the blood glucose to be transported from the blood into the cells. The cells can then use the glucose as energy to carry out its functions. Once transported into the cell, the blood glucose level is returned to normal within hours. Insulin causes liver cells, muscle cells and fat tissue to take up glucose from the blood and store it as glycogen in the liver and muscle. Contrary to this if insulin is lacking, blood glucose remains in blood and cells becomes starved of energy and symptoms of diabetes develops. Cells then start utilizing fat as energy source for emergencies and in later stage it starts producing ketones. Ketones may act as poison and kill the cells and leads to serious illness and coma.

In year 1921, Canadian Scientists Frederick, G. Banting and Charles H. Best successfully purified insulin from dog's pancreas. Then insulin was extracted from pancreas of cattle and pigs and purified. The chemical structure of insulin in these animals is slightly structurally different in 1-3 amino acids between the animal insulin and human insulin. However, it functions so well in human body but some time negative immune system or allergic reactions may takes place. Biotechnological tools were invented to synthesize the human insulin with more accuracy. Today insulin users increasingly moved to a form of human insulin created through recombinant DNA technology. But isolation of insulin from slaughtered animals is still relevant and used for the purpose.

Pancreas is a good source of insulin and produced from β-cells of pancreas called islets of Langerhans. Pig pancreas is most suitable for insulin production because only one amino acid is differ from human insulin while beef insulin is different in 4-5 amino acids from human insulin. but bovine pancreas can also be used for the purpose. It is highly perishable gland and requires immediate chilling and freezing to prevent the destruction of insulin by proteolysis. It is noticed that insulin is easily destroyed at room temperature within 2-3 hrs by own enzymes. It is evident from research that one kilogram of fresh bovine or pig pancreas can produce 150 mg of crystalline insulin with an activity of 25 IU/ mg insulin. Insulin can be extracted from pancreas by acidified ethanol or by enzymatic cleavage. Recently insulin can be produced by bacteria coded with human DNA genome by recombinant DNA technology.

Routine insulin extraction process

Step	Process description
Collection of pancreas	Fresh pancreas should be collected from animals like cattle, pigs etc. as soon as possible after slaughter of animal. Otherwise insulin will be destroyed by pancreatic enzymes.
Chilling	Individual pancreas should be collected in vessel covered with ice but always avoid direct contact of ice with gland otherwise insulin will leach to water.
Freezing	Immediately after chilling pancreas should be freeze to avoid insulin destruction.
Grinding	Freezed glands are grinded in acetone and alcohol to prevent proteolytic destruction of insulin or acidified methanol can be used for insulin extraction.
Concentration	Extracted insulin is concentrated at 40^{0}C and fat is removed.
Salting	Crude insulin is slated by brining and floated part contains insulin is separated in form of salt cake and purified.
Washing	Crude insulin is then washed with alcohol as well as with ether and solid mass is collected.
Purification	Insulin can be purified by crystallization using a solution containing small amount of zinc salt or picric acid.
Precipitation	Supernatant is precipitated with absolute ethanol. Discard the supernatant and collect the precipitate as insulin.
Storage	Best condition of insulin can be maintained for a year under freezing condition but for short time storage insulin can be preserved in refrigeration. Pure insulin can be obtained by gel filtration technique.

Insulin extraction and precipitation from camel pancreas (Elamin et al., 2014)

Step	Process description
Collection of pancreas	Collect fresh pancreas from animals like cattle, pigs etc.
Homogenization	Homogenization of pancreas in a solution containing acid: ethanol: water (1.25:80:20).
Centrifugation	Centrifuge the bland in refrigeration centrifuge at 600 x g for 15 minutes at 4^{0}C. It separates the content into

	pellet and supernatant. Supernatant is allowed to refine and adjust the pH 8.0 and keep for further use.
Washing	Pellet is washed with solution of acid: ethanol and water(1:60:40)
Centrifugation	Centrifuge the mass at 600 x g for 10 minutes at 4°C and mass will be separated into pellet and supernatant. Discard the pellet and collect supernatant and adjust the pH 8.0. Mix the supernatant with previously prepared supernatant.
Centrifugation	Centrifuge the mass at 600 x g for 10 minutes at 4°C and again discard the pellet and collect the supernatant.
Rotary evaporation extraction	Fractionate the supernatant extract with CH_2Cl_2 with rotary evaporation extractor and separatory funnel into aqueous phase and organic phase. Discard the organic phase and collect aqueous phase. Aqueous phase extract is then added with 20% NaCl and stored at 4°C.
Centrifugation	Centrifuge the extract at 10,000 x g for 20 minutes at 4°C and separate supernatant and precipitate. Discard the supernatant and collect precipitate.
Washing	Precipitate is washed with 20% NaCl.
Acidification	Precipitate is dissolved in 75% ethanol and acidified to pH 3 with AcOH.
Centrifugation	Centrifuge the extract at 10,000 x g for 20 minutes at 4°C and separate supernatant and precipitate. Discard the precipitate and collect supernatant.
Precipitation	Supernatant is precipitated with absolute ethanol. Discard the supernatant and collect the precipitate as insulin.

Heparin production

Heparin or phosphatide can be obtained from liver, lungs and lining of small intestines. It is a good quality anticoagulant and thins the blood. So it is widely used in prevention of blood clotting during surgery and organ transplantation. It also prolongs the clotting time of blood.

Production process

Step	Process description
Collection of liver or lung or lining of intestine	All the raw materials should be collected separately in fresh and sound condition.
Tissue mincing	Collected tissue should be minced separately.
Autolysis	Tissue is autolysed at 30^{0}C for 24 hrs in presence of toluene to prevent tissue spoilage.
Extraction	Crude heparin is extracted by heating at 50^{0}C for one hour in presence of ammonium sulphate and sodium hydroxide. Intestinal heparin can be extracted by salt solution.
Precipitation	Precipitation should be done with alcohol for twenty hours in case of liver and lungs while saline solution with acetone precipitation is preferred in intestinal heparin.
Hydrolysis	Crude heparin is enzymatically hydrolyzed with trypsin.
Centrifugation	Hydrolyzed material is centrifuged at 600 x g for 10 minutes to clear the solution.
Precipitation	Clear solution is then precipitated with double volume of alcohol.
Purification	Purification by gel filtration technology.
Assessment	Heparin can be assessed for biological activity by sheep plasma assay.

Liver extract

Liver can be utilized in various forms by human beings. It is a good source of vitamin-B_{12} and helps in cure of pernicious anaemia. Liver taste sweet due to high glycogen content and can be used as source of energy. Injectable form of liver can be used in treatment of sprue- a type of catarrhal dysentery. Liver can be utilized in form of extract, desiccated liver, paste, liver powder or granules. Desiccated liver can be produced in unfitted or defatted form and can serve the purpose of nutritional supplement. Nutritional supplementation can also be obtained by addition of liver paste, concentrate, liver protein etc. Liver extract added with folic acid can be injected in humans to control the anaemia. Liver extract, granules or powder can be produced using vacuum drying or freeze drying process and may provide 54 mg of riboflavin per kg of product.

Step	Process description
Collection of liver	Liver should be collected in fresh and sound condition without damage.
Mincing	Mincing should be done in meat mincer and suspend the minced liver in hot water maintained at 85^0C.
Digestion	Suspended liver mince is digested with pepsin for at least 3 hrs at neutral pH.
Heating	Digested liver is heated to 90^0C for 30 minutes to inactivate the enzyme and coagulate the liver protein.
Filtration	Liver material is filter pressed to separate clear filtrate and suspended material.
Concentration	Clear fluid is concentrated to a syrupy mass.
Drying	Concentrated liver mass is dried or granulated by vacuum or freeze drying.
Storage	Dried powder is stored in air tight container for further use.

Heart valve for xenografting in humans

Porcine heart is an important by-product which can be utilized in xenografting of heart valves in human beings. Porcine aortic valve can be utilized as biological plastic or bioprosthetic heart valves in case of human heart failure and disorders. The detailed procedure of porcine heart valve preparation for xenografting is given under. Pericardial tissue of cattle can be utilized after heart surgery and prevents adhesions of replaced heart with myocardium and sternum. It can also be processed using glutaraldehyde processing.

Processing of porcine heart valve for human heart valve replacement

Step	Process description
Collection of heart	Fresh and sound porcine heart is collected in ice in Styrofoam containers as early as possible after pig slaughter.
Inspection	Heart is thoroughly inspected for conditions before dissection.
Harvesting of aortic valve	Aortic valve from porcine heart is harvested aseptically by series of five cuts.
Preservation	Fresh aortic valves are placed in buffered saline solution and preserved under refrigeration.
Dissection	Fresh dissection of aortic valve to a proper size and septal shelf. There are three steps are generally followed:

	i. Scissor cleaning to separate myocardium and adventitia. ii. Turning of valve inside out to judge the architecture. iii. Turn to natural position by blade cleaning.Following blade cleaning coronary arteries are sutured and valve is fixed with fixation valve holder.
Fixation	Fixation of valve for few days transform the fresh tissue into biological plastic or bioprosthetic heart valve using 0.2% solution of glutaraldehyde. In the process of fixation additional collagen crosslinks are added to provide the strength to valve.
Orificing	Fixed valves are checked for capacity of orifice to bear high pressure (82 mm Hg) or low pressure (1.5 mm Hg) recirculating fluid pressure system depending on choice of valve.
Fixed dissection	Fixed valve is inspected by eyes and stereo-microscope for physical anomalies. Sizing of annulus and trimming of aorta followed by removal of adventitia if any by forceps.
Mounting bias	Valves are mounted on appropriate sized stents aseptically.
Sizing and alignment	Valve is checked with sterio-microscope and if necessary extra parts are shaped.
Holder attachment	Stented valve is stitched with annulus by square knot and pulmonary conduit by surgeon's flat knots. Inflow and outflow of valve is check for accuracy and extra parts are trimmed if necessary. Complete first step of bias by purse string stitches and second by ticked tissue and stent. Hold the valve on valve holder by suturing.
Sterilization packaging	Valve is placed in glutaraldehyde in sterilized package.
Final quarantine	Valves are finally quarantined and check for abnormalities and fitness.
Shipping	Heart valves are ready for shipment for human implantation

Bile

Bile is a dark, golden greenish viscous fluid obtained from gall bladder. It is very bitter in taste and alkaline in nature. The specific gravity of bile is 1.020 to 1.025. Chemically bile is a mixture of conjugated bile acids (70% of cholic and deoxycholic acid), bile pigments, fatty acids, phospholipids, proteins, cholesterol and other minor components. Cholic and deoxycholic acid are used in synthesis of corticosteroids. Bile salts are responsible for emulsification of fats in intestine and play an important role in absorption of fatty acids. In natural form bile is perishable and putrefies easily. For its better and prolong use as liquid, bile is diluted and acidified and filter precipitated with mucins. Bile can also be converted syrup or powder to reduce the volume. Liquid bile after dilution with water in a ratio of 1:5 can be utilized as detergent. Dried bile can be utilized in secretion disorders. It can be obtained by using acidification of bile with acetic acid followed by mucin precipitation and concentration into syrup. Finally it can be dried by vacuum drying and converted into powder.

Gallstones

Gallstones are precious products can be collected and processed by drying. The highest priced gallstones are reddish brown stones. Special care is required in collection of gall stones from spleen because of brittleness and discolouration on sunlight. For high quality stones recovery they are placed separately and drying should be done in trays with wire gauze. After drying they should be packaged in tissue paper or cotton wool followed by paper. Shipment of gall stones can be done in cardboard or wooden boxes.

Organs and glands are very useful in human life if processed properly. The technologies and awareness about the importance of organs and glands are needs to be made available to the butchers and slaughter personnel. The facilities and technical staff training is utmost important to cater the high value organs and glands for medicinal and pharmaceutical uses.

References

1. Elamin, B.A., Al-Maleki, A., Ismael, M.A., Ayoub M.A. (2014). Purification and functional characterization of pancreatic insulin from camel (*Camelus dromedarius*). Saudi Journal of Biological Sciences, 21: 574–581.

2. Kondaiah, N., Anjaneyulu, A.S.R., Lakshmanan, V. (1993). Incorporation of chicken by-products in mutton nuggets. J Food Sci. Technol., 30(2):143–144.

3. Liu, D.C. (2002). Better utilization of by-products from the meat industry 2002-10-01. Extension Bulletins. Food and fertilizer Technology Center for the Asian and Pacific region (FFTC publication database)

4. Ockerman, H.W. and Hansen, C.L. (1988). Medicinal and pharmaceutical uses of by-products. *In:* Animal By-Products Processing, Jointly Published by Ellis Horwood Ltd., Chichester, England and VCH, Weinheim, New York (USA), Pp 176-201.
5. Sharma, B.D. (2003). Glandular by-products. *In:* Modern Abattoir Practices and Animal By-products Technology, First Edition, Jaypee Brothers Medical Publishers,New Delhi. Pp 129-134.

Chapter **20**

Abattoir and Meat Plant Effluent Treatment

Abattoir is a structure meant to recover the edible portions of slaughtered animals for human consumption. These structures are used to cater the need of domestic purposes as well as some of them are utilized for export purposes. The demand of Indian meat and meat products is increasing day by day not only in our country but also around the globe. Therefore, millions (about 15 million cattle and buffalo and 1 million sheep and goat) of food animals are slaughtered every year to meet the current demand. Such large scale slaughter of food animals generates huge amount of wastes but due to lack of proper sanitary measures in majority of slaughter houses of our country their wastes not only deteriorate the hygiene of meat and meat products but also pose a potential threat to the environment. Therefore, it is an urgent need for safe and proper disposal of slaughter house and meat processing waste for food safety and human health. It is also important to protect the environment and to improve the quality and hygiene of meat and meat products.

Abattoir and meat processing plant generates significant quantities of waste materials including organic and inorganic solids. The solid waste mainly comprised of non edible left over's viz. leather, hair, wool, hooves, waste of the rumen and intestines, bones, undigested ingesta, bladder as well as womb and occasionally aborted foetuses whereas, blood, urine, water, dissolved solids and gut contents are the major components of liquid wastes. It is general thinking that abattoir activities are responsible for the pollution of surface and underground waters as well as air quality which indirectly affect the health of residents living within the vicinity of abattoirs. In addition, primary producers in affected water bodies may be destroyed by such pollutants, which may directly affect fish yield, with serious consequences on diet. In general, large animal (cattle and buffalo) slaughter house produces 12.6 kg blood and heads, 8.0 kg intestinal contents, 6.4 kg waste tissues and 11.8 kg bones per animal slaughtered while small animal (sheep and goat) slaughter produces 0.72

kg blood and head, 1.25 kg intestinal content, 0.80 waste tissues and 2.06 kg bones after per head slaughter. The major sources contribute in abattoir effluents are lairgae, slaughtering and bleeding, dressing, paunch, rendering, processing and cleanings. Basically there are two types of materials are generated from abattoir-solid waste and liquid waste. The ideal solid waste generated is less than 7.5 kg per 500 kg of live weight while ideal water waste is less than 5000 litres/ 500 kg of live weight.

Indicators of pollution in abattoir

Slaughterhouse effluents are considered detrimental worldwide due to its complex composition of fats, proteins, and fibers, as well as the presence of organics, nutrients, pathogenic and non-pathogenic microorganisms, detergents and disinfectants used for cleaning activities, and pharmaceuticals for veterinary purposes. Therefore, the treatment and disposal of wastewater from slaughterhouses and meat processing plants are an economic and public health necessity. To define the pollution level in meat industry certain indicators are used like effluent, affluent, biological oxygen demand (BOD), chemical oxygen demand (COD), total organic carbon (TOC), total suspended solids (TSS), total nitrogen (TN) and phosphorus (TP) etc.

i. *Effluent* is generally defined as the material exited from abattoir while *affluent* means material enters in the abattoir.

ii. *Biochemical oxygen demand* (BOD) is a measure of readily biodegradable material in an effluent and can be defined as the amount of oxygen required during first 5 days to decompose organic matter at 20^{0}C by aerobic process. It is a measure of readily biodegradable material in an effluent. It is generally used to determine the concentration of pollutant remaining after treatment and prior to discharge effluent in water source. The average BOD value for poultry meat plant is 1000-1200 mg/litre, pig meat plant is 1500-2000 mg/litre and cattle/sheep meat plant is 1400-3200 mg/litre while BOD value of domestic sewage is 250-300 mg/litre which is comparatively quit low than meat plant effluent. Chicken and turkey manures have BOD concentrations in excess of 40,000 mg/kg on an as excreted basis. So it should be managed properly in poultry slaughter house. Blood is an abattoir waste has ultimate BOD of 405,000 mg per litre and requires special attention.

iii. *Chemical oxygen demand* (COD) can be defined as a measure of oxygen required for oxidation of all organic matter in a known volume of effluent using standard technique. It is used to determine the oxygen requirements of an effluent before treatment. Slaughter house or meat processing plant has COD value in the range of 2000-10000 mg per litre.

iv. *Suspended solids:* suspended solids are the solid materials produced in slaughter house or total non-filtrable residues retained on filter. In slaughter house suspended solids are mainly dependant on efficiency of intestinal content and paunch disposal. If it is higher than 300 mg per litre then sewage or effluent is considered as strong sewage.

v. *Dry matter (DM) or total solids (TS):* it is a final weight of known amount of effluent that has been dried to constant weight at 105^0C over 24 hrs. it is usually measured in gram per litre or mg per litre.

vi. *Chloride:* chloride is a measure of salinity in effluent.

vii. *pH:* pH is a measurement of alkalinity or acidity. Too much alkalinity or acidity is not desired in effluent for proper disposal. The pH of effluent should be near neutral for disposal suitability.

viii. *Grease, fat and oil (FOG):* these are immiscible substances with a lower specific gravity which cause them to float. They hamper the treatment system and measured by extraction with hexane or Freon.

ix. *Nitrogen or total Kjeldahl nitrogen (TKN):* it is the amount of nitrogen present in effluent. It is present in form of nitrate in aerobically treated effluent and high nitrate encourages the growth of algae and other plant growth. The maximum level of nitrate in effluent should be 0.5 mg per litre. The presence of ammonia in effluent is toxic to aquatic life. So the maximum discharge of ammonia in sewage should not be beyond 40 mg per litre.

Characteristics of abattoir or meat plant effluent

Meat plant effluent is constituted by a large amount of highly polluting waste waters, semi-solids such as blood, stomach content and manure etc. and solids (up to 10 percent). Abattoir or meat plant waste is called strong sewage because it contains very high values of biochemical oxygen demand (BOD) and chemical oxygen demand (COD) and high amount of solids. So it should not be discharged directly to the domestic sewage system without prior treatment. Effluent produced in abattoir or meat processing plant can be categorized in four broad categories:

i. Non toxic and none directly pollutant but liable to disturb the physical nature of receiving water.

ii. Non toxic and pollutant due to organic matter content of high oxygen demand.

iii. Toxic containing highly poisonous materials.

iv. Toxic and pollutant due to organic matter of high oxygen demand and toxic in addition.

Some of the major features of abattoir effluent can be describe as:

i. Abattoir or meat plant effluent contains up to 10% solids while municipal sewage or domestic sewage contains about 2% solids.

ii. Abattoir or meat plant waste is typically organic in nature and a high percentage of it is capable of being decomposed.

iii. It also contains grease, fat and oils and these substances tend to coat treatment systems, block pipes, pumping systems and screens. They reduce oxygen transfer and can seriously reduce the efficiency of aerobic treatment systems.

iv. In meat plant effluent or abattoir, nitrogen existed in three forms: organic nitrogen, ammonia salts and dissolved ammonia gas. Nitrogen as nitrates are found in aerobically treated effluents. The presence of ammonia in meat plant effluent is toxic to aquatic life and its maximum discharge limit to sewers is 40 mg/litre. Similarly high nitrate concentrations (above 0.5 mg/litre in potable water) in natural water encourage algae and other plant growth and block water courses.

v. Meat plant or abattoir effluent must be treated according to temperature, pH, turbidity and colour of treated water before release to a water source. Effluent before discharge to water source should have colourless and clear appearance with effluent temperature equal or few degrees above the receiving water in order not to disturb the natural biocycle and almost neutral pH.

vi. Abattoir or meat plant effluent also contains methane and sulphur dioxide.

Common characteristics of slaughterhouse wastewater

Pollution indicators	Values
BOD (mg/l)	410-4635
COD (mg/l)	1250 - 15,900
TOC (mg/l)	100-1200
TSS (mg/l)	300 - 2800
pH	4.90 - 8.10
Ca (mg/l)	32 - 316

K (mg/l)	0.01 - 100
Na (mg/l)	62 - 833
Pb (mg/l)	0.21 - 34 4
TN (mg/l)	50 - 841
TP (mg/l)	25- 200

Source: (Bustillo-Lecompte *et al.*, 2016)

Waste disposal and treatment

Waste material generated from slaughter house and meat processing plant requires immediate action for its disposal. It is because improper disposal of meat plant waste leads to serious threat to human and animal health. These wastes also provide good breeding ground for mosquitoes and flies as well as for several kinds of parasitic larvae. Therefore, it is utmost important to take certain measures for management of slaughter house waste with the following objectives:

i. Proper disposal and treatment of waste helps in elimination of public health hazards and threat of a diseases.

ii. Effluent if treated properly can be transformed into readily reusable resource thus conserve both water and nutrients.

iii. Efficient treatment of wastes is essential to ensure safe discharge of waste into water source or sewage with recommended discharge limits.

Golden rules in disposal of slaughter house or meat processing plant

The disposal of slaughter house and meat processing plant waste should be efficient to minimize environmental hazards and improve the hygienic quality of meat and meat products. It can be achieved by following certain golden rules:

i. There should be the efficient water management system to conserve the utilization of water in abattoir and meat processing plant. It can be achieved by placing the pressurized self-closing water nozzle for washing.

ii. There should be the system for reutilization and recovery of materials like fat, protein, blood and bones but minimum water should be utilized for plant operations.

iii. The solid waste generated in meat plant should be recycled by composting or biomethanation. Composting is a process of decomposing the wastes into valuable compost through microbes which can be utilized as soil conditioner. However, in biomethanation organic solids are converted into biogas (methane and CO_2) and slurry. It is generally utilized as a clean source of energy while slurry is used in agriculture fields.

iv. There should be the separate handling of solid and liquid waste. Solid waste can be achieved by screening while liquid wastes are subjected to primary treatment where chemical and electro-coagulation used to settle down the organic solids. In further treatment remaining liquid wastes is settled and treated with microbial degradation of organic matter in the effluent by biological means in septic tanks.

v. There should be the modern facilities to utilize plant waste on priority basis. It is necessary to utilize the solid and liquid separately into valuable products. It can help the plant to reduce the environmental pollution and minimize the bacterial load in the premises.

vi. It is basic necessity that illegal slaughtering of animals must be curbed to minimize water pollution, clogging of drains and generation of huge volume of waste.

Management of solid wastes

Solid waste generated from abattoir is usually disposed by burial, landfill and burning which may lead to the environmental pollution and contamination of water. So to maintain the meat quality and proper sanitation in meat plant, solid wastes must be collected twice in a day. Generally, slaughter house solid wastes are high in moisture (85-90%) and organic in nature. They can be easily biodegraded into valuable products. Solid waste generated from slaughter house or meat processing plant can be categorized into three classes-1, 2 and 3 according to European Union categories. Among which class 2 and 3 waste can be utilized in form of compost or anaerobic digestion in approved biogas plants while, category- 1 waste cannot be disposed by these methods. The common methods adopted for solid waste management are:

i. *Burial and land filling:* burial and land filling is an oldest method of waste disposal and mostly applied for domestic waste in most of Indian cities. It is not a recommended method of slaughter house or meat plant waste disposal because of risk of contamination to surface and ground water, soil and air. For burial or land filling always prefer the approved site and after burial waste should be immediately cover to a depth of at least 60 cm and not less than 100 meter from the abattoir.

ii. *Burning or incineration:* in routine practice solid waste is collected in a place near by the slaughter house and burned over fire. This practice usually lead to environmental pollution and health hazard to living beings. So for effective utilization of solid waste, incineration (controlled thermal destruction) process may be a good alternative. It is because thermal destruction most effectively destroys the potential pathogenic microbes of high risk organic waste.

iii. *Manuring:* the slaughter house solid waste particularly digestive content and excreta can be utilized as manure. It is usually collected in a place near slaughter house and dried under uncontrolled conditions in open environment in traditional system. This practice of manure production lost most of the nutrients such as nitrogen by evaporation and soluble substances like potassium and phosphorus by leaching during rains. So some shot of protection and covered environment to the manure production protect all these nutrients. Such manure may be a good source of nitrogen, potassium and phosphorus to the soil and may be helpful in enhancement of soil fertility.

iv. *Composting:* composting is an inexpensive and environmentally acceptable method for disposal of slaughterhouse wastes (both organic and inorganic) into organic manure by microbes. Compost produces high quality manure which can be utilized as organic manure for soil. Generally, there are two methods are applied for compost production i.e. *windrows and in-vessel system. Windrows* method is generally preferred over in-vessel system for slaughter house waste management. It is because windrows composting achieves higher temperature which helps in reduction of pathogenic microbes. However, *in-vessel system* requires less space, provides better control and offers high process efficiency. The cool zone of in-vessel system where no turning is applicable encourages the microbial growth which is not desirable in good quality compost.

v. *Rendering:* rendering is a process of recovery of fat from slaughter house waste and conversion of rest material into carcass meal and water. It can be achieved by heating like cooking, evaporating and drying, as well as solvent extraction followed by mechanical process such as grinding, mixing, pressing, decanting and separating. The solid waste particularly trimmings and discarded parts of animal body and dead carcasses are rendered to transform it into valuable products. The materials which may pose the health hazards must be rendered at 133^{0}C for a minimum 20 minutes at 20 bars pressure. The rendered material yields various types of meals which can be utilized in animal feed or as fertilizers whereas, fat obtained in this process can be used in animal feed, industries and as a fuel. However, currently the feeding of meat-bone meal to animals is totally banned in several countries including India due to risk of spread of BSE. However, India is producing more than 21 lakh tonnes offal and bone per annum in abattoirs. By proper utilization of such solid wastes, good quality feed can be produced for pigs, poultry, fish, dog cat etc.

vi. *Biomethanation or anaerobic digestion:* biomethanation is a biological process in which organic matter is decomposed in absence of air producing sludge for land application and biogas (methane and CO_2) as a source of energy. Thus dependency on fossil fuel can be reduced and CO_2 emission can be declined. Biomethanation process consist of four major stages i.e. hydrolysis, acidogenesis, acetogenesis and methanogenesis through which solid wastes containing high amount of protein and lipid are broken down into methane and CO_2 by fermentative and methanogenic bacteria. It is an effective method of slaughter house wastes management because thermophylic process produces higher methane and better inactivation of pathogenic organisms as well as reduced foul odour. Several meat plants are running biomethanation for slaughter waste management like Al-Kabeer Exports Pvt Ltd, Hyderabad and Hind Agro Industries, Aligarh, Uttar Pradesh. They are collecting solid wastes in dissolution tank and mixed properly with mixer. After homogenized waste goes to macerator for reducing the particle size for effective biodegradation. The material is then proceeding for anaerobic digester for biomethanation and produced biogas is stored in gasholder and is utilized as energy source. Similarly digested sludge is collected in buffer tank and pumped to filter press to dewater the residue which is utilized as bio-manure.

vii. *Alkaline hydrolysis:* alkaline hydrolysis is comparatively new technique for disposal of animal carcasses and other infectious materials generated in slaughter houses. It is an effective technique for transformation of slaughter house wastes containing proteins, nucleic acids, carbohydrates, lipids, etc. into a sterile aqueous solution consisting of small peptides, amino acids, sugars, and soaps using sodium or potassium hydroxide as catalyst for hydrolysis. In routine practice alkaline hydrolysis is carried out at 100^0C and 103 kpa for 3 hours and destroys most of the pathogenic microbes. But for prions destruction carcass material must be heated at 150^0C at 486 kpa for 6-8 hours.

viii. *Co-digestion:* co-digestion process is completed in anaerobic digestion plants. In which manure and slaughter house wastes like blood, fat stomach and viscera as well as rendering plants residues are subjected for digestion. Co-digestion process is actually helps in dilution of toxicants and maintains nutrients and proper moisture.

Management of effluent or liquid wastes

Effluent or liquid wastes generated in slaughter house mainly due to washing of slaughtering line, cleaning of the guts, carcass washing, cleaning and sanitizing of equipment and facilities, and for cooling of mechanical equipment such as compressors and pumps. In poultry scalding and defeathering is also added the liquid waste while pigs slaughter requires water for scalding. Effluent or liquid waste generated from slaughter house falls under high strength waste water having about 45% soluble and 55% coarse suspended organic matter. Effluent contains organic matter such as faeces, fat and lard, grease, undigested food, blood, suspended material, urine, loose meat, soluble proteins, excrement, manure, grit and colloidal particles is major pollutant. Liquid waste generated from a typical abattoir contains 200-1500 mg/l suspended solids, 3700-4600 mg/l total solids, 1000-4100 mg/l biological oxygen demand (BOD), 2000-10000 mg/l chemical oxygen demand (COD), 6 -7 pH and 70%-75%, moisture. Due to all these pollution indicators higher than normal sewage, it must be treated before its final disposal in domestic sewage. Liquid waste also contains high chloride content from salted skin or hide.

Treatment of effluent or liquid waste

Liquid waste or effluent generated from slaughter house is usually discharged to sewer which is generally treated by municipal treatment plant. Sometimes it is utilized in land application for irrigation. But most effective way of waste water treatment is on site treatment in which waste water treatment plant is installed in abattoir premises. For convenience waste streams lines should be separated into sanitary lines, grease and non grease waste stream, blood line and stockpen line. Each line can be handled separately according to the need like sanitary line can be directly discharge to sewage; blood can be utilized for blood meal etc and grease can be trapped and rendered. In stockpen manure is hauled as solid waste and liquid can be used as filed irrigation etc. Modern effluent treatment plants consist of various sections like preliminary treatment, primary treatment, secondary treatment and tertiary treatment.

1. *Preliminary treatment:* preliminary treatment of effluent is a combination of operations including screenings, catch basins,

equalization and settlers. The effluent is then passed through these chambers for recovery of proteins and fats. Section wise *screens* are used to separate suspended solids and remaining water is reutilized. *Catch basins* or *settling tanks* are based on principle of gravity separation and removes grease and fine suspended solids. Settling tanks are generally used to remove the scum and grease with the help of skimmer while scrappers are used to remove sludge from bottom. Preliminary treatment helps in reduction of biological oxygen demand (BOD), dissolved solids and fat by 25- 40%, 50-70% and 80-90% respectively. Quantitively BOD reduction is up to 200-250 mg/litre.

2. *Primary treatment:* primary treatment of effluent mainly comprises of dissolved air flotation technique. This technique is applied to separate very fine particles within a short period of time by using air bubbles at the bottom of floatation tank. These air bubbles help in floatation of light solids with grease and fat to the surface as scum. Developed scum is then removed with the help of skimmer. For better performance certain chemicals viz. coagulants (Alums) and flocculants (Polymers) are mixed before floatation which easily clump and precipitate proteins and improve fat floatation. This combination technique reduces the chemical oxygen demand (COD) by 32- 90% as well as Total COD (TCOD) and Suspended COD (SCOD) reduced up to 67%. In recent days electro-coagulation technique is applied in which electricity is passed through aluminium electrodes. This technique settles down the dissolved solids with in a shorter period of time. Cationic (Fe^{3+} and Al^{3+} salts) and anionic (sodium hexametaphosphate, lignosulfonate and sodium alginate) coagulants at appropriate pH precipitate and agglomerate protein and other organic materials into larger particles which can easily recovered by dissolved air floatation technique. Cationic coagulants helps in precipitation of phosphorus while anionic coagulants helps in separation of haemoglobin which makes major portion of soluble organic load in meat plant waste. Primary treatment helps in separation of dissolved solids from liquid wastes and remarkably reduces quantum of fat, suspended solids and BOD of effluent.

3. *Secondary treatment:* secondary treatment of effluent is a controlled biological treatment in which microbial cultures are used to remove organic compounds from effluent. This treatment system is capable to remove more than 90% pollutants from waste water. There are two systems of secondary treatment are generally in practice - anaerobic and/or aerobic treatment.

A. *Anaerobic treatment:* anaerobic treatment is a system in which organic matter is digested in absence of oxygen under closed system. Generally anaerobic system is suitable for waste containing high amount of organic matter and BOD level beyond 2000 mg/litre. Basically anaerobic digestion is a stage fermentation process in which volatile fatty acids are formed which are utilized by methanogenic bacteria to produce methane and CO_2 along with biologically stable sludge as a by product. It is a high efficiency process because of reduction of total solids by 50-80%, BOD and COD by 50-90%. It is low operating cost system because of low sludge production and less energy requirement. Methane can be utilized as a clean source of energy and sludge as a soil conditioner. However, system is not capable to remove nitrogen and phosphorus and maintaining of pH around 7.0-7.2 is very important. There are two systems are usually applicable for degradation of organic matter by anaerobic process.

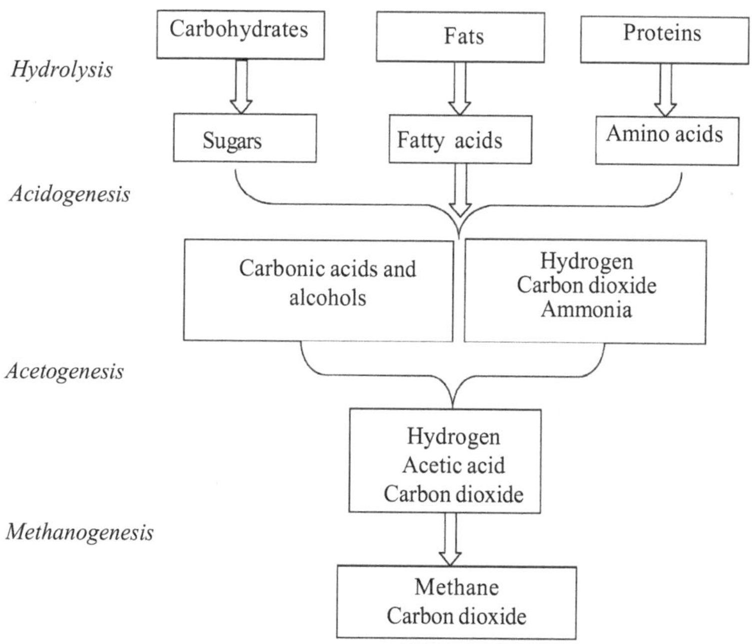

Anaerobic fermentation process

i. *Low rate system:* low rate system of effluent treatment basically comprises anaerobic lagoons. These lagoons are constructed with the depth of 3-5 meters and retention time of effluent in these lagoons is 5-10 days. In this system agitation takes place with gas mixtures and mechanical agitation is not allowed. The scum formation is on the surface which ensures the anaerobic conditions and minimizes heat loss. Low rate system of effluent treatment or anaerobic lagoon system is capable to reduce BOD by 97%, suspended solids by 95% and COD by 96%.

ii. *High-rate systems:* high rate system of anaerobic treatment is suitable for high throughput which actually accelerates the treatment process and requires less area for operation. There are five systems generally falls under this category:

   a. *Upward-flow anaerobic sludge blanket (UASB) reactor:* UASB reactor is a three phasic reactor which separates solid in form of sludge, liquid and gas particularly CO_2 and CH_4. In this process effluent enters in reactor through digester located at base. Then flows upward through a compact layer of bacteria called 'sludge blanket'. Ultimately it goes out through an outlet situated at top. UASB reactor is capable to reduce COD by 80-85% and produces biogas even at low temperature. It is suitable method for effluent carrying organic load in between 2.7-10.8 kg COD/m^3/d. It is also capable to treat 3000 litres waste water and can produce about 147.67m^3 of biogas/day which may generate 294 kWhr/ m^3/ day electricity.

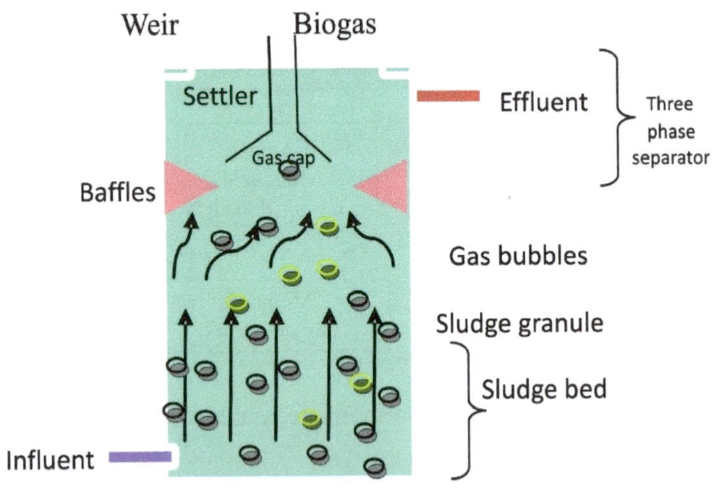

UASB Reactor

b. *Anaerobic sequencing batch reactor (ASBR)*: ASBR system comprises of feeding, settling and decanting operations to be performed in a single vessel. In this operation intermittent mixing is done in cycle but complete mixing is generally discarded. It is suitable method for handling effluent containing organic load of 2.07-4.93kg/m^3/day. It generally works at 30^{0}C and hydraulic retention time is 2 days. It requires low initial investment and operating cost with minimum daily maintenance. ASBR is capable to reduce COD by 90-96% and produced biogas contains around 75% methane which can be utilized as source of energy.

Steps	Detail
Wastewater feeding	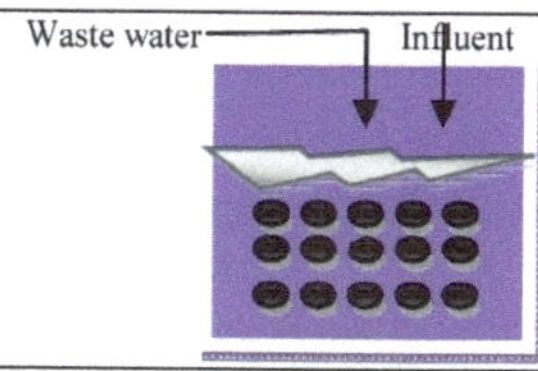
Reaction time	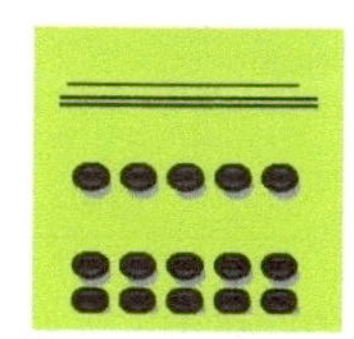
Settling and clarification	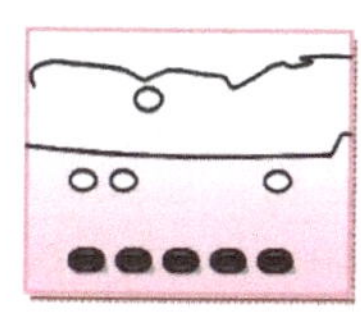
Removal of treated waste water	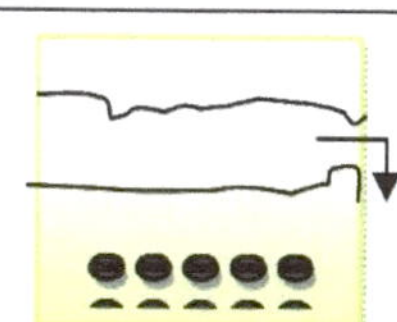
Waste sludge removal	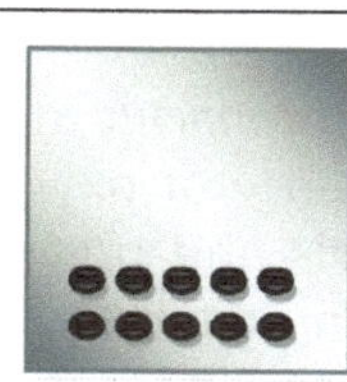

c. *Anaerobic fixed film reactor (AFFR):* anaerobic fixed reactor is an important system for pre-treatment of waste with high organic load. In the process cylindrical or rectangular tanks with built-in devices are used to retain the microbes. They help in degradation of organic material present in effluent. It is suitable method for effluent treatment contains organic load of 1.4kg/m^3/day. AFFR is also capable to reduce COD up to the level of 76-95%.

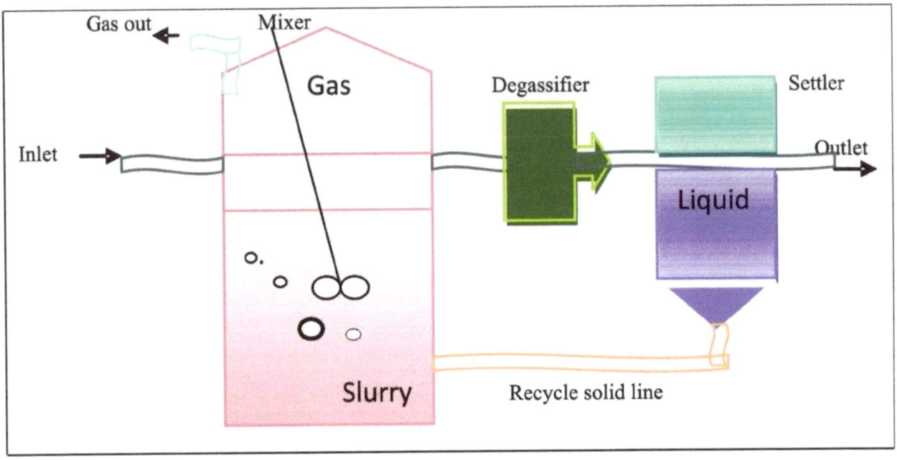

d. *Anaerobic filters (AF)*: anaerobic filter consists of column. These columns are usually filled with various types of media and operate as a fixed film reactor. The efficiency of effluent treatment in this system is basically based on temperature and hydraulic retention time. It is a suitable technique for effluent treatment containing organic loads up to 22-25 kg COD/m^3/d and can remove COD by 80-90%.

e. *Expanded granular sludge bed reactor (EGSBR):* EGSBR system is most practical method to treat the effluent containing organic load of up to 15 kg COD/m^3/d. This system effectively treats effluents at 35^{0}C and hydraulic retention time is 5 days. It is capable to reduce COD by 67%, fat by 85% and suspended solids up to 90%.

B. *Aerobic treatment:* in aerobic treatment of effluent, aerobic bacteria in presence of oxygen utilize organic matters for their own cell synthesis and organic carbon is converted into carbon dioxide, nitrogen or nitrate ions. Aerobic treatment is capable to reduce odour and pathogens in effluent thus it is necessary to treat anaerobically treated waste water with aerobic treatment before its final discharge. Aerobic treatment is also capable to remove most residual BOD and suspended solids as well as it oxidize NH_3 and H_2S into less harmful nitrate and sulphate. The systems used in this process are aerobic lagoons, activated sludge processes, extended aeration, complete mix, oxidation ditches, sequencing batch reactors (SBRs), and trickling filters and rotating biological contactors (RBCs).

i. *Trickling filters*: a trickling filter is simply a bed of stones or slug or honey combed plastic cellular modules from 3-10 feet deep through which the effluent passes. In this process effluent is applied to filter either through a network of pipes laid on or beneath the surface or by spraying from rotating horizontal pipes which trickles downward through the media to which micro-organisms are attached. Trickling filters can achieve upwards of 90% reduction of BOD and removal of suspended solids.

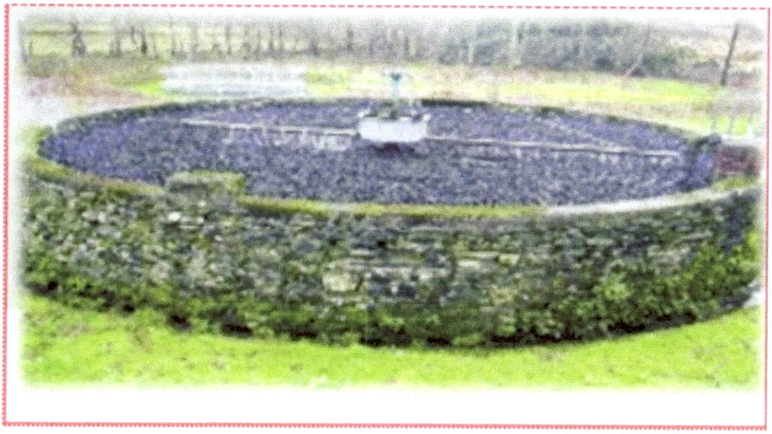

ii. *Activated sludge process*: activated sludge process is mainly comprised of two tanks: the aeration tank and the final clarifier cum settling tank. Process start with the feeding of primary treatment waste stream into aeration tank where mixing and aeration are uniformly provided by mechanical mixers and/or pressurized air diffusers. It is then passes to clarifiers cum settling tank to separate clear supernatant which can be discharged to the receiving water after chlorination while concentrated sludge is collected separately. After that in start of continuous process, a portion of about 30% activated sludge from final settling tank is brought to aeration tank which speeds up the action of aeration tank. It is because the activated sludge contains activated bacteria which actively convert organic matter into harmless inorganic matter.

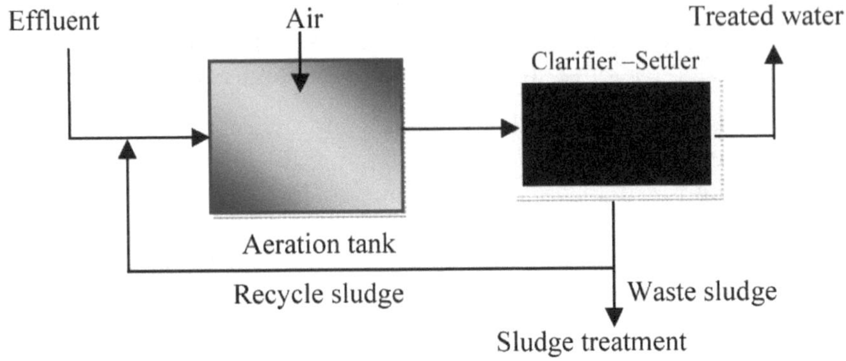

Activated sludge process

iii. *Lagoons*: lagoons are commonly used method for meat and poultry plants effluent where low cost land is available. Generally warm, clear and sunny conditions are favourable for successful operation of lagoons. Basically lagoons are scientifically constructed ponds usually 3 to 5 feet deep in which sunlight, bacteria, algae and oxygen interact. Depending on the availability of dissolved oxygen, lagoons can be aerobic or anaerobic.

Aerobic lagoons recommended dimensions of aerobic lagoons are generally 3-4 meter depth with embankment slopes of 1" to 2". It is usually lined by butyl rubber or similar masonry material to protection erosion and scours in embankments and lagoon bottom. Lagoons are basically dependant on algae for source of oxygen but it is supplemented with mechanically floating surface aerators. It is because algae can not produce sufficient oxygen required for proper functioning of lagoons particularly in winters. The exposure time in aerobic lagoon is 2-6 days depending on temperature. The sludge produced in aerobic lagoons contains high BOD and need to be removed before the effluent is discharged into a water course or used for irrigation. So series of maturation ponds are required for settling of effluent. The retention time varies for 5-10 days and number of ponds depends on reduction of faecal bacteria. Aerobic lagoons can reduce BOD and suspended solids by 90%.

Anaerobic lagoons: anaerobic lagoons are required particularly in winters when scum of grease and other floatable material forms on the top of the lagoon which facilitate insulation. In this process anaerobic decomposition of organic matter is resulted into production of methane and hydrogen sulphide but treated effluent requires oxidation before final discharge. Anaerobic lagoons are capable to reduce BOD and suspended solids by 70-80%.

The combination of *aerobic lagoons* as well as *anaerobic lagoons* is most suitable for meat industry effluent. It is because combination of both systems reduces BOD by 99%, suspended solids and grease by 98%.

4. *Tertiary treatment:* tertiary treatment is mainly comprises of biological treatments or physico-chemical treatment through which suspended or dissolved nutrients like nitrogen and phosphorous are removed. However, it is costly means of slaughter house effluent treatment so generally not recommended in routine practice.

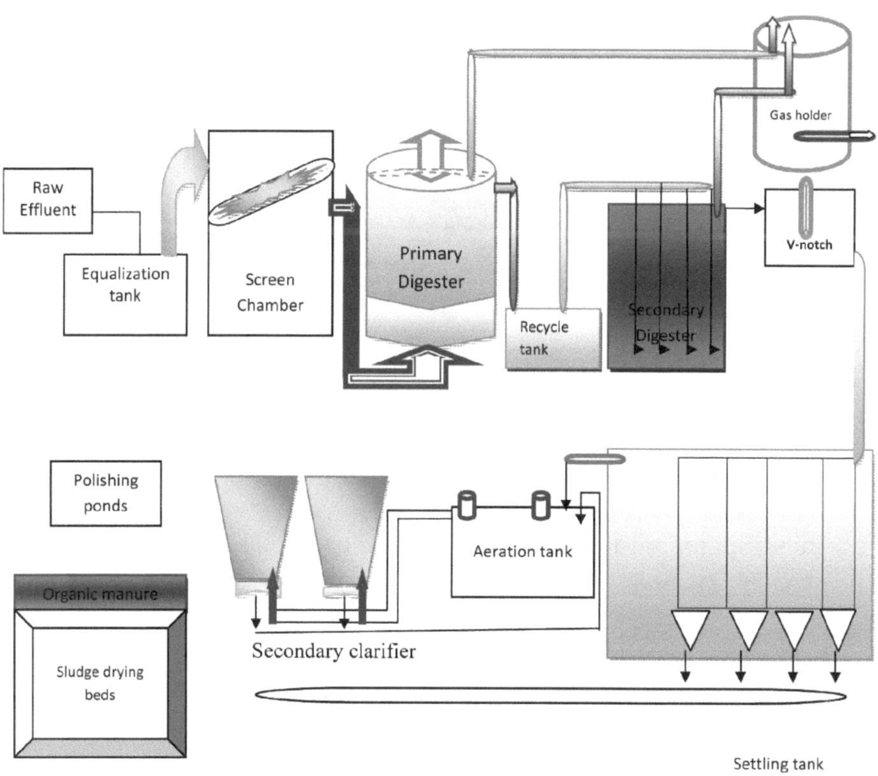

Schematic Diagram of effluent treatment plant

Novel methods for slaughter house waste treatments

In recent days many innovations has been done in treatment of effluent from different sources. Similarly some of the modern methods are also recommended to treat the effluent generated from abattoir or slaughter house.

1. *Electrocoagulation*: in electrocoagulation method of effluent treatment current is passed to facilitate the degradation of organic matter present in abattoir effluent. It is easy in operation; shorten retention time and sludge precipitate or sediment rapidly.

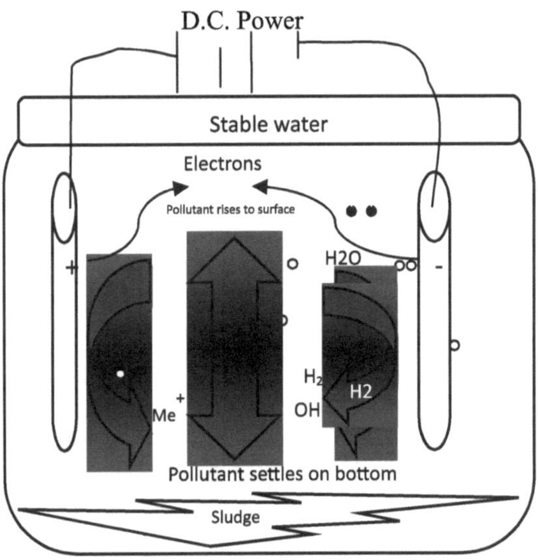

2. *Membrane separation:* there are various types of membrane filtration techniques are used now days to produce valuable substances. For example ultrafiltration is used to separate fat, oil and grease while reverse osmosis and nanofiltration for water purification, desalination and disinfection. Microfiltration is a technique used to recover or to concentrate the particulate material from slurries or liquid.

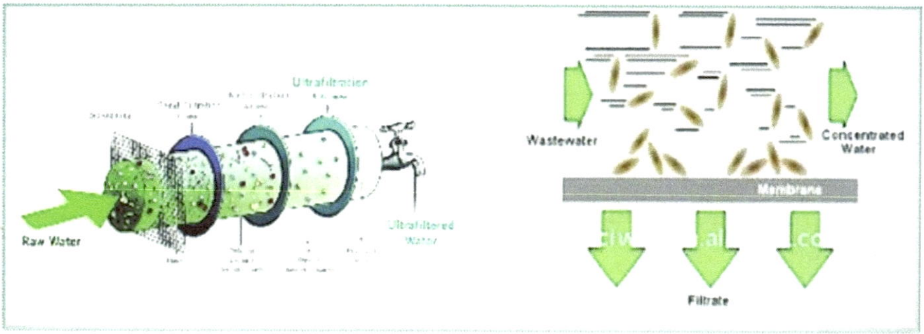

Recent trends in slaughter house waste management

Quality meat production requires effective management of slaughter house wastes. By the effective utilization of waste hazards can be minimized and hygienic quality of meat and meat product can be achieved. Some of the strategies in waste management in plant may be helpful in reduction of waste and reduces the cost of plant maintenance.

i. Water conservation in meat plant is utmost important and it can be achieved by the construction of pressurized water and fitting of self closing nozzles.

ii. Waste generation can be minimized by maximizing the recovery and reutilization of useful materials such as fat, protein blood and bone and minimum utilization of water for cleaning the floors.

iii. Solid waste generated in meat plant can be recycled by composting or biomethanation. It can convert the waste into valuable organic materials for agricultural purposes and biomethanation produces biogas (methane and CO_2) which can be utilized as source of energy.

iv. There should be the provision of separation of solid with liquid waste. Accordingly they should be managed.

v. There should be the modern infrastructural facilities development in abattoir and meat processing plants. So that most of the waste generated can be utilized and converted into valuable products.

vi. There should be the astringent rules to control the illegal slaughtering procedures. So that definite strategies can be formulated for utilization of generated waste.

v. There should be the strict provision for installation of waste treatment plant in abattoir and meat processing plant. The biogas produced through biomethanation can be utilized as alternative source of energy for plant operations.

Recommended minimum effluent standards

Parameters	Effluent utilization mode		
	Direct discharge to surface water	Used as restricted irrigation	Used in unrestricted irrigation
pH	6-9	-	-
BOD_5 (mg/l)	50	-	-
COD (mg/l)	250	-	-
Total suspended solids (mg/ml)	50	-	-
Oil and grease (mg/ml)	10	-	-
Total nitrogen	10	-	-
Total phosphorus	5	-	-
Colour	colourless	-	-
Temperature (^{0}C)	Same as sewage	-	-
Faecal coliforms (per 100 ml)	<5000	<5000	<100
Algae (per ml)	<1 lakhs	-	-

Biogas Production

Biogas production may be a good alternative as an energy source from slaughter house waste. For biogas production, animal waste along with ingesta and digestive tract content is digested aerobically. In this process raw materials are collected in airtight tanks called digesters where anaerobic digestion takes place and gas is produced. This gas then compressed in tanks and allowed to distribute for consumption. The fuel is then burnt for steam production which forces the turbines to generate electricity. Alternatively, it can be utilized for cooking, heating, lighting and even energy source for car engines. In large plants, it may fulfill the need of energy and electricity and residual part or sludge can be utilized as good source of organic fertilizer.

Biodiesel Production

Biodiesel is actually a substitute of diesel fuel produced from renewable sources such as vegetable oils, animal fats and recycled cooking oils. Biodiesel is biodegradable, non-toxic and on burning produces fewer emissions than petroleum based diesel. It may be a good alternative of fossil fuel. The fat extracted from wastewater may be a good source of biodiesel. The extracted fat can easily be converted into biodiesel by trans-esterification process. Biodiesel produced in this way has approximately 33.3 mega joules per litre gross calorific value and 0.88 kg per litre density. It is used worldwide as source of energy and blended in diesel in same way as blending of ethanol with petrol. Biodiesel can be blended successfully in diesel in a ratio of 20 percent biodiesel and 80 percent diesel.

The waste management may play key role in quality meat and meat products development besides management of environmental pollution. It may also be helpful in generation of revenues and enhancement of meat industry image. But the need is to explore and utilize the improved and economically viable techniques in disposal of slaughter house wastes. They may be helpful in generating the eco-friendly environment in the meat industry and clean source of energy can be utilized for plant operations.

References

1. Aniebo AO, Wekhe SN, Okoli IC (2009). Abattoir Blood Waste Generation in River State and its Environmental Implications in the Niger Delta. Toxicol. Environ. Chem. 91:619-625.
2. Arvanitoyannis IS, Ladas D. (2008). Meat waste treatment methods and potential uses. Int J Food Sci Tech., 43:543- 559.
3. Gracey, Collins and Hue (1999). Meat hygiene, 10th Edition, W.B. Saunders Company.
4. Hui, Nip, Rogers and Young (2001). Meat Science and Applications. Marcel Dekker Inc.
5. Masse,D.I. and Masse, L. (2000). Treatment of slaughterhouse waste water in anaerobic sequencing batch reactors. Agriculture and Agri-Food Canada. Contribution no. 659.
6. Ranken (2000). Handbook of Meat Products Technology. Blackwell. www.fao.org
7. Sindhu, R. and Meera, V. (2012). Treatment of slaughter house effluent using upflow anaerobic packed bed reactor. International Congress on Informatics, Environment, Energy and Applications-IEEA 2012 IPCSIT vol. 38, Singapore.

Chapter **21**

Sanitation of Abattoir and Meat Processing Plant

The *sanitation* word is derived from a Latin word *sanitas*, meaning "health." In true sense sanitation is the creation and maintenance of hygiene and healthful conditions in abattoir or meat processing plant. So that produced food provides full nutrients with minimal contaminations and hazards to the human health. It creates the aesthetic environment in the workplace which ultimately enhances the work efficiency and satisfaction to the workers. It helps in maintenance of clean environment, less pollution, proper waste disposal and improves ecological balance. It is a prerequisite of food safety, good hygienic practices and total quality management.

Necessity of Sanitation

Sanitation is a way of life and must come within the people. The old adage, "Sanitation doesn't cost, it pays," is more realistic today. It is because of enhancement in working efficiency and acceptability of the products by consumers. There are number of benefits can be attained by maintenance of good sanitary conditions in abattoir and meat processing plants. Some of them can be highlighted as:

1. Sanitation is the baseline to achieve the goals of hazard analysis critical control points in plant operation.
2. It enhances the shelf life of products and helps in avoidance of off flavour, taste and spoilage to the product.
3. It enhances the profit of plant owners by reducing the losses, packaging cost, pilferage losses, microbial contaminations and by enhancing the aesthetic appearance of products.
4. It enhances the morale of workers, faith of regulatory agencies and consumers. Thus enhances trust on products and confidence in the producers.

5. Prevent public health hazards and helps in reduction of pollution in environments. Thus meat processing plant and abattoir gets acceptability in that locality and society.
6. All these facts enforce the owner to make necessary provisions of sanitary requisites and install the facilities to reduce waste generation and waste maintenance.
7. Moreover, by the adoption of sanitary measures consumers get wholesome and safe food products.
8. Sanitation reduces the quantity of waste generated from plant thus helps in enhancing the profit.

Sanitary laws, regulations and guidelines

There are number of laws, regulations and guidelines are formulated and enforced by various agencies to maintain the sanitary and phytosanitary status in a plant. All these provisions are actually not static but change in response to sanitation, public health, and new scientific and technical information regarding biological, chemical, and physical hazards and other important issues brought to public attention. Some of these agencies may be discussed who are responsible for maintenance of sanitary conditions in abattoir and meat processing plants:

1. *Food and Drug Administration Regulations*: Food and Drug Administration Regulation is governed by food, drug and cosmetic act. This act mainly deals with the adulterations in foods which may cause health hazard to the consumers. Under this act adulterated or misbranded products that are in interstate commerce are subject to seizure. There are number of chemicals and their appropriate dose can be designated by this act.
2. *Good Manufacturing Practices*: Good Manufacturing Practice (GMP) regulations were published first time on April 26, 1969 by Food and Drug Administration. It primarily deals with the sanitation in manufacturing, processing, packing, or holding food. Overall GMP includes cleaning and sanitizing of equipment and utensils; storage and handling of clean equipment and utensils; pest control; and the proper use and storage of cleaning compounds, sanitizers, and pesticides.
3. *Good Hygienic Practices (GHP)*: GHP is basically a group of combined measures (physical, biological and chemical) to be taken to obtain a full proof GHP system. It is mainly governed by Schedule 4 of Food Safety and Standards (Licensing & Registration of Food Businesses)

Regulations, 2011. It controls the contamination at animal themselves, personnel, buildings, equipments, tools, water and soil. GHP is necessary to produce quality meat, reduce microbial contamination, preserve freshness and to enhance shelf-life.

4. *Total quality management*: Quality is the degree of acceptability which can be maintained by the comprehensive operations. To obtain quality products each and every operation related to processing and product development must be taken care. Total quality management is the joint responsibility of management and employees working in a plant for productivity enhancement, cost reduction, product uniformity and acceptability. Effective sanitation programme can be implemented by employees training and managemental participation and belonginess.

5. *Hazard Analysis Critical Control Points*: HACCP is a food safety management system in which seven principles are generally employed. All these principles works together to produce safe food to the consumers. HACCP principles are established by Codex Alimentarius Commission (CAC) and National Advisory Committee on Microbiological Criteria for Food (NACMCF). The seven principles of HACCP are hazard identification, identification of critical control points, establishment of critical limit, programme implementation and monitoring, implementation of corrective measures, verification and validation, record keeping and maintenance. The meat and poultry plants requires establishment of a programme at every stage of operation so that hazards can be minimized in products.

6. *U.S. Department of Agriculture (USDA) Regulations*: USDA has the provision of control in food processing through Federal Meat Inspection Act, the Poultry Products Inspection Act, and the Egg Products Inspection Act. All these inspection activities are regulated by Food Safety and Inspection Service (FSIS) established in 1981. In India, similar regulations are innacted by Food Safety Standards Authority (FSSAI) of India implemented in year 2011.

7. *Environmental Regulations:* The environmental protection agencies have the provision of enforcement of various act and statutes. Some of them are pollution control act implemented by pollution control board. Some others are resource conservation and recovery act, residual control acts etc.

Terminology commonly used in sanitation

Antimicrobial: antimicrobial are the substances which prevent proliferation of microorganisms.

Antiseptic: antiseptic are the chemical substances which interfere or inhibit the growth of certain microorganisms.

Cleaning: cleaning is a process of removal of soil from floors, equipments and objects for proper functioning and prevention of contamination in plant.

Contaminant's: contaminants are foreign and unwanted materials which can infect or contaminate the foods and hazard to the human health.

Coving: coving is a structural provision in which curved sealed edges are installed between floor and wall to facilitate cleaning and retarding insect harborage.

Cross-contamination: cross-contamination is a transfer process in which microorganisms are transferred from one food to another through a nonfood surface, such as equipments, utensils, or human hands.

Deflocculation: deflocculation is a process through which aggregates are breaks into individual parts.

Detergent: detergents are chemical cleaning agents similar to soaps but they are chemically different. They assist in cleaning by reducing the surface tension. Thus reduces the amount of mechanical energy for cleaning.

Disinfect: disinfect is a process through which potentially pathogenic microorganisms are removed from food processing plants, equipments and environment.

Disinfectant: Disinfectants are those chemicals which are capable to destroy the growing forms of potentially pathogenic microorganisms but not necessarily the spores.

Dispersion: dispersion is sometimes called deflocculation in which mass is converted into fine particles that are suspended in solution.

Endotoxin: endotoxins are those toxins produced within a microorganism and liberated when the microorganism is disintegrated.

Exotoxin: exotoxins are those toxins excreted by microbes into the surrounding medium.

Germicide: germicides are the chemicals which posses the ability to kill certain microbial cells.

GRAS substances: food additives that are designated as "Generally Regarded As Safe" for use in foods.

Hygiene: hygiene is a state to maintain good health by providing safe food, environment and working atmosphere.

Ionic: substances used in sanitation with electrical charge are ionic substances.

Nonionic: substances used in sanitation with lack of electrical charge through a balance of negatively and positively charged compounds.

Pollution: pollution is the condition in which foreign or unwanted materials are accumulated in environment and causes nuisance or a danger to the human health.

Potable: potable term is generally used for water suitable or safe for drinking.

Sanitary: sanitary is a condition in plant which is free from disease causing microorganisms and other harmful substances.

Sanitation: Sanitation is maintenance of conditions good for health and environment.

Sanitization: sanitization is a process of destruction of all pathogenic and almost all non pathogenic micro-organisms from floor, equipments and objects to make safe production.

Sanitize: sanitize is a condition in which plant is treated with heat or chemicals to reduce the number of microorganisms to a safe level.

Soap: soap is a compound of fatty acids and alkalies used for cleaning purpose.

Sterile: sterile is a condition in plant, equipments or objects which is free from all living microorganisms.

Sterilization: it is absolute term through which all living organisms are destroyed by physical, chemical or any other means.

Pre-requisites of meat and poultry plant sanitation

Food safety is a prime concern today which can be achieved by proper sanitation. Proper sanitation is also necessary to prevent the food borne illnesses, to enhance the sale, reputation, consumer confidence and to meet out the legal standards. To achieve these objectives following parameters are to be taken care:

1. There should be a definite cleaning and disinfection plan in a plant.
2. All buildings, fixtures, and other physical facilities of the plant should be maintained in a sanitary condition.
3. All portions of the operation must be thoroughly cleaned then sanitized.
4. There should be pest control and employee training programs. So they may be aware about the sanitary practices.
5. Always avoid the cross contaminations for plant, food, food contact surfaces and food packaging materials.
6. Always use the good quality cleaning agent and disinfectant with proper concentration and exposure time.
7. There should be the judicial use of insecticides and rodenticides with certain precautions.
8. The equipments used in plant should always be maintained in proper sanitary conditions and their design should be suited for cleaning and disinfections.
9. Employees who appear healthy should be allowed to work in food contact areas. Any person who is known to have, or appears to have, an illness, open lesion, including boils, sores, or infected wounds, or any other possible contamination should always be avoided.
10. Plant and exterior surroundings should be kept in a sanitary manner to protect against possible contamination due to rodent infestation.
11. There should be facility of sanitary equipments, facilities and basic amenities like brushes, pails, scrapers, cleaners, sanitizers and high pressure equipments.
12. Always handle raw as well as processed foods in a platform which has gone through proper cleaning and sanitization.
13. There are number of organisms responsible for contamination to the carcasses. They are *Salmonella* and *Campylobacter, Aermonas hydrophila, Listeria monocytogenes* etc. *Campylobacter* can cause serious threat to the human beings while *L. monocytogenes* is a challenge for meat processors because it is very difficult to eliminate this pathogen from the processing plants. So they must be considered during sanitation and carcass decontaminations.

Cleaning of meat and poultry processing plant

Cleaning term is generally applied to remove dust, dirt and organic substances such as fat, protein particles etc. from plant structures like walls, floors and equipments. Cleaning helps in providing the clean environment to the workers and removes 90 percent of micro-organisms. However, biofilms of micro-organisms cannot be removed simply by cleaning. For removal of these biofilms there are certain chemical compounds are required. They should call as cleaning agents. The effective cleaning can be obtained if the compounds used for cleaning possess following quality characteristics:

1. Cleaning compounds should not impart salt deposition over equipments. They should also have good compatibility with chelating or sequestering agents or sequestrants.
2. They should have action similar to detergents to decrease the surface tension thus facilitates dislodging of soil from walls, floors and equipment surfaces.
3. They may have the capacity to break the fat and protein particles into physically small size than original.
4. They should have the peptizing ability means alkaline solution when used with proteinous material may form the colloidal solution from partially soluble materials.
5. They must have good rinsibility means they should wash easily with water with minimal residual levels.
6. They should have good saponification property means they can convert insoluble material such as crude fat into soluble crude soap.
7. They should have the good wetting property so that they can dissolve the materials easily.

Cleaning steps

To remove all visible particles from the equipments and facilitues generally seven cleaning steps are followed in manual cleaning. They may be summarized as:

1. Dry cleaning of plant surface and areas followed by picking up scraps of meat and other materials.
2. Scrapping of equipments and machineries by using rubber scrapper to reduce the contamination as much as possible.

3. Rinsing of all surfaces with hot water maintained at 40-50^{0}C.
4. Cleaning of surfaces using alkaline cleaning agent.
5. Rinsing with hot water maintained at 80-85^{0}C.
6. Sanitization of the equipments and objects using chemical sanitizers.
7. Drying of the equipments and surfaces using drip drying or clean rubber scrapper.

Cleaning process is generally adopted to remove all visible materials adhered with equipments and facilities. It also reduces number of bacteria but not necessarily all. So cleaning is always supplemented with sanitization to remove all pathogenic micro-organisms. In meat plant, chlorine and iodine are the most commonly used sanitizers. Chlorine is used for sanitization in the strength of 100-200 ppm while iodine in the strength of 12-25 ppm. The recommended contact time for effective sanitation for these compounds is about 30 minutes.

Cleaning compounds

There are number of cleaning compounds are used in abattoir or meat processing plant. They are broadly classified as alkaline (pH 7-14), acidic (pH 0-7), neutral (pH 7) etc. Most of the cleaning agents used in meat plant for removal of fat, oil, grease and proteins belong to alkaline solutions. The acid cleaning agents are good to remove encrusted surface materials and dissolve mineral scale deposits. However, better results can be obtained with the combination of alkaline and acidic in alternate way serve the purpose better. Synthetic detergents are also used to emulsify the fats, oils and grease and also added the property of lower the surface tension of solution which promotes wetting particles, deflocculation and suspension of soil particles.

Major group of cleaning agent	Minor group of cleaning agents	Examples	Optimum pH	Qualities	Uses
Water	Potable water	Soft water	Neutral	Water is a universal solvent. So generally used for rinsing but it is capable to dissolve and float the soil. Hot water (80-90^{0}C) or steam (100^{0}C) is more effective. But hot water polymerizes the fat and denatures the protein and bind with surface and soil. So for better results water can be added with detergents and sanitizers. Water is also known as natural detergent but has poor wetting and surfactant property due to higher interfacial tension.	Rinsing of floors, walls, equipments and objects.
Alkaline cleaning agents	Strong alkaline cleaners	Sodium hydroxide (caustic soda) and silicates	>11	Highly germicidal activity, protein dissolution, and deflocculation/ emulsifying properties and can be used for removing heavy soils. No role in mineral deposits. But corrosive so limited in use particularly for manual cleaning.	Generally 0.2-2.0% concentration is used. It is most suitable for cleaning of commercial ovens and smokehouses.

	Heavy duty alkaline cleaners	Sodium metasilicate (good buffering agents), sodium hexametaphosphate, sodium pyrophosphate, sodium carbonate, and trisodium phosphate	>11	Good soil-emulsification activity. Excellent for removing fats but have no value for mineral deposit control. Slightly corrosive.	Commonly used cleaning agents for CIP, high pressure and in other mechanized system used in meat and poultry plants. They can be used as good buffering agents and can tie with chelating agents.
	Mild Alkaline Cleaners	Sodium bicarbonate, sodiumsesquicarbonate, tetrasodium pyrophosphate, phosphate water conditioners (sequesters) and alkyl aryl sulfonates (surfactants).	8-10	Good water-softening capabilities No value for mineral deposit control.	Good for hand cleaning of lightly soiled areas.
	Chlorinated Alkaline Cleaners	-	-	Cleaners to peptize the proteins for easier removal	Good for cleaning in-place (CIP) of pipes, tanks, and vats and remove effectively fats, oils, grease, and proteins.
Acidic cleaning	Strong acid cleaners	Hydrochloric, hydrofluoric,	4-6	Capable to remove the encrusted surface matter and mineral scale.	Good for steam-producing

agents		sulfamic, sulfuric and phosphoric acids.		Nitric and sulfuric acids are not used in manual cleaning because of its corrosive properties.	equipments, boilers, and some processing equipment.
	Mild acid cleaners	Levulinic, hydroxyacetic, acetic, and gluconic acids	>6	Effective against encrusted material. Less corrosive.	Suitable for manual cleaning
	Cleaners with active chlorine	Sodium or potassium hypochlorite	-	Efficiently removes carbohydrate and/or proteinaceous soils.	Suitable for meat plant cleaning.
Detergents or surfactants	Soapy detergents	Made by heating of vegetable or animal fat with alkali (caustic soda)	-	Reduces surface tension and effectively works with water.	Rinsing of equipments, floor, walls and objects.
	Soapless detergents	Made from mineral oils with sulphur trioxide by sulpho-nation process.	-	Available in powder and liquid form.	Rinsing of floor, walls and objects.
Synthetic detergents	Cationic wetting agents	Quaternary ammonium compounds	-	Producing positively charged active ions in an aqueous solution.	Detergents are poor wetting agents but strong bactericidal.
	Anionic wetting agents	Sodium salt of various complex organic materials	-	Producing negatively charged active ion in solution.	Most commonly used wetting agents because of good compatibility with alkaline cleaning

					agents and good wetting qualities.
	Nonionic wetting agents	Teepol	-	Producing no charge in an aqueous solution.	Good wetting agent in both alkaline and acidic conditions and not affected with hard water. But produces foam which is not desirable. The ratio of anionic and nonionic detergent in a ratio of 2:1 is most effective for meat industry.
Enzyme-based foam cleaners	*Bacillus* based cleansers	They contains a number of enzymes like proteases combat protein-based stains, amylases work on carbohydrates and starches while lipotases break down fats or lipids.	-	They are proteases because they break down protein and work best on the alkaline side at 60°C or lower.	Break soil into smaller pieces and aid in its removal by destroying bacterial attachment sites.

Types of cleaning

Cleaning is basically of two types-dry and wet cleaning.

Dry cleaning is generally used as first step in floor and equipment cleaning. In dry cleaning scraps such as coarse solid particles are physically removed using dry brush or broom and shovel. It is necessary step before wet cleaning because it reduces waste water and avoids the chances of clogging the drains.

Wet cleaning is generally utilized water of sufficient quantity to remove the dirt and organic substances from the premises of abattoir and meat processing plant. In small plants *manual cleaning* is performed but modern plants requires *high pressure cleaning system.*

1. *High pressure water cleaning system*: the high pressure system is generally used 30-70 bar pressure through a spray nozzle. For fatty surfaces and places where fat is handled requires high pressure system with hot water (at least 55°C temperature) facility. It is an efficient technique of cleaning floor and walls of meat processing plant particularly for the removal of small solid parts, blood, dirt, meat and fat particles. It can also be effectively used for removal of meat and fat as well as protein particles from equipments. However, better results can be achieved when supplemented with dry cleaning and by the use of hot water.
2. *Pressurized steam cleaning:* the effectivity of cleaning can further be enhanced by using pressurized steam at 100^{0}C. But production of intense fog and aerosols leads to spreading of microbes and high humidity with condensation. So pressurized steam technique is generally not preferred in meat industry.
3. *Chemical cleaning system*: the presence of sticky or encrusted layers of fat and proteins in meat plant cannot be effectively removed by water and steam system. These materials actually require certain chemicals to remove it completely. Traditionally *alkali* solutions such as sodium carbonate, washing soda are effectively used to dissolve organic dirt, fat and protein residues. But these chemicals have corrosive effect on equipments above pH 11. *Acid* cleaning agents are effective against encrusted residues of dirt or protein or of inorganic deposits or scales such as waterstone, lime etc. *Neutral* cleaning agents are not as effective as acid or alkaline solutions but can be utilized for manual cleaning of smooth surfaces without encrusted dirt. So in modern day's combination of chemicals are used for cleaning in meat industry as alkaline for routine practice

and acid for cleaning of encrusted substances. The cleaning agents are sometime added with *surfactants* or *detergents* because they decrease the superficial tension of water and act as surface active agents to loose the dirt. Detergents also have additional cleaning components such as chlorine, silicate or phosphate.

4. *Foam cleaning system*: in today world, modern plants are preferred to use foam cleaning system in large plants. In this system water foam containing detergents and other cleaning agents such as alkaline or caustic foam, chlorinated and acid based foams or neutral foams and gels are sprayed on wet walls, floors, ceilings, piping, belts, equipment surfaces and storage containers. The generated foam produces long lasting effect and after impact period of 15 minutes foam is washed with high pressure water spray. Foam is quite effective method of cleaning and saves labour and time. It is safe to use, biodegradable and produces less effluent problem.
5. *Gel cleaning system*: gel cleaning system works on the same principle as high pressure system but gel is the cleaning medium rather than sprays. It is because gel is more effective cleaning agent and clings with the surface to remove soil. It is effective cleaning method for packaging equipments.
6. *Foam and gel cleaning system*: in foam and gel cleaning system cleaning agents are adhered with soil and break them by chemical reaction. It can be removed easily by rinsing. The system is operated by compressed air or sometime with electrically operated compressor. In this system expansion of solution is quite high (15-20 times) and about 45.4 litre solution can be expanded to 727-909 litres which is capable to cover about 55.7-92.9 square meter area within 15-20 minutes. Gel cannot collapse easily and produces long lasting effects when added with foam. Gel is also effective on hot surfaces and can remove even very thin layers of fat and proteins. It also has all the benefits mentioned in foam cleaning system.

Automated systems of cleaning

1. *Cleaning –in-place (CIP) system*: in CIP system, cleaning agents are circulated through the pipes and clean all the internal surfaces attached with each other. In this system cleaning, rinsing and sanitization takes place automatically under closed system. It is most suitable method for liquid industry particularly liquid milk plant. Though CIP can also be utilized for foods which are processed in liquid form. It can be utilized in cleaning and sanitization of vacuum thawing chambers, pumping and brine circulation lines, pre-blend

or batch silos and fat rendering. CIP can be utilized in cleaning of mixers, choppers, tanks and other equipments. In poultry plants CIP can be utilized in washing of shackles, rollers and chains.

2. *Central cleaning system (CCS)*: CCS cleaning system is a preferred method of cleaning in meat plant. In this system cleaning is performed using a centrally located pump system. The centrally located pump is capable to maintain a pressure of 35-49 bars and can spray about 136-181 litres water or cleaning agent to distant locations in meat plant. It can mix the detergents as well as cleaning agents at centre point and supply to different locations of meat plant for effective cleaning and rinsing. Alternatively, detergents can supply separately using a cleaning gun and water can be used separately for rinsing.

3. *Self-contained system(SCS)*: SCS cleaning system contains various units at a place like water pumping system, chemical spray system, foam generation unit, hot/steam and cold water supply system. The system can also be utilized as portable system and failure of one unit can not affect another unit.

4. *Cleaning-out-of-Place (COP)*: COP system consists of a cabinet with oscillating spray bars. Spray bar facilitates the cleaning in all areas with high pressure volume. System has limited use in meat and poultry industry. However, it can be utilized in washing of equipments, racks, returnable containers. The recycling of water and detergent can be done so it saves the cost of cleaning. The complete process of washing and rinsing takes about 5-20 minutes depending on the nature and amount of soil adhered with the equipments.

Disinfection and sanitization

Disinfection or sanitization terms are most of the time used as synonyms. They can define as a process of complete elimination of surface micro-organisms or contaminations. Traditionally there are two methods of plant disinfections- hot water or steam disinfection and chemical disinfection. The efficiency of disinfection is basically depends on proper cleaning because it helps in removal of microorganisms embedded in encrusted dirt, protein and fat which cannot be properly dissolved by disinfection chemicals. The most commonly used sanitizers in meat industry are hot water, chlorine, iodophors, and quaternary ammonia compounds. Disinfection can be achieved by stationary equipment or by mobile spray units. Stationary equipment is generally used for small plant while mobile spray unit is preferred for large plant units. For best results disinfectant solution should have the temperature up to 50^{0}C and exposure time should be at least 30 minutes. The effective rinsing is another prerequisite for best disinfection plan. The combination of organic acids, surfactant {alkylbenzene sulfonates (detergents), (fatty acid) soaps, lauryl sulfate foaming agent), di-alkyl sulfosuccinate (wetting agent), lignosulfonates (dispersants) etc} and peroxide compounds (sodium peroxide or bleaching agent) can also serve the purpose in much more effective manner.

The basic aim of disinfection in abattoir or meat processing plant is to kill all the pathogenic micro-organism. There should be a definite plan of cleaning and disinfection of various equipments used in meat and poultry processing plant. Hand tools, meat saws and cutting boards should be cleaned and disinfect several times in day using hot water and suitable chemicals. Grinders, fillers, stuffers and other dismantled equipments should be disinfected daily while some equipments, floors and walls of processing and chilling rooms should be disinfected on weekly interval.

The sanitization of carcasses can be achieved by using acidified sodium chlorite, hydrogen peroxide, trisodium phosphate, cetylpyridinium chloride alone or in combination. Electrochemically activated solution is a mixture of sodium hypochlorite and peroxides can also be used for wide range of microorganisms. The combination of organic acids and hydrogen peroxide can use for carcass washing. To inhibit the *Clostridium perfringens* 2 percent sodium citrate or sodium lactate can successfully be used. But inhibition of *L. monocytogenes* can be achieved by using citric acid with irradiation. Carcasses can be decontaminated from Salmonella using combination of cetylpyridinium chloride, lactic acid and sodium tripolyphosphate.

Group of disinfectant/ sanitizers	Examples	Qualities	Uses
Halogen or chlorine containing compounds	Sodium or calcium hypochlorite Gaseous chlorine and hypochlorous acid	Effective against a wide range of bacteria and act by penetrating the cell walls. Chlorine when mixed with water produces hypochlorus acid and hypochlorite ion depending on pH. At low pH hypochlorous acid is produced more which is quite effective for	130-220 ppm strength is good for plant sanitation while for carcass washing maximum strength should be 100 ppm.

		sanitization of water. Corrosive effect on equipments.	
Quaternary ammonium compounds (QUAT)	Cetyl trimethyl ammonium bromide (CTAB), lauryl dimethyl ammonium chloride (LDAC)	They are cationic detergents and can be used as disinfectant and act on cell walls It also posses cleaning properties and can act as surfactant. Odourless and non corrosive.	Good cleansing agent but not suitable for meat industry as disinfectant because of bacteriostatic property only against G+ve bacteria and inactivated by organic matters. Combination of acid sanitizers and QUAT can be effectively used to control *L. monocytogenes* and mould growth.
Amphoteric compounds	Long chain substituted amino acids or betaines	Surface active agents. Compatible with other detergents and sanitizers. Not affected with hard water.	Not common in food industry due to high cost.
Organic acids	Acetic, butyric, propionic, valeric acid, citric acid.	Destroy micro-organisms effectively. Corrosive in nature.	Not commonly used in meat industry as sanitizer.The combination of sodium chlorite and citric acid is commonly used as antimicrobial in meat and poultry plant.
Oxygen releasing substances	Peroxide compounds (H_2O_2) & Per acetic acid	Effective against most of the micro-organisms, spores and viruses. Odourless	Used for decont-aminsation of carcasses.

		Corrosive above 1% concentration.	
Combination of disinfectants	Organic acids + surfactants + peroxide compounds	Commercially used combination of disinfectant. Organic acid acts as sanitizer and helps in lowering the pH, surfactants or surface active agents are helpful in penetration of organic materials. The peroxide compounds have direct antimicrobial effect by coagulation and denaturation of proteins (virus) and penetration through cell walls causing cell destruction (bacteria).	Effective sanitizers for meat plant.

Ideal cleaning and disinfection plan

1. *Pre-cleaning*: pre-cleaning of abattoir and meat processing plant should be done with dry sweeping followed by potable water of 40-50^{0}C under 20-30 bar pressure.
2. *Cleaning*: cleaning should always be performed daily with alkaline cleaning substance (pH about 12) in a 1.0 percent concentration at 40-50^{0}C with the exposure time of at least 20-30 minutes. It is always advisable to clean the plant in a monthly interval with 1.5% acid cleaning substance (pH about 1.8) maintained at 40-50^{0}C with the exposure time of at least 20-30 minutes.
3. *Rinsing*: rinsing should be done under pressure (5-10 bars) with potable water maintained at 30-50^{0}C.
4. *Drying*: plant and equipment surfaces are allowed to dry for sufficient period of time.
5. *Disinfection*: disinfection of plant can be done twice in a week with suitable disinfectant (pH about 5.7) in a concentration of 0.5 percent. The temperature of disinfectant should be 30-40^{0}C with the exposure time of at least 30 minutes. For best results it should also be disinfected with another disinfectant (pH about 10.2) in a concentration of 1.0 percent thrice in a week. The temperature of disinfectant and exposure time should be similar as mentioned in previous disinfectant.

6. *Final rinsing*: final rinsing should be done under pressure (5-10 bars) with potable water maintained at 30-50^{0}C.

Sanitation in meat and poultry plant is utmost important operation to produce quality meat and products. It can be achieved by making a plan and their proper implementation. The use of cleaning agents and sanitizers is basically depends on the area of sanitization, type of equipment used and their ultimate utilization as well as the nature of soil. The cleaning agent's mostly alkaline cleaning agents are used to remove soil and mineral depositions from the plant. The sanitization can be done using chlorine or iodine. But best results can be obtained by using combination of cleaning and sanitization techniques.

References

1. Gracey, J.F. and Collins, D.S. (1994). Meat plant construction, equipments and operations. *In:* Reprint of 9th Edition, Meat Hygiene, ELBS, The Bath Press, Avon. pp 117-139.
2. Marriott, N.G. (1990). Meat sanitation guide II. American Association of Meat Processors and Virginia Polytechnic Institute and State University, Blacksburg.
3. Marriott, N.G. and Gravani,R.B. (2006). Meat and Poultry Plant Sanitation. *In:* 5th ed. Principles of Food Sanitation, Springer Science and Business Media Inc. 295-325.
4. Singh,V.P. and Sharma, B.D. (1998). Sanitation in meat processing plant. Processed Food Industry, 1 (12): 16-18.
5. Stanfield, P. (2003). Seafood processing: Basic sanitation practices. *In:* Food plant sanitation, eds. Y.H. Hui, et al., 543. New York: Marcel Dekker, Inc.
6. Walstra, P., Wouters, J.T.M. and Geurts, T.J. (2006). Fouling and sanitization. *In:* Dairy Science and Technology, 2nd edition, Taylor and Francis, Pp 399-410.

Chapter 22

Glossary of Terms in Wool Industry

Animal Fibers	The animal materials like wool, hair, fur, mohair and silk used for weaving, knitting or felting into a fabric are generally termed as animal fibers. Animals used for the purpose are sheep, goat, llama, alpaca, camel, vicuna and silk worm.
Apparel wool	Wool used for preparation of clothes or apparel fabrics except carpet and pulled wool is called apparel wool.
Bale	Wool packs containing a specified minimum weight of wool. In common term one bale weighing 100-200 kg wool.
Ball	The unit of large quantity of processed wool in which wool fibers are wound around its own middle and form a solid mass of wool.
Batt or Batting	The sheets or rolls of fibers or carded wool or cotton or mixture thereof which is normally used for spinning, felting, quilting, stuffing , padding etc.
Bellies	The wool obtained from belly region of sheep which are usually short and often defective is termed as bellies.
Blacks or Black Wool	Sheep fleece of grey, brown or black colour is called blacks or black wool. It is considered low value fleece than white but can be classified as fine, medium and coarse.
Blanket	The term blanket was evolved on the name of English Flemish weaver Thomas Blanket who used a cloth first time in 14th century as a covering for warmth and sleeping.
Blend	Blend term is generally used for textile containing two or more different fibers or variants of the same fiber with different colors and grades.
Blood	The terms blood in wool industry is generally applied in American grading system of wool which indicate degree of fineness. It is actually indicative of Merino blood present in native sheep.

Bold	Bold is a term indicated well-grown wool of good character.
Braid	Term Braid is applied in United States for long, lustrous and coarsest wool while in Canada for course wool.
Break	Break is a condition during growth of wool fiber in which wool becomes marked thin and weak at a point in staple. The condition arises mainly due to sudden change in pasture, feed, water, diseases, faulty dipping, bad lambing etc.
Breech or Britch wool	Coarse and hairy fibers on lower hind legs. It is coarsest in the fleece.
Broadcloth	Term is generally applied for elegant cloths produced by compact weaving and contains smooth nap, velvet projections and high lustre.
Brushing	Brushing is a process of raising nap during knitting and weaving.
Bucks or Buck wool	Term used to the wool obtained from rams. It has characteristic smell and high shrinkage than ewe wool.
Bump	Bump is a unit of larger quantities of processed wool measurement in which a hole is present in middle and fiber is wound into cans at the end of combing.
Burling	Burling is a process of removal of objectionable matter during dry finishing.
Burr	Term burr is referred to the vegetable matter like twigs, straw etc present in wool.
Burry wool	Wool with burr. It has high shrinkage and requires carbonizing before use.
Carbonizing	Carbonizing is a process of removal of vegetable matter such as burr and seeds by chemical treatment (acids particularly sulphuric acid) by inducing little damage to the wool fiber.
Card	Card is a machine used for separation of wool by opening the locks and tufts.
Carding	Carding is a process in yarn manufacture in which fibers are brushed up, makes parallel and free from foreign matter and converted into manageable form known as *sliver*.
Carpet wool	Course, harsh and strong wool suitable for making carpet is termed as carpet wool.
Carroting	Carroting is a process of treating the rabbit wool tips or ends by chemicals to stiffen or soften in order to induce artificial crimp.

Chaffy wool	Wool with small particles of straw and hay is called chaffy wool.
Character	Character is a term used in wool industry to denote uniform and distinct crimp in wool fibers.
Clean wool	Scoured wool after removal of vegetable and foreign material is termed as clean wool. It contains 12% moisture and 1.5 % alcohol extractable matter.
Clip	Clip is a slot of total wool produced either from one flock or total annual national or world total.
Clothing wool	Short wool less than 5 cm in length used for manufacturing of woolen cloths.
Coarse	In Canadian system wool of 36s-40s is considered as course wool. It is equivalent to braid in American system.
Combing wool	Wool above 6.5 cm long fibers which are arranged in parallel fashion is called combing wool.
Combing	Combing is a process of making the longer fibers parallel and removal of short fibers (noil), broken ends, tangled naps and larger vegetable particles. It is intermediate process in worsted yarn preparations subsequent to carding. Combed yarns are comparatively finer, cleaner, stronger and more lustrous than carded yarns.
Condition	The term condition is referred as the amount of grease and dirt present in wool. More the condition more will be the shrinkage on scouring.
Conductivity	Conductivity is an insulating value of fiber through which wool fibers holds body heat and keeps heat out.
Cortex	Cortex is a body of fiber lying within the cuticular scales surrounding the medulla.
Cotts or Cotted fleece	Term is generally applied for fleeces in which fibers are matted or felted together while on sheep. It is due to unfavourable weather, sickness and lack of yolk to protect fiber etc. It is generally observed in coarse wool.
Cotted wool	It is reject grade wool in which fibers are felted together due to matting or cotting. This condition arises due to sickness or lack of grease.
Cotty wool	Wool that is matted or felted on sheep's body due to lack of grease.
Count	Count is a numerical expression of degree of fineness of wool fiber.
Course wool	Wool that is normally used for floor coverings and sometimes in coarse wearing apparel.

Crease retention	Crease retention is the ability of a fabric to retain a pleat or a fold which has been made deliberately.
Crimp	The term crimp is generally referred as natural waviness in wool fibers. Crimp is the indication of fineness of wool, more is the crimp higher will be the fineness of wool.
Crimpiness	Crimpiness is the ability of wool fiber to make crimps. The number of crimps vary in wool from 2-12 per cm depending on quality or fineness.
Crimp recovery	The crimp recovery is the ability of a yarn or fiber to return to its original crimped state after being released from a tensile force.
Crinkle	The term crinkle is expressed as waviness of each individual fiber on separation from a lock. It has irregular pattern and responsible for elasticity.
Crutching	Crutching is the act of shearing wool from udder, breech area and hind legs prior to lambing. It is done to enhance the wool clip and reduce lamb losses.
Dags	Term dags is indicative of staples or locks of wool on breech area heavily coated with dung.
Dead wool	Wool obtained from dead sheep is called dead wool. It is low value wool and has strong odour. It has more shrinkage, softness and less strength than live wool. Murrain wool of decayed carcass has no value.
Defective wool	Wool with heavy burr, highly damaged with insects, disease, fire or water and gives lower scouring percentage is termed as defective wool.
Delaine wool	Fine wool with long staples is termed as delaine wool.
Dingy	Dingy term is applied to the wool lacks brightness or lustre which could be due to excessive yolk, unfavourable environment, or presence of external parasites.
Domestic wool	Wool produced on farm is termed as domestic wool.
Down wool	Medium type wool produced by the sheep's originated in downs of England.
Dyebath	Dyebath is generally referred to the solutions usually contains water, dyes, dyeing assistant and other necessary ingredients.
Dyeing	Dyeing is a process of applying permanent colour to the wool fiber, yarn or fabric by using dyes. Wool fiber is easy to dye because it allows penetrating different colours.
Elasticity	Elasticity is a property of wool to return to its natural form after release of stretch or compression.

Felt	Felt is a firm dense material or non-woven sheet of matted material developed from wool, hair or fur. It is created by entanglement of fiber mass on the application of heat, moisture and pressure. It can be utilized in manufacturing of outerwear, sportswear, accessories, trim and other industrial articles.
Felting	Felting is a process of interlocking the wool fibers by action of heat, moisture, chemicals and friction. It is caused by directional friction effect of scales on the fiber surfaces.
Fiber	Fiber is a unit of fundamental component used for making textile yarns and fabrics and having length at least 100 times its diameter or width.
Fiber length	Total length of the fiber after removal of crimps or waviness by straightening wool staple.
Fine wool	Fine wool is obtained from fine wool breeds of sheep like merino of sub breeds. It is high in crimps and used for making the fine fabrics.
Flannel	Flannel term is generally applied to lightweight, soft woolen or worsted cloths developed by plain weave with a slightly napped finish. Examples are coats, suits, sportswear's and dresses.
Fleece	The term fleece is generally applied to entire coat sheared from an animal at one time.
Frowsy or Mushy wool	Term used to dry, weathered and wasty wool.
Fulling	Fulling is a process of shrinking the woven or knitted cloths in both directions by moisture, heat and friction to make the compact and solid mass and giving the appearance of felt.
Fur	Term fur is used for undercoat of mammals other than the sheep, goat or camel families.
Greasy wool	Term greasy wool is generally referred to raw wool which is shorn from the sheep and does not subjected to washing and cleaning.
Guard hair	Guard hairs are long, stiff, usually coarse fiber projects on wooly undercoat of pelt.
Hand or Handle or Texture	It is expressed as general tactile feel of fiber related to the combination of all the fiber characteristics. It include the characteristics like dull, lustrous, wooly, stiff, soft, fine, coarse, open or closely woven etc.
Handspun	Term handspun is used to spun the yarn by hand using spinning wheel or electric spinner.

Hank — Hank is a unit of fiber measurement which contains a definite length of textile material. It varies according to the fiber type like one hank of wool is 560 yards, cotton and silk is 840 yards and linen is 300 yards.

Heterotype — Heterotype denotes the type of fibers present in fleece of indiscriminately bred sheep. These fibers are of different length, physical structure and posses characteristics of both wool and hair.

Hogget wool — Term is generally applied to first fleece of a sheep which has not been shorn as a lamb.

Hunger wool — Hunger wool is the wool produced from under nourished ewes and normal in length but less in diameter and fibers are brittle in nature.

Inflammability — Wool is inflammable and slow in burn. On burning it gives pungent odour and forms bead on ceasation of burning.

Jersey — Term Jersey is applied to the plain knitted fabric made on circular, flat or warp knitting machines.

Kemp — Coarse hair like fibers growing with wool around the hind quarters on legs and about the head. They are characterized by chalky white, lusterless, hard, brittle, opaque, medullated fibers and much shorter than normal wool fibers. They are categorized under reject grade but more valuable than hairs.

Knits — Term Knits is generally used for fabrics made by interlocking series of one or more yarn loops. Example are Jersey or circular knit and tricot or warp knit produced in a variety of plain, stockingette, rib and novelty stitch patterns.

Lamb's wool — Wool obtained from lambs up to seven months of age. It is very soft and possessing superior spinning properties.

Lanolin — Term is used for wool grease. It is sometimes called yolk and is a secretion of sebaceous glands of sheep. It can be utilized in cosmetics and lubricant industries.

Lock — Term lock is used for small approximately finger-size bit of wool which tends to stay together at shorn of sheep.

Long wool — Long sized wool obtained from certain English breeds like Lincoln, Leicester and Cotswold.

Loom — Loom is a device or machine used for weaving cloths.

Lumpy wool — In wool rot infestation in skin of sheep, sores heal but growing wool carries the scabs away in fleece. Such wool is called lumpy wool.

Lustre — Term luster indicates the ability of wool to reflect light. It is exhibited in form of shine and gloss. Wool with lustre takes better dye and gives brighter appearance than lusterless wool. Normally coarse wool with fewer scales has more luster than fine wool because of smooth fiber.

Medulla — Medulla is a hollow rounded cell present in center of fiber and run continuously along the length of the fiber.

Medullation — Medullation is a process of development of hollow space in the center of wool fibers.

Mohair — Highly resilient, lustre and strong fibre obtained from Angora goat.

Nap or Pile — Term is used for fiber ends which are raised from yarn body for development of fibrous surface in cloths.

Nep — Term Nep is used for small knot of tangled fibers consist of short, dead or immature fiber.

Noils — Noils are short, tangled and broken fibres in wool which may contain vegetable matter. Noils are usually removed during combing and utilized in development of woollen and felt trade.

Off wools or Off sorts or Reject — These terms are used for undesirable fleece or its parts.

Pelt — Term is used for sheep skin contains wool.

Picking — Picking is a process of fiber opening and/or removal of foreign matter.

Plucked or Pulled wool — Terms are used to remove loosen wool from the skin of slaughtered carcasses or lamb's.

Ply — Term Ply is usually used to express one of any number of single yarns twisted together to form a yarn.

Poplin — Poplin is a durable plain-weave fabric with fine cross ribs developed from warp yarns. They are considerably finer than the filling yarns with heavier rib and resemble to broadcloth. They are generally used for manufacturing of dresses, draperies, shirting and uniforms.

Raw wool or Grease wool — Raw wool is obtained from sheep body by shearing and contains grease, salts and dirt.

Resilience or Memory — It is an ability of wool fiber to recover to its original shape and size after release of external forces like strain, crushing and wrinkling.

Scales or Cuticles — Scales are outer layer of cells of wool or hair fibers enclosed with cortex. It is hard, flattened, unevenly orientated with surface overlaps. Scales are pointed towards fiber ends and provide friction effects and felting to wool fibers. Scales are used for identification of fibers but size and shape of fiber vary with species.

Scouring — Scouring is a process of dirt, grease, and foreign matter removal from raw wool with the use of lukewarm solutions of soap and sodium carbonate followed by a rinse.

Scouring yield — Scouring yield is a percentage of clean wool obtained after scouring. In this process some loss of weight and volume is observed. So scoring percentage can be calculated as 100 -shrinkage percentage.

Sebaceous gland — Sebaceous gland or wax gland is present at the root of wool fiber.

Second cuts — Term second cuts are used to recover short pieces of wool by cutting the staple twice in shearing.

Semibright — Term is used for subclass of wool. It lacks brightness due to environmental factors during growth phase.

Semi worsted spinning system — Semi worsted spinning system is similar to worsted spinning system but combing is eliminated.

Shearling — Shearling is an English term used in place of yearling sheep after shearing.

Shrinkage — Term shrinkage is generally used for loss of weight and volume of wool by scouring. It is expressed in percentage and loss is mainly due to removal of grease, sweat and foreign matter.

Skirting — Term skirting is generally practiced in Australia. It is a process of removal of stained, unusable or undesirable portions of a fleece to improve clip quality.

Sliver or Roving — Term is used to make the fibers parallel to one another during processing of carded wool. It is achieved by drawing wool through a tube which rolls the wool together and pulls it out.

Softness — Softness term is used for fabrics with soft touch. It is due to numerous scales and their loose fitting over one another.

Sorting — Sorting or grouping of fibers or fleece is done on the basis of comparable quality and characters.

Soundness — Soundness of wool fiber is the expression of strength of fiber and freedom from breaks and tenderness.

Spinning — Spinning is the final process of conversion of fiber into yarn in which twisting of sliver or roving is done.

Spinning count or Yarn count	Terms are used in English system of grading which describes number of hanks of yarn that can be spun from a pound of wool. More number of hanks that can be spun indicates fine wool. In other words hank of yarn that can spun from 450g of clean wool is considered spinning or yarn count. One hank is considered equivalent to 512 m of length.
Stained wool	Wool stained with urine cannot be converted into white fabric and considered as low value wool.
Staple	Staple is a synonym of fiber which may contain lock or tuft of wool.
Staple length	Term is used for total length of a fiber in natural condition without stretching or disturbing the crimp.
Staple wool	Term is applied for combing wool or bundle of wool fibers that cling together naturally in fleece. It has minimum 5 cm length.
Strawy	Wool with straw is called strawy.
Style	Term style is used for combination of crimp and crinkle in wool.
Suede cloth	Term is used for luxurious woven or knitted worsted fabric napped for a tanned leather appearance. It can be utilized for manufacturing of coats, suits and dresses.
Suint	Suint is a dried sweat secretion of sudoriferous or sweat gland of wool. It is water soluble fraction of yolk and hygroscopic mixture of potassium salts of organic acids such as oleic and stearic acids as well as inorganic salts such as the carbonates, chlorides, phosphates and sulfates of calcium, sodium, potassium and magnesium.
Tags	Term is used for broken or manure-covered locks of wool and other wastes of floor sweep in shearing areas.
Tag locks	Term is used for torn, ragged or discoloured parts of fleece.
Tartan	Term is used for woollen fabric with number plaids and colours. Each of which belongs to a specific Scottish clan.
Tare	Tare is applied during settlement of wool in which weight of wool sacks is deducted before settlement.
Tender wool	Term is used for wool staple with weak places in fibers due to illness, excessive weather or poor nutrition. So it is suitable for carding rather than combing.
Tensile strength	Term is used for the ability of fiber to withstand against pulling, stretching and breakage.
Tippy wool	Term is applied for wool containing considerable amount of grease, dirt and debris and tips of wool dye differently

	from rest of fleece. The condition is mainly due to exposure of bad weathers.
Top	Top is a continuous strand of partially manufactured wool in the processing of worsted yarn. Such wool has already gone through scouring, carding and combing.
Top knot	Term used for wool shorn from crest or poll of sheep.
Trading	Trading is the trend of ultimate use of wool. Wool is basically classified into clothing trade and carpet trade. Both are entirely processed and management is entirely depends on staple length, fiber diameter, fiber soundness, colour and state of contamination.
Twig	Wool with very small thin branches of tree or shrub.
Twill	Twill is a type of fabric usually woven with a pattern of diagonal parallel ribs. Twill fabric is generally used for the production of chino, denim, gabardine, tweed and serge.
Twist	Twist is generally expressed as turns per inch in a yarn or textile strand.
Vegetable matter	Term is used for the plant origin materials like burrs, stickers, chaff and seed heads present in fleece.
Virgin wool	Term is used for wool which has not been processed to develop fabric previously in any way, shape or form.
Warp	Term warp is used for threads running along the length of a piece of cloth.
Wasty wool	Wasty wool is a type of wool lost during manufacturing steps like carding and combing. The loss is due to vegetable matter, weakness or tenderness or shortness or tangleness of wool fiber.
Weaving	Weaving is a process of cloth manufacturing by interlacing yarns at right angles according to a predetermined pattern.
Weft	Weft is threads running side to side at right-angles to the warp in a piece of cloth.
Wool	Term wool is used for fibers present on outer covering of skin in sheep. However, it also includes fleece of a sheep, angora goat, undercoat of a cashmere goat, and specialty fibers of alpaca, llama, vicuna, and guanaco.
Wool ball	Term is used for mass of wool tangled into ball through swallowing of mothers fleece while suckling. It stuck in stomach of lamb and blocks the passage leads to death.
Wool blindness	Term wool blindness is a condition or a type of traumatic eye disease occurs in sheep with heavily woolen face.

	Such wool causes continuous irritation in eye tissues, injury and obscuring the vision. It can be managed by periodic trimming of wool around the eyes in head region.
Wool classing	Term is generally used in Newzealand and Australia for grading of skirted fleeces and pieces before packing in shearing sheds.
Woolen	Term is used for yarns or fabrics manufactured with uncombed wool by woolen spinning system.
Woolen spinning system	Woolen spinning system is consisting of only two steps carding (2-3 times) and spinning but combing step is eliminated. System can utilize wool of different types, length and characters. However, preferences are given to short wool with more crimps and better felting qualities.
Wool fat or Wool grease	Terms are used for waxy or greasy substances secreted from fat glands of sheep skin. These substances are usually clings or coats the wool fibers and used for ointment base because they absorbed easily in skin.
Wool maggots	Wool maggots are called fleece worms, especially of black blow fly, the blue and green bottle fly. They laid their eggs on wool present at rump and thigh of sheep contaminated with faeces and urine. They may also contaminate other parts of sheep which are soiled and moist as well as wool stained with blood.
Wool rot	Term is used for fungal infection caused by *Dermatophilus dermatonomu* which causes irritation to the sheep skin in wet weather and develops hard yellowish scabs. These sores heal after sometime but growing wool in these areas carries scabs away in fleece.
Wool sorter or Wool stapler	Terms are used for persons engaged in wool sorting.
Wool sorter disease	The infection of Anthrax in human beings is termed as wool sorter disease.
Wool sorting	Term is used for separation of wool fleece into different parts based on fineness and length. Wool sorting and grading terms are used in different sense because in later division of fleece is usually not done.
Worsted	Term is used for yarn or fabric made with combed wool by worsted spinning system.
Worsted spinning system	It is a design of system used for production of compact, smooth, even and strong yarn from medium or longer wools measuring 2.5 to 7 inches fiber lengths and other fibers. The process steps are opening, blending, cleaning, carding, combing, drawing and spinning.

Yarn	Yarn is a continuous strand of textile fibers made by twisting of endless filaments or shorter fibers.
Yield	Term yield is used in different sense such as amount of wool fiber in original fleece while in processing it is used as scouring yield, top yield or even yarn yield.
Yolk	Yolk is a natural secretion (grease +suint) of sebaceous and sudoriferous glands of sheep skin.

References

1. Bergin, W.V. (1968). Physical properties of wool. *In:* Wool handbook, Vol-1, Inter Service Publishers, London, 142-157.
2. Feldtman, H. D., Leeder, J. D. and Rippon, J.A. (1983). The role of fibre structure in wool fibre and fabric performance. In: Postle, R., Kawabata, S. and Niwa, M., Objective Evaluation of Apparel Fabrics, Japan, The Textile Machinery Society of Japan, 125–134.
3. Leeder, J.D. (1984). Wool - nature's wonder fibre, Ocean Grove, Vic.: Australasian Textiles Publishers,
4. Simpson, W. S. and Crawshaw, G. H. (2002). Wool: Science and Technology, The Textile Institute, Woodhead Publishing, Pp 202-317.
5. Wani, S.A., Malik, A.H., Salahuddin, M., Pal, M.A., Sofi, A.H. and Kirmani,M.A. (2008). Laboratory manual for animal fiber technology, Division of LPT, SKUAST, Srinagar, Pp 1-70.

❑❑❑

Chapter 23

Introduction to Wool, Fur, Pelt and Speciality Fibers with Respect to Processing Industry

India is one of the chief carpet wool producing and exporting countries of the world. A large quantity of carpet wool is exported to the developed countries. Wool production in Indian subcontinent is mainly dependant on distinct type of sheep producing wool in a particular geographical area. For example small and course wool is produced by Bikaneri breed in North Western India, course wool by Deccani breed and hair type breed by Mandya breed in Peninsular India and fine wool is produced in Himalayan region. In general, tropical breeds of sheep are mainly producing course wool which is highly suitable for carpet manufacture. Most of the Indian sheep breeds are producing low fleece yield. The annual total yield of greasy wool is in the range of 1-1.5 Kg. Overall great quantity of wool is produced in southern hemisphere but consumption is in northern hemisphere.

Wool is an important animal fiber produced over sheep body as protective covering. It is thick, wavy, fibrous, elastic and has an excessively scaly surface. It has felting qualities and serrated fibers tend to interlock and cling together. Elasticity and interlocking of wool fibers allows wool to be readily spun into yarn for weaving. The outside surface of wool fiber consists of a series of serrated scales, which overlap each other much like the scales of a fish. Wool fiber is naturally grow on sheep and mainly composed of protein substance called *keratin*. Wool is a unique animal fiber contains sulfur besides the presence of carbon, hydrogen, nitrogen. The wool fibers are known for spongy feel and create insulation for wearer due to presence of crimps or curls and create pockets. Wool fiber consist of basically keratin (insoluble protein) (33%), dust (26%), suint (28%), fat (12%) and mineral matter (1%).

Wool is basically used to manufacture the cloths and fine wool is more suitable for the purpose while course wool is used to develop the carpet, blankets and floor coverings. So the overall quality of wool is important and good quality wool must have minimal losses at the time of combing, carding, spinning, felting, weaving, knitting etc. The good quality wool is mainly dependant on fineness, or diameter of the fiber, length or staple, strength, elasticity, crimp, softness, pliability, uniformity, colour, luster, felting property, spinning and working properties.

Quality of raw wool and wool impurities

Raw wool is also known as grease wool and obtained directly from sheep after shearing. Raw wool contains keratin along with other impurities. Basically there are three types of impurities are generally encountered in raw wool i.e. natural, acquired and applied. Natural wool impurities includes grease or wool and suint while acquired impurities are mixed in wool during pasture and inhabitation like dust and dirt (mineral impurities), straw, burrs, twigs, grass (vegetable substances) etc. However, impurities comes through application of drugs to control diseases and insects such as dips, identification mark, tar and paints etc. are applied impurities. So the material usually found in raw wool can be categories as:

Wool constituent (%)	Wool type			
	Fine wool	Medium wool	Carpet wool	Hair
Wax	20-50	15-30	5-15	2-10
Dust	5-40	5-20	5-20	5-20
Vegetable material	0.5-2.0	1-5	0.5-2.0	0-1
Moisture	8-12	8-12	8-12	8-12
Wool fibre	20-50	40-60	60-80	60-80

1. *Wool wax*: Wool wax is also termed as wool fat or grease. These are basically the fatty secretions of wool and chemically more suited to the term wax because it is a mixture of esters but comprises of no glycerine in fatty acids. Cholesterol is present in wool in good quantity. Other compounds noticed in wool wax hydrolysates are water insoluble alcohols and higher fatty acids, 23 different aliphatic alcohols and 36 different aliphatic acids. Wool wax also shows the presence of 5 different sterols, 6 different iso-cholesterols and small amount of hydrocarbons. Wool sterols have great importance in pharmaceutical industry. Lanolin is purified form of wool wax and

can be utilized as emollient. It is helpful in maintenance of human skin as smooth and soft even in most adverse conditions. There is a direct correlation between wool quality and wool wax and finer wool has higher wax content.

Quality wise wool wax is yellow to pale brown in colour, density at 15^0C is 0.94-0.97 g/cm^3, refractive index at 40^0C is 1.48, and melting point is 35-40^0C, free acid value is 4-10%, free alcohol is 1-3%, iodine value is 15-30 wijs, saponification value is in the range of 95-120, molecular weight range is 790-880 and proportion of fatty acid is 50-55%.

2. *Suint*: Suint is basically a dried residue secretion of sudoriferous or sweats glands. It is usually 2-15 percent of the wool composition. Suint consists of aqueous extract of sweat, nitrogen, sulphur, mixture of potassium soaps of fatty acids, ranging from valeric to palmitic acids. The small quantity of lactic, hippuric, and succinic acids, urea, and lanaurin is also present in suint. On burning of suint over fire potassium salt is converted to carbonate and principal component observed is potassium carbonate (70-80 percent of the suint ash).
3. *Ash:* Wool ash is 0.5 percent of the scoured wool. It consist chiefly water soluble sulphates. The basic components present in Lincoln wool are potassium oxide (31.1%), sodium oxide (8.2%), calcium oxide (16.9%), aluminium oxide (12.3%), silica (5.8%), sulphur trioxide (20.5%), carbonic acid (4.2%) and traces of ferric oxide, phosphoric acid and chlorine.
4. *Chemical elements:* Wool fibre basically contains five chemical elements like carbon (50%), oxygen (22-25%), nitrogen (16-17%), hydrogen (7%), and sulphur (3-4%). Among all elements first four are the constituents of amino acids while sulphur is a component of cystine and methionine.

Quality characteristics of wool

Wool is an animal fiber having some special quality characteristics. The major one is colour, fiber length, fiber diameter and clean dry yield. These characteristics jointly account nearly 80 percent of wool value.

1. *Colour*: colour is an important criterion to select the wool because pigment present in wool decides the acceptance of dye. The ideal colour of wool is white or creamery white with conspicuous lustre. It is because white coloured wool can take any dye while wool fibre with darker hue can receive only dark colour dye. The major

problem encountered in Indian wool is coronary staining or yellowing of wool. It is due to bacterial action at higher pH and presence of low grease. The larger quanity of lanaurin pigment in suint of wool leads to development of abnormal yellow colour of some fleeces.

2. *Fibre diameter*: fibre diameter is the diameter of cross section of a wool fibre. Fineness of wool is directly related to the quality of wool as higher the fineness, better is the quality. Fine wool has diameter between 17-18 mμ while course wool fibre diameter is 35-38 mμ which is just double to the fine wool diameter. Wools less than 30 mμ fibre diameter and non medullated are only suitable for clothing in textile industry. Fibre diameter indicates the average thickness of wool fibre. It is directly related to the quality of wool. More is the fineness, better is the quality.

3. *Clean dry yield*: clean dry yield is an indicative of purity of raw wool. Higher the yield higher will be the profit in wool industry. Clean dry yield of fine wool is 65-70 percent while medium wool is 70-75 percent and carpet wool is 80-90 percent.

4. *Moisture*: wool is capable enough to absorb moisture and naturally it contains about 12-17% moisture. It provides flexibility and lustre to the wool.

5. *Staple length*: staple length is a total length of a fibre in its natural condition. It is obtained by measuring the natural staple without stretching the crimps out of the fibre. Staple length is generally decides the ultimate use of wool. Longer wool of about 51 mm length is called combing wool that is processed to worsted yarn while short stapled wool is profitable to produce the woollen cloths.

6. *Fibre length*: fibre length is average total length of fibre after removal of crimps by straightening wool staple. It is important parameter for spinning. In general, fine wool is less than 6 cm in length whereas wool more than 10 cm is called coarse wool.

7. *Crimpiness:* crimpiness refers to the waviness of the wool fibre and crimp number varies from 2 to 12 per cm depending upon the quality. Crimpiness has great importance in spinning and increases the elasticity of the yarn and fabric. More the crimps greater the fineness of wool.

8. *Elasticity:* elasticity is a natural property of wool through which wool returns to its natural form after stretching. Wool elasticity helps wool in resisting, wrinkling, bagging and tearing.

9. *Kemp:* kemp is chalky, white, lustreless and dad fibres grow with the wool. They are not desirable in good quality wool.
10. *Heterotype:* heterotypes are the fibres mixed with hairs as well as wool and have different length, physical structures and characteristics. However, good quality wool requires uniform quality.
11. *Lustre:* lustre is a typical quality of wool to reflect light. Wool with lustre produces brighter appearance on dyeing than wool without lustre. Coarse wool with fewer scales has more lustre than fine wool because of smoothness of fibre.
12. *Strength:* wool fibres should have sufficient strength to withstand on processing. Good quality wool is strong enough and durable.
13. *Conductivity*: good quality wool fibre should be capable to retain body heat and keep external heat out. It is due to insulating nature and poor conductivity of wool to heat.
14. *Dyeing property:* wool is a natural animal fibre which can dye in any colour by using dilute acid dyes. But wool fibre is fragile to alkaline dye.
15. *Softness:* wool contains numerous, small scales which are overlapped with one another loosely and produce fabrics which are softer to touch.
16. *Inflamability:* wool is naturally slower to burn, and on burning, it gives pungent odour and form bead.

Factors affecting quality of wool

The quality of wool, particularly macro and micro elements of wool in sheep is affected by many factors. These factors may be direct or indirect but most common are genetic and environmental factors. Wool quality and quantity is also affected by some bacterial, viral, fungal and especially parasitic diseases. Some additional factors are exogenous chemicals, hormones, weather and photo period.

1. Physiological and Environmental factors

a. Factors affecting wool fibre in foetal and early post natal life:

i. *Nutritional factors:* the follicular development is affected by the nutritional status of sheep. The malnutrition or under nutrition during advance pregnancy or in lambs within few months of life adversely affect the follicle growth development. The major observed effect is in initiation and maturation of secondary follicles during the latter third of pregnancy, when the nutrient demands for growth of the foetus are greatest.

ii. *Birth capacity of ewe:* the ewe born in twin or reared a twin has less annual clean fleece yield in comparison to the single born or reared ewes. It might be due to restricted nutrient supply in uterus and during early lactation.

b. Factors affecting wool fibre in adult life:

i. *Nutrition*: supply of nutrients to follicle greatly influences the rate of fibre production and the characteristics of the fleece.

ii. *Diseases and health status:* diseased or unhealthy sheep's has lower wool production than healthy herd of sheep's.

iii. *Rearing and grazing:* free range reared sheep and maximum grazing exposure to sheep facilitates wool production.

iv. *Hormones*: fibre growth is markedly hormone dependent and pituitary hormones, including thyroid stimulating hormone, adrenocortico-trophic hormone which act on target glands and growth hormone, exert a controlling influence on wool growth. In normal sheep, growth hormone stimulates wool growth by stimulating secretion of polypeptides known as somatomedins.

v. *Physiological state*: age and sex are the major physiological parameters affect the wool production. In general, less wool is produced in young animals and maximum in sheep between three to five years of age. It is probably due to per unit of feed intake and competition for nutrients between follicles and other tissues. Rams tend to produce more wool than wethers and ewes, due mainly to their greater size and the better feeding given to rams and state of reproduction. Reproduction, pregnancy and lactation also adversely affect the quality and quantity of wool. Overall, reproduction usually reduces annual fleece growth of ewes by 10 to 14% but greatest reduction is observed in ewes rearing twins.

vi. *Exogenous chemicals:* a number of exogenous chemicals such as thallium salts, cyclophosphamide, analogues of cortisol (dexa methasone and flumethasone), and mimosine and related compounds are responsible to influence the fibre growth; fleece shedding etc. These compounds do not act specifically on wool follicle but inhibit cell division.

vii. *Parasites and diseases:* there are number of microbial infections and external parasites are responsible to reduce the wool quality both qualitatively and quantitatively. The effects are higher in young sheep's than aged. These effects sometimes may be permanent because of specific effects on protein metabolism associated with loss of blood proteins at sites of infection. The major effect observed is damaged wool due to Fleece rot and mycotic dermatitis. Copper deficiency in sheep leads to steely wool.

viii. *Weather and photoperiod*: weather conditions like temperature, seasons, photoperiods etc greatly influences wool quality and quantity in sheep's body. Normally weather condition has no adverse effect on wool quality except newly shorn sheep's. The effects of high temperature are very little on wool except unphysiologically high while cold temperature retards the wool length and growth. The effects are mainly due to reduced blood flow and hence nutrient supply. The composition of wool is altered in summers due to alteration in water quality as pond water shows higher carbonates and bicarbonates in summer. Photoperiod particularly day length controls the seasonal cycle of moulting and annual rhythm of wool growth. It is due to hormonal secretions, most likely from the pineal gland. Sulphur content in wool is also affects by seasons and winter wool contains higher sulphur than summer wool.

2. Genetic factors

The maximum contribution in production of wool or hair by sheep or other animals is dependent on genotype. As a result different breeds of sheep has differing capacity to grow wool and in various fleece characteristics. For example, Merinos have much greater follicle density than Down and long wool breeds. The variation in growth and quality can also be observed in between strains and individual sheep. In the Australian Merino, clean fleece weight associated with increased fibre diameter, staple length and body weight. Genetically high-producing Merino sheep have follicles which are usually straighter and deeper in the skin, grow wool of a lower sulphur content and have a lower concentration of cystine in plasma than low-producing sheep. There are various characteristics of fibre and follicles are highly heritable and significant changes can be made by selection for the desired characteristics. The heritability of wool traits such as greasy or clean wool weight, number of follicles per unit area of skin, S/P follicle ratio, fibre diameter, staple length and crimp frequency are in the region of 0.3 to 0.6.

The effect of breeds of sheep can also be observed The wool growth of Merino sheep will respond to changes in nutrition throughout the year, but breeds with a large inherent rhythm in wool growth rate, such as the Cheviot or Scottish Blackface, show little or no response to changes in nutritive status during winter.

Hair

Hairs are natural fibres produced by number of animals other than sheep like cow, goat, camel, llama, horse etc. Both hairs and wool are similar in composition. Hairs are necessarily contains medulla and developed from primary follicles. Hairs are generally used with course wool to manufacture the carpet, blankets and other floorings. Hairs are usually straight, smooth (lack of scales), wavy or curly while wool contains crimps. Some of the basic differences in hair and wool can be summarized as:

Wool	Hair
Wool is mainly obtained from sheep.	Numbers of animals are utilized to produce hairs.
Wool contains crimps and is more elastic and flexible.	Much less elastic and straight.
Wool fibre surface is with scales and rough.	Hair fibre is smooth due to absence of scales.
Wool scales are loosely attached with cortex.	Wool scales are very closely attached to cortex.
Wool is felting due to interweaving the fibres and keeps them together.	Felting is not present in hairs.
Wool is readily spun into yarn for weaving.	Hair is difficult to spun into yarn.
Wool is solid in cross section due to absence of medulla.	Hairs are air filled and hollow in centre due to presence of medulla.
Cuticle is irregular.	Cuticle is regular and smooth.
Good insulators and poor heat conductor.	Less insulator and comparatively good heat conductor.
Secondary follicles are generally used to develop wool fibres.	Grow mainly from primary follicles.
Wool contains irregular mosaic scale pattern.	Hair contains regular mosaic pattern.
Wool fibers are mostly circular in cross section.	Hair fibres are either circular or elliptical in cross section.

Wool fibres are small in diameter.	Hair fibres are typically long and straight with large diameter.
Softness, elasticity, lustre and heat retention is more.	All these qualities are comparatively less.
Moisture retention capacity is 12-17 percent.	Moisture retention capacity is 7-12 percent.
Dye retention is permanent.	Dye retention is temporary.
Inflammability is less.	Inflammability is comparatively more.

Pelt

Pelt is a wooled sheep skin. Pelt is an untanned hide or skin in which skin or fur remains attached. Pelt is generally obtained by slaughtered animals.

Fur

Fur is a speciality fibres obtained as outer covering of different animals like Angora rabbit, common rabbit, muskrat hairs, Beaver hair and lately reindeer hair. However, Angora rabbit is mostly used for fur production in textile industry. Fur can also be produced from fox, rabbit, mink, otters, sable, seals, cats, coyotes, chinchilla and possum.

Angora rabbit is a native of France but commercially they are produced in England, Netherland, Belgium etc. It is white rabbit sheared four times in a year and yields 7-14 ounce fur annually. In winters shearing is done by leaving half inch fur from body while in summers shearing is done close to the skin. Microscopically, Angora rabbit contains two types of fibres i.e. fine fur fibres and guard hairs. These fibres contain ladder shaped medulla which appears as series of evenly spaced dark patches. In cross section fur fibres are angular and scale pattern is irregular petal to chevron shaped. Fur fibre length is 0.5-3 inches while its diameter ranges from 10-18 μ. The affinity of water or regain moisture in fur is less than wool which is 2% in fur than 12-17% in wool. The specific gravity of fur is in the range of 1.28-1.30.

Processing steps

Softening	Pelt with fur is churned with damp saw dust to make soft after rotation for 30-60 minutes.
Opening	Opening by removal of grease from skin by churning with raw dust or other cleansing material.
Stretching	Stretching by feeding machine.
Pulling	Pulling and clipping of guard hairs.

Carroting	Fur fibres are treated with nitric acid and hydrogen peroxide to enhance the felting property of fur.
Cutting	Separation of fur with skin by cutting machine.
Blending	Mixing of fleece with other fur in separator.
Blowing	Elimination of guard hairs and dust by air blow.
Processing	Fur can be converted into boiled fur or bleached fur as per the demand. Boiled fur is a least expensive fur and obtained by boiling rabbit skin in sulphuric acid. But white fibres are in high demand which can be produced by bleaching of fur fibres with iron salt and hydrogen peroxide.

Specialty fibers

Specialty fibers are those fibers which are produced other than the sheep. It is obtained mostly from goat and camel family animals. Though, rabbits, cow and horses are also used to produce the specialty fibers.

Classification of specialty fibers

Animal Family	Type of fiber produced	Quality of fibers
Goat family	Mohair by Angora goat	Highly resilient, strong and durable fibre with lustre. Kid mohair is better than adult mohair. Used in home decorative and garment fabrics including tropical worsted.
	Cashmere from Kashmir goat	Soft hairs used for weaving or knitting of fine garments. They can also be blended with silk, cotton, or wool.
	Goat hairs	Circular to flat in cross section. Medulla is ribbon like lattice, unbroken interrupted or fragmentary. Used in manufacturing of chief felts and carpet.
Camel family	Camel hairs	Extremely soft and fine hair production. Bactrian (double humped camel) produces softest and finest camel hairs. Dromedary (single humped camel) produces short and course camel hairs.

		Camel hair is made up of two layers-outer and under coat. Outer coat is 15 inch in length, course, tough and wiry while under coat is 1-5 inch in length, soft, smooth and fine. Hair contains interrupted medulla and fainty visible scales. Diameter of camel hair is 10-40μ and cortical cells length is 140 μ. Camel's hair can be utilized alone but for best quality fabric production they are often used with fine wool for manufacturing of overcoats, topcoats, sportswear and sports hosiery. Most of the time camel hairs are used in its natural colour.
Llama family	Llama hairs	Hairs are mixture of fine, course and kemp. Fleece is brown, black, white or mixture of all. Staple length is 3-10 inches with 4-8 crimps per inch. Hair is with interrupted medulla and epidermal scales are distinctly visible.
	Guanaco fibres from Guanaco	One of the luxury fibres. Fibre diameter is 18-24 mμ. Medullation percentage is >50.
	Alpine hairs from Alpine	Hairs are with superimposed fleece. Smooth fibres with semi coronal scale patterns like wool.
	Vicuna fibres from Llama Vicugna. It is small and wild animal and generally killed to obtain the fleece. So it is protected by rigorous conservation measures.	Vicuna wool is rarest and finest fibre in world. It is softest coat cloth in the world. It is very expensive and costing several hundred dollars per yard. It is intermingled with 10% beared hairs with fine wool. Fibre diamter is 13-14μ and length is 0.5-2.5 inches. Fibre scale is coronal in pattern and tensile strength is 15000-17000 pounds per square inches.
	Alpaca fibre from Alpaca	Rich with silk fibre with considerable lustre.

Rabbits	Angora wool from Angora rabbit	Soft fibre used in manufacturing of sweaters, mittens and baby clothes.
Miscellaneous sources	Cow hairs from cow Horse hairs from horse	These specialty fibres are course and used in production of carpets, blankets and other types of floor floorings along with course wool.

Mohair

Mohair is a main specialty fibre. It is long lustrous fibre coat or covering of Angora goat. Angora goat was originated in Asia Minor but native of Turkey. Commercially they are cultured and produced in Turkey, South Africa and USA. South African mohair is called 'Cape'. The kemp removal from mohair is a necessary step in quality mohair production. Mohair fibres are basically classified into tight fleece, flat fleece and fluffy fleece. Tight fleece produces extremely fine mohair while flat fleece gives heavy shearing weight and satisfactory quality mohair. However, fluffy fleece is inferior mohair and can easily break on processing. Mohair fibre grows at the rate of 2.5 cm per month and fineness is bearing with age. Kid's mohair is better in terms of fibre and yarn than mohair obtained from aged animals. Mohair is more durable and stronger than cashmere. Turkish mohair can be classified as principle mohair and secondary mohair. Principle mohair can again be classified as kids-I, kids-II, best average mohair, good average mohair, fair average mohair, kastambol average mohair, konua mountain mohair, konia plain mohair and gingerline mohair.

Quality characteristics

1. Raw mohair is brown in colour due to presence of foreign matter, dust, sand and grease. Physically mohair contains 6% grease, 1.5% suint, 7% sand and dust, 0.25% vegetable material and clean dry yield of mohair is 85%. Sulphur content in Texas mohair is 2.92% while in Turkey mohair is 3.58%.
2. Male Angora rabbit mohair fibre is 22.7 μ in diameter; 7.9 cm in staple length, medullation percentage is 5.2 with 4.5 percent kemp while females' mohair fibre is 23.3μ in diameter, staple length is 8.2 cm with 6.6 medullation percentage and 7.6 percent kemp. Clean yield percentage wise females mohair (82.3%) is better than males' mohair (81.3%).
3. Microscopically epidermal scales of mohair is fainty visible and hardly overlap and tie close to the stem provides smooth appearance.

The scale length is 18-22 μ and numbers of scales are five in 100 μ area of mohair while 9-11 in fine wool. Mohair contains less crimp (one per inch) than wool due to presence of ortho cells in cortex of mohair. Number of medullated fibres in well bred mohair is only 1%.

Pashmina

Pashmina is a softest, finest and costliest animal fibre of textile industry. It is obtained from Pashmina goat (*Capra hircus*) of Asia and its parent breed is Kel of Kashmir. Pashmina is also produced from Chegu and Changathangi breeds. But sub zero temperature is essential for the growth of Pashmina fibre. Pashmina fibre is generally obtained in mountainous region, high plateaus of Asia, Himalayan region and outer magnolia. Generally male goat produces higher yield of Pashmina than females. Yield increases in between 1- 4th fleece and declines thereafter. Pashmina is usually soft structured fibre, weaker and less durable than Mohair and wool. It is obtained by combing and selected and sorted on the basis of colour, length, diameters and percentage of guard fibres. The felting property as well as heritability and repeatability of Pashmina fibre are not very good but insulating property is three times higher than wool.

Quality characteristics

1. Physically Pashmina is white to brown coloured, 13-18 μ in diameter and 3-12 cm in fibre length. Pashmina fibre is basically influenced by sex, season, age, and purity of dam etc. It contains actually 10-40 percent hairs and scouring yield is around 64 percent.
2. Microscopically Pashmina fibre is short, soft, non medullated and scales are cylindrical but long than wool. Cut ends are usually not observed in Pashmina fibres.

Marketing of wool and specialty fibres

Indian wool industry is mainly based on carpet wool and India is a major exporter of carpet wool. Different regions of the country contributing different types of wool depending on rearing of sheep breeds in different parts of India but major share of wool is confined to Punjab and Rajasthan. As per the record India is having 257 organized woolen units. Among them 36 are purely spinning units, 195 purely weaving and 26 composite units. Indian wool is comparatively inferior in quality and fetches low prices. In India, wool with highest fineness (15-25 μ in diameter), longer fibre length, less shrinkage, higher elasticity and crimps, white colour etc is more valuable and sale price is comparatively higher than other type of wool. On the basis of domestic demand, wool can be classified into five broad classes:

1. Spinning of yarn for cottage scale.
2. Wool for manufacturing of country blankets, including spinning and weaving.
3. Carpet and floor rugs manufacturing by hand or machine.
4. Wool for modern mills to prepare clothing material and knitting purposes.
5. Wool for industrial manufacturing of shawls, towels, lohis using indigenous methods.

References

1. Bergin, W.V. (1968). Physical properties of wool. *In:* Wool handbook, Vol-1, Inter Service Publishers, London, 142-157.
2. Feldtman, H. D., Leeder, J. D. and Rippon, J.A. (1983). The role of fibre structure in wool fibre and fabric performance. *In:* Postle, R., Kawabata, S. and Niwa, M., Objective Evaluation of Apparel Fabrics, Japan, The Textile Machinery Society of Japan, 125–134.
3. Leeder, J.D. (1984). Wool - Nature's wonder fibre, Ocean Grove, Vic.: Australasian Textiles Publishers,
4. Simpson, W. S. and Crawshaw, G. H. (2002). Wool: Science and Technology, The Textile Institute, Woodhead Publishing, Pp 202-317.
5. Wani, S.A., Malik,A.H., Salahuddin, M., Pal, M.A., Sofi, A.H. and Kirmani, M.A. (2008). Laboratory manual for animal fiber technology, Division of LPT, SKUAST, Srinagar,Pp 1-70.

Chapter **24**

Basic Structure of Wool Fiber and Development of Wool Follicle

Wool is a thick and wavy animal fiber makes fibrinous protective covering of sheep. There are 170 different types of proteins are found in wool but the major and foremost protein is keratin. It is insoluble in nature and forms most of the part of wool. True wool fiber is basically modified hair that is not shed like the hair of most farm animals and medulla is absent in true wool. Wool contains excessively scaly surface but hair surface is mostly smooth, less elastic. The matured keratinized fiber extruding above the skin is considered dead tissue. Wool fiber is basically originated from follicle situated in dermis or middle layer of skin. Wool fiber is elastic, hygroscopic, retains warmness, durable, non inflammable and transmits ultra-violet light. Wool has felting quality because serrated fibers interlock and cling together. So the felting property and elasticity makes the wool a suitable fiber for spun into yarn by weaving. All the typical qualities of wool are due to its typical structure.

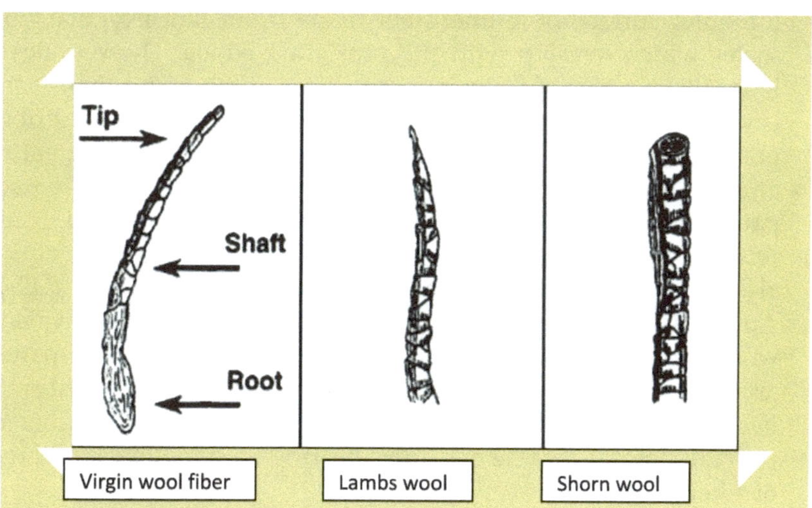

Structural components of wool fiber

A. Physical structure of wool

Typical wool fiber consists of three distinct morphological components arranged from outer to inner are cuticle or skin, cortex and medulla. The centre part medulla is found only in hairs and course wool while it is absent in true or fine wools.

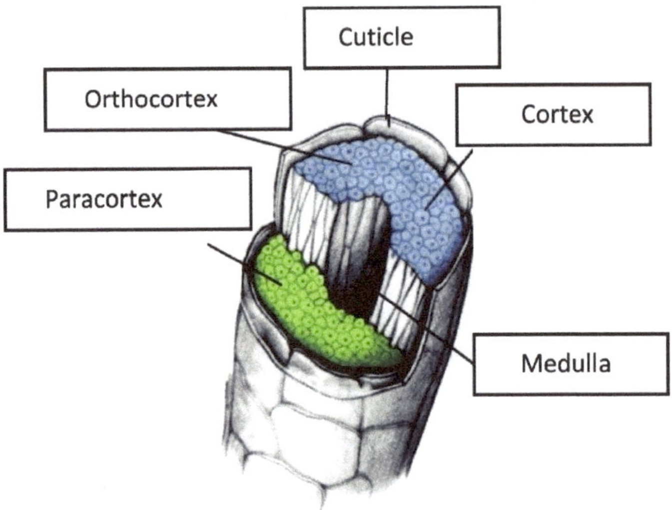

Source: spinningshepherd.blogspot.com

1. ***Cuticle:*** wool cuticle is also termed as epidermis or skin. It is actually the outer surface of animal fiber made up of flat, irregular horny scales which overlap with the projecting edges. These scales are looks like a series of funnels set inside each other and their fashion is similar to the fish scales. The free end of scales in animal fiber is pointing towards the fiber tip. There are number of scaling patterns and external edge margins are observed. There are three scale patterns are generally observed in wool fibers like coronal, coronal reticulate and reticulate patterns. The external edge margins are also of different types such as *smooth, crenate, rippled* and *scalloped*. Among all external edge margins, smooth form is most prevalent in wool while scalloped type is rare in textile fibers. These patterns are responsible for various quality characteristics of wool fiber. The basic function of cuticle is to protect the main part of fiber and provide rigidity. Cuticle has direct bearing on smoothness and lustre of fiber.

Structure and pattern of scale in cuticle

Scale pattern	Description	Location in animal fiber
Coronal pattern	In this pattern, scales form a complete ring around the fiber. They are arranged in such a way that top of one scale overlap with the bottom of next like a column of the flower pots set into one another.	Found in very fine animal fibers like merino wool fiber.
Coronal reticulate pattern	In this system edge of scales forms a band around the fiber but each band contains more than one scale. The lateral or axial overlapping gives transverse appearance to bands at fiber axis or they run diagonally across the fiber.	In course Merinos and in some kemp fibers.
Reticulate pattern	Scales are arranged in irregular network over the surface of fiber.	In course fibers.

The scale patterns present in cuticle of wool fibers can be utilized as a tool to distinguish certain fibers such as fine wool with Cashmere and medium wool with Mohair. The visible scale length is another criteria used for identification of fibers. The average visible scale length of fine wool fiber is 8-10 μ while greater in coarser wool. The scale length observed in cashmere is 14-16 μ and in Mohair 18-22 μ. The composite structure of hair comprises of three distinct layers i.e. epicuticle, exocuticle and endocuticle. The epicuticle is non proteinaceous in nature. It is readily damaged mechanically but highly inert to chemicals. The body of scales is mainly composed of exocuticle and endocuticle. In which exocuticle is less resistant to enzyme digestion as compared to endocuticle.

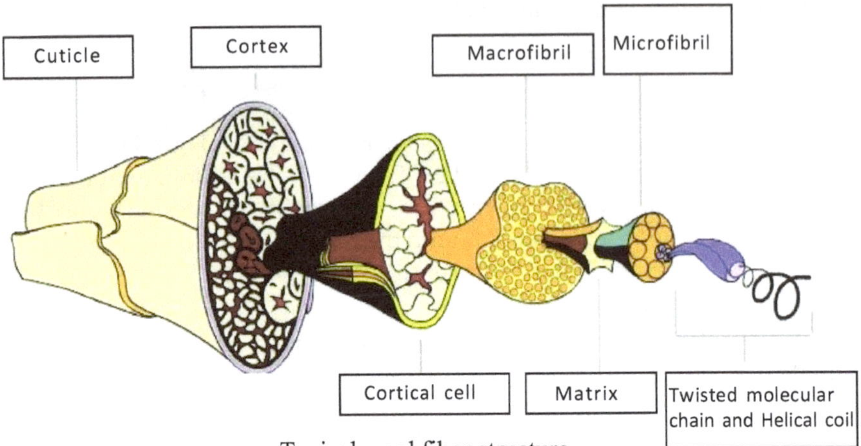

Typical wool fiber structure

Source: textilebd-yarn.blogspot.com

2. ***Cortex***: cortex is the body or main portion of wool fiber and comprises approximately 90 percent of the fiber. Cortex is made up of elongated cells lying parallel to the fiber axis and cortical cells are held together by the cell membrane complex. Cortex cells are long, slightly flattened and twisted spindle shaped. Cortical cells are about 100μ in length and 2-4μ in width. In cross section fibers may be circular but mostly they are elliptical, irregular and polygonal. The cortical cells are basically made with longitudinally oriented fibril and residue of the cell nucleus at centre. These fibrils are further split up into smaller units' fibrillae. Cortical cells can be obtained by digestion of fiber with chemical and enzymatic degradation.

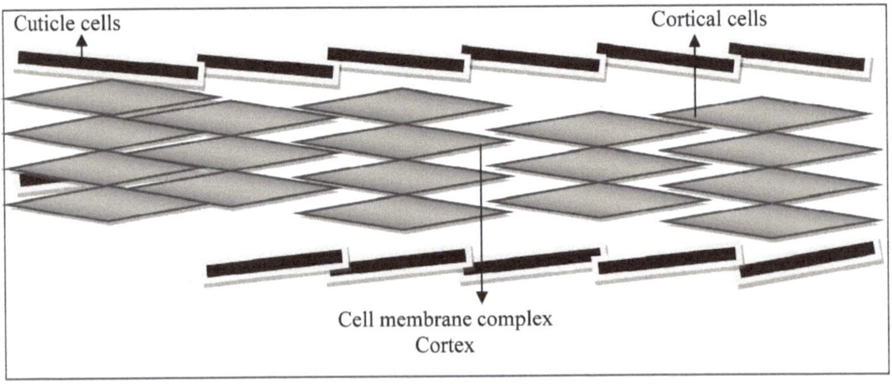

In fine wool fiber cortex is made up of two distinct structures namely *Orthocortex* and *Paracortex*. In general, Orthocortex is less stable and ordinary portion of cortex while Paracortex is stable part of cortex. These two components differ in characteristics like dye reception, swelling with alkali and birefringence after exposure to alkali etc. The bilateral form of cortex is always found only in fine or crimped fibers such as Merino and Rambouillet wools. Kid Mohair consists of chiefly ortho cortex while human hair indicates the presence of paracortex. In fine wools, cortical cells like orthocortex and paracortex are arranged in semi cylinders wound around each other helically in phase with fiber crimp. The orthocortex is always located on outer convex side while paracortex is in concave fashion of crimp curvature. Orthocortex is considered as more reactive part or has greater sensitivity part of cortex to alkali while Para cortex is less reactive to chemical reagents. In general cortex has tendency to swell to about two halves of the cortex on alkali treatment. So on treatment of fine wool fiber with aqueous solution of one percent sodium hydroxide produces curling and coiling in fiber. Basically the difference in cortical structure originates in follicle but bilateral structure appears in fiber after its keratinization. The fine structure is more distinct in the paracortex than in orthocortical cells. Cortical cells like Orthocortex and paracortex are surrounded and held together with cell membrane complex. It contains protein and waxy lipids and runs through the whole fibers. These complexes are facilitator of dye molecules to the animal fiber.

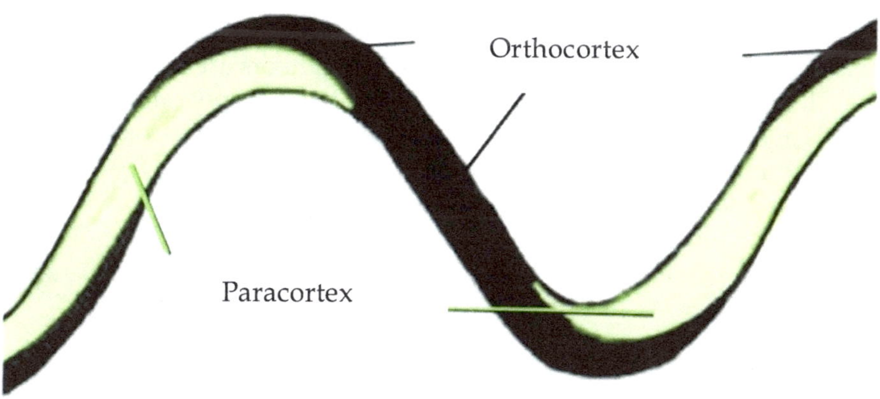

Source: spinningshepherd.blogspot.com

Another structure evident in microstructure of cortex is macrofibril, matrix, microfibril and twisted molecular chain and helical coil. Macrofibrils are long filaments found inside the cortical cells in which microfilaments are embedded in matrix. Matrix is a high sulphur proteins which attracts water molecules and provides absorbent property to wool (wool can absorb upto 30% water to its weight). Matrix is also responsible for wool properties like dye absorption, fire resistance and anti-static properties. Microfibrils which are usually 60-65 A° in diameter imbedded in amorphous matrix of cortical cells. They are made up of serial segments like X and Y zones and always arranged in a definite order following hexagonal or a whorl pattern. Both X and Y segments have differences in their reactivity. Twisted molecular chains are protein chains coiled in helical shape and works like a spring. So to make them stiff hydrogen and disulphide bonds are found in protein chains which are linked to helix coil and prevents stretching. The smallest structure in wool fiber is helical coil which are responsible for wool flexibility, elasticity and resilience. It is also provides definite shape and wrinkle-free structure to fabric.

3. ***Medulla or core***: medulla is a honeycomb like core or network of air filled cell walls or sometime hollow tube in the centre of fiber structure. Medulla is generally found in fibers having thickness more than 30μ with the exception of Lincoln and Leicester wool. These sheep breeds are coarse type but having small proportion of medullated fibers. Essentially medulla is present in hair fibers while course wool fibers are partially medullated and medulla is totally absent in fine wool. Thus fine wool fibers are generally made up of only two structures- cuticle and cortex. Medulla present in hairs and course wool is responsible for higher volume and body of fiber and provides thermo-regulatory properties due to presence of air space within medulla. Heavy medullated fibers are tend to increase light reflection and seems chalky white in appearance. Medulla appears black under microscopic examination but on filling of mounting medium it becomes transparent. Generally medullated fibers are showing four types of medulla structures- fragmented, interrupted, continuous and discontinuous or ladder type. Last pattern of medulla is generally observed in rabbit fur.

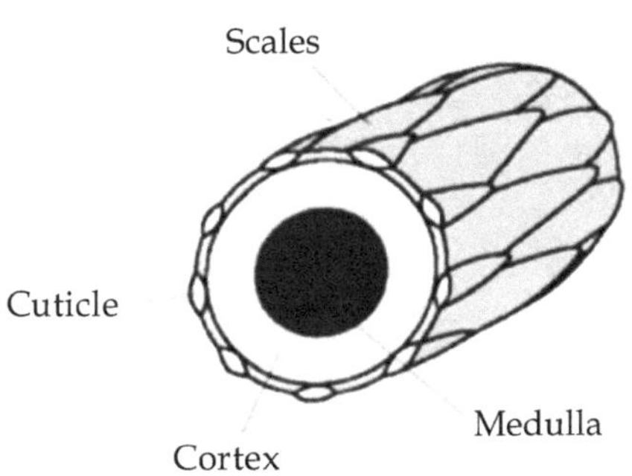

On the basis of presence and absence of medulla, wool fibers can be classified into three broad categories i.e. solid wool fibers, hairy or medullated fibers and Kemp fibers. Term *solid wool fiber* is usually designated to fine wools in which medulla is absent and core is solid type. *Hairy or medullated fibers* are course fibers with hollow or air filled space in center. They are less pliable, cannot be molded into desired directions, resistant to twist in spinning and absorption of dyes. They are also showing rough feel, less elasticity, uncoiling and less durability. Kemp fibers are heavily medullated with the 90 percent medullation percentage with the exception of tip and root, coarse and brittle fibers with fine tip. They are actually hair like fibers found around hind quarters and exhibited the properties like chalky white appearance, lusterless and poor spinning. Kemp fibers appear dumbbell in shape. Kemp wool is a type of reject grade wool but having value greater than hairs.

B. Chemical structure of wool

The chemical structure of wool fiber is quite complex and involves number of combinations of amino acids and cross links of basic and acidic groups. However, some of the salient features of wool fiber can be explained as under:

1. It is general consideration that wool contains about 170 types of different proteins but major wool protein is keratin protein.
2. All these proteins are distributed unevenly in wool fiber and specific proteins are located at specific regions of wool fiber. Such unevenness of proteins makes the wool fiber heterogeneous and decides the physical and chemical properties of wool.
3. Wool proteins are generally made up of amino acids which are 18 in number and are basically made up of basic amino (-NH) and acidic carboxyl (-COOH) groups. Amino acids are joined together to form long polymer chains called polyamides because each structural unit is joined with amide group. The repeat unit of amide groups is called polypeptides. The individual polypeptides chains are joined together to protein formation by a variety of chemical or covalent bonds called cross-links and non-covalent physical interactions.
4. The most important cross link is sulphur containing disulphide bonds by keratinization in fiber growth phase. The process is responsible for keratin development which is insoluble and quite stable protein against physical and chemical reactions. These bonds are important for finishing of wool and provide smooth dyeing property of wool fabric.

5. Another cross link of wool fiber is called isopeptide bond which is developed between amino acids containing acidic or basic groups.
6. Besides chemical bonds some other interaction are also visible in wool fiber. These are hydrophobic interactions between hydrocarbon side groups and ionic interactions between groups that can exchange protons. The ionic interactions forms salt linkages between acidic or carboxyl and basic or amino side chains and is most important among non-covalent interactions. This interaction provides wool the amphoteric or pH buffering properties and controls the dyeing behaviors of wool fiber by interaction with negatively charged dye molecules.

Development of wool fiber

The follicle responsible for development of wool fiber in sheep begins to start in unborn lambs or in two months old foetus. So it can be explained that most of the wool follicles responsible for mature fleece development are already present before birth of lamb. Basically the skin of lamb is made up of two distinct layers- dermis and epidermis. Dermis is under skin structure while epidermis is outer skin. These two layers of wool fiber are always remains identical from start of follicle development to maturation of follicle. A highly active layer of cells called basal layer present in epidermis is the key structure take part in follicle development. It remains growing and dividing continuously from start of development in prenatal stage of lambs' life till its maturation. The wool follicle development into wool fiber can be explained as under:

i. Basal layer present in epidermis becomes thicken at certain places and start growing towards dermis and converted into a sort plug in cell tissue. This plug structure is the base for development of wool follicle and accessory structures.

ii. Plug continues growing towards downside and appears in two growth structures on the same side. These growth structures are rudiments of bilobed wax or sebaceous gland and sac like or coiled seat gland or sudoferous gland.

iii. Plug which is bulbous in primary stage is now turned into dome like structures called papilla by actively dividing cells. Basal layer at this stage is continuous over dome of papilla and supplied with the small blood vessels.

iv. The dividing cells gradually elongate and form cuticle and cortex as well as inner root sheet around the fiber.

v. The cells responsible for development of orthocortex and paracortex are predetermined in the germinal layer of papilla.

vi. In hairs, course wool and Kemp, a hollow tube or structure appears which is developed by individual cells of basal layer at the apex of dome of the papilla. These cells pass upward into the centre of growing fiber and form a hollow tube like structure called medulla. To develop the hollow structure or canal in wool fiber, these cells completely separated from rest of the fiber during keratinization.

vii. The tip of growing fiber along with inner root sheath is pushed upward through the follicle plug by the pressure of new growing cells. These new growing cells continue growing from dome of papilla and creating continuous pressure. In this growth phase papilla is directed towards one side of follicle and provides shape of golf club. The orientation of papilla and shape of follicle is directly related to the crimpness and waviness of fiber in later stage.

viii. Skin is comprises of two types of follicles such as *primary* and *secondary follicles*. These follicles are responsible for development of wool. These follicles contains roots which grows downward to give rise the wool fiber in skin.

ix. *Primary follicles* are called '*trio*' because of presence of all three accessory structures present in mature wool fiber. These structures are sebaceous glands, sweat gland and arrector muscle. Sebaceous glands are responsible for secretion of grease to fleece for lubrication and glossy appearance. Sweat glands are responsible for production of dried sweat or suint of fleece. The secretion of both sweat glands (suint) and sebaceous glands (grease) jointly produces yolk of fleece. Third structure is commonly termed as erector muscle which helps the hair to stand on end. These primary follicles start growing on 15th -18th day of pregnancy. Basically primary follicles are part of British mountain breeds and some hairy breeds in other countries. The developmental pattern of primary follicle is definite which begins from head, legs, trunk and ends on the back of the sheep. The follicle density usually observed in course wool or hairy fiber is in the range of 3000-4000/sq.cm of skin surface.

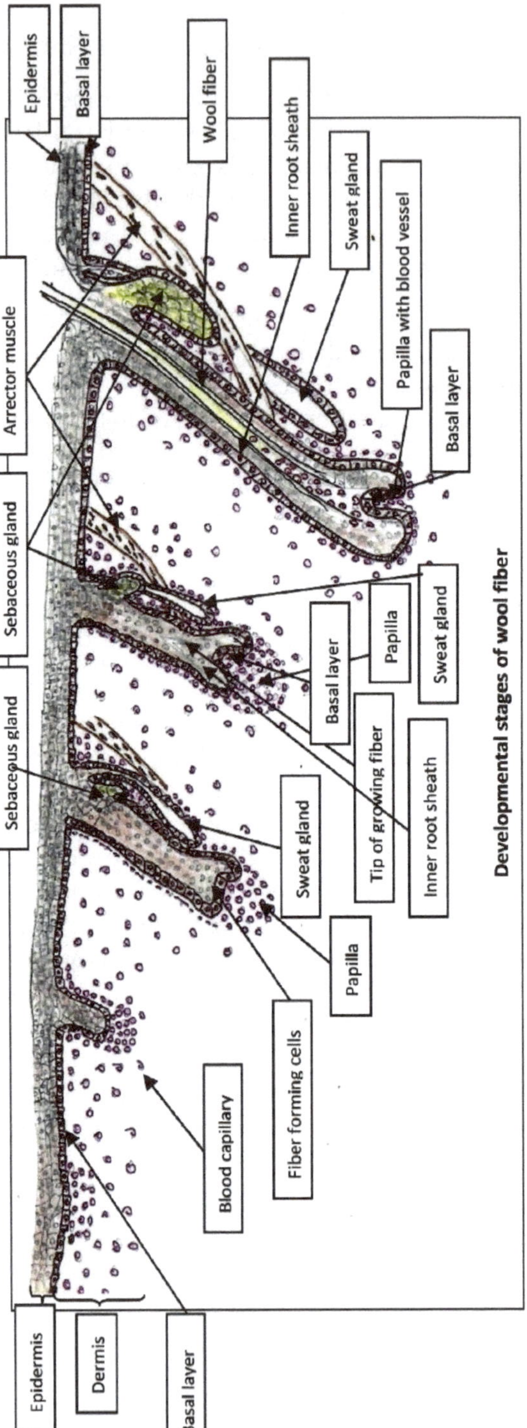

Developmental stages of wool fiber

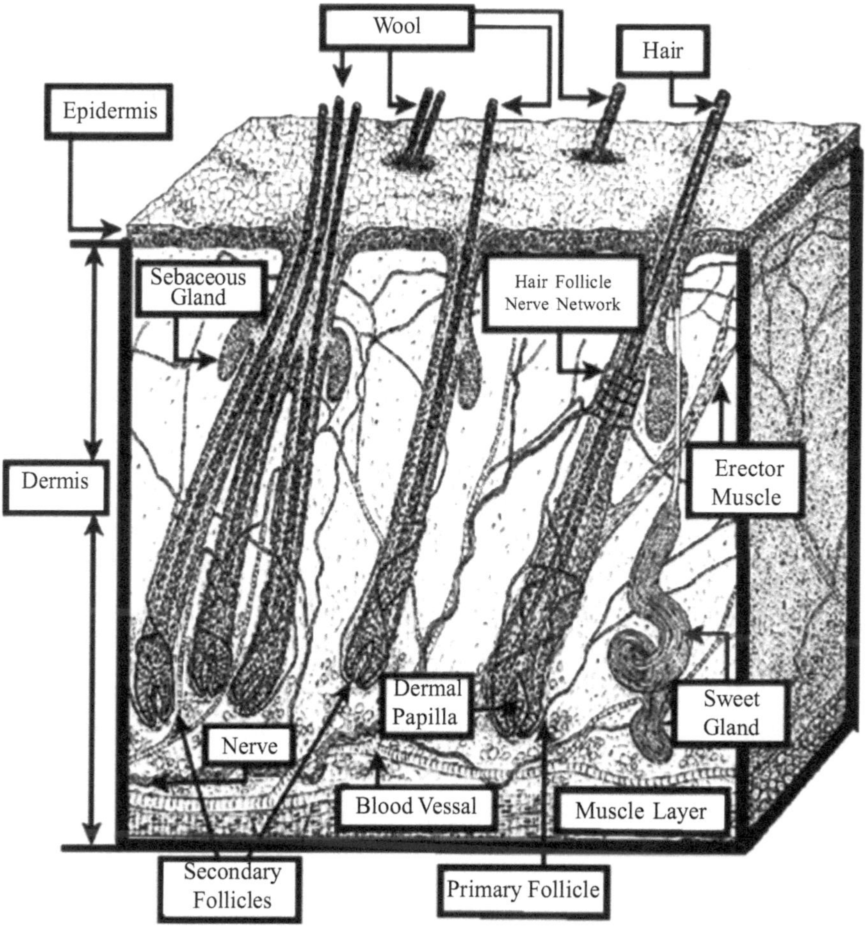

x. The later grown follicles are known as *secondary follicles* which start growing on day 85th of pregnancy in sheep. As per another opinion these follicles initiated at the time of birth. These follicles are mainly responsible for development of true fibers. These follicles contain only sebaceous glands and other structures such as sweat glands and erector muscle are usually absent. These follicles are smaller in size but follicle density is more than 10000/sq.cm area of skin. Secondary follicles are mainly found in wool fibers of Merino sheep.

xi. Another structure found in wool fiber is follicle bundles. They are separated with each other with connective tissue bands. Actually primary and secondary follicles in various combinations give birth to the follicle bundles such as trio with secondary follicles or one or two primary with secondary bundles.

Fiber growth and follicle arrangement is important to know how about the fleece structure and wool yield in sheep. The ratio of primary and secondary bundles is significant to access the wool quality in lamb before and after birth. The structural development may also be helpful in planning of breeding policy for the production of a particular type of wool breeds and culling of animals.

References

1. Bergin, W.V. (1968). Physical properties of wool. In: Wool handbook, Vol-1, Inter Service Publishers, London, 142-157.
2. Leeder, J. D. (1984). Wool - nature's wonder fibre, Ocean Grove, Vic.: Australasian Textiles Publishers,
3. mdpi.com
4. Morton, W.E. and Hearle, J.W.S. (1993). Physical Properties of Textile Fibres, 3rd ed., Manchester, UK. The Textile Institute.
5. Rippon, J. A. (1992). The Structure of Wool; Chapter 1, *In:* Wool Dyeing, Lewis, D.M. (Ed.), Bradford (UK): Society of Dyers and Colourists
6. Rippon, J. A. (2003). Wool. *In:* Encyclopedia of Polymer Science and Technology, New York: Interscience Publishers.
7. spinningshepherd.blogspot.com
8. textilebd-yarn.blogspot.com
9. what-when-how.com
10. Wildman, A.B. (1954). The Microscopy of animal textile and wool. Industries Research Association, Leeds, 566-589.

❑❑❑

Chapter **25**

Classification, Grading and Quality Characteristics of Wool

Wool is a fibre basically composed of amino acids and have excellent absorbency, moisture regain capacity, tend to warm the human body if used in form of cloths and others, good in elasticity and resiliency but poor in resistance to alkali but acid tolerance is good. To get better utilization of wool, they may be classified into various categories based on their origin, fleece quality, fineness of wool fibres etc.

A. Wool classification based on their origin

Class	Wool type	Qualities
Class-1	Merino wool	Merino wool has greatest number of crimp and maximum number of scales which provide merino wool high quality warmth and spinning. Merino wool fibres are strong, fine, elastic and relatively short from 1-5 inches in length.
Class-2	English, Scotish, Iris and Walis sheep wool	Good crimp wool and present number of scales per inch area. Wool fibres are comparatively strong, fine, elastic and 2-8 inches in length.
Class-3	United Kingdom sheep wool	Less crimpy, coarser, fewer scales and wool fibre is 1-18 inches in length. Wool fibre is smooth, lustrous, less elastic, and resilient but can be utilized in good clothing.
Class-4	Mongrel sheep wool or half breeds wool	Wool is least elastic, strong and less crimpy with few scales. Wool fibres are smooth, more lustrous, course and hair like with the length of 1-16 inches and mostly used for production of carpets, rugs and low grade clothing.

B. Wool classification based on fleece

Wool type	Age of sheep and kind	Quality of wool
Lamb's wool/ fleece wool/ first clip	First time sheared wool of 6-8 months old lambs	Natural, tapered and soft wool.
Hogget wool	Wool obtained from shearing of 12-14 months old but not been previously shorn	Fine, soft, resilient, mature with tapered ends. Used mainly for warp yarns.
Wether wool	Wool obtained from > 14 months old sheep	Soiled, dirty and greased wool.
Pulled wool	Wool obtained during slaughtering of sheep for meat	Low quality wool.
Dead wool	Wool obtained from dead sheep	Inferior in quality.
Cotty wool	Wool obtained from sheep exposed to severe weather	Poor grade, hard and brittle.
Tag locks wool	Wool obtained from fleece which is torn, ragged and disclоured	Inferior quality wool

C. Wool classification based on fineness

Wool type	Fibre diameter (mμ)	Clean dry yield (%)	Quality of wool
Fine wool	17-20	65-70	High quality, light weight and used for woollen cloth knitting.
Medium wool	22-24	70-75	Good quality, heavier wool and used for cloth manufacturing.
Course wool	25-32	80-90	Inferior quality wool and mainly used for manufacturing of carpet, blankets etc. Course wool generally used for carpet with wool fibres and hairs in a ratio of 65:25 by weight but kemp should not exceed >4%.

D. Classification of Indian wool

Wool type	Fibre diameter (μ)	Percentage of Indian Production
North India Superior Clothing White	≤ 30	4.9
North India Clothing White	30 - 42	44.7
North India Rug White	43 - 46	12.4
North India Carpet Type	≥ 46	10.0
South India Blanket Type	43 - 46	23.5
South India Tannery Type	≥ 46	4.5

E. Wool classification based on location in sheep body

Location in sheep body	Quality of wool
Top knot	Kemp, course and broader wool
Back	Poor quality wool
Fleece	Good quality wool
Flank	Very good quality wool
Shoulder	Choice quality wool
Britch	Kemp and stained wool
Belly	Skirting which is poor quality wool.
Arms and shank	Hairy wool

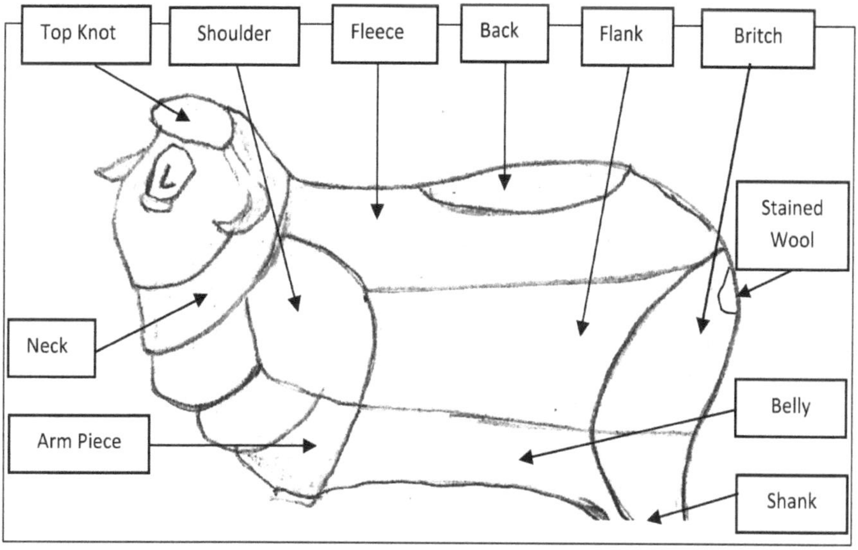

Sheep showing parts of the fleece

Wool grading

The grading of wool is important to merchandise and to segregate different type of wool for ultimate use. It is usually done by a trained grader after skirting in which objectionable parts such as tags, leg pieces, neck pieces, bellies, locks and stained portions from the body of the fleece are removed. There are different grading systems in various countries or even within the country.

Systems of wool grading

1. *FAO/UNDP grading*: Grading of Indian wools was initiated under FAO/UNDP project based or wool quality, length, colour and vegetable fault (content of vegetable matters, e.g burr, and seed). About 90 types were prescribed.

2. *Indian Standard Institution (ISI) grading (IS 2900: 1979):* The Indian standard institution (IS 2900:1979) evolved a grading system of wool based on micron value. It can be done on the basis of visual appraisal of length and fineness. It prescribes 120 grades and above system is hardly operative. The major grades can be classified as:

Grade	Fibre diamtere (μ)	Burr percentage	Colour
A	34.4 μ or below	< 3.0	White
B	34.4 – 37.4 μ	3.0-5.0	Tinged white
C	37.4 – 40.0 μ	>5.0	Light yellow
D	40.1 μ and above	-	Heavy yellow

3. *British system*- it is based on the spinning count of fleece.

Wool grade	Fibre length (cm)	Fibre diameter (μ)	Spinning count
Fine wool	2.5 to 12.5	17-21	60-80
Medium wool	4-12.5	22-24	50-62
Coarse wool	10-12 cm	25-32	30-40

4. *American system or blood system*: This is the oldest system and developed in United States. The grades were developed using the merino fleece as the standard fine wool or on the percentage of merino blood.

5. *The spinning count or Bradford system or English system*: It was developed in England and is based on the fineness of fiber.

6. *Micron count system*: Actual measurement of the diameter of fiber in micron, which is the unit of measurement.

1 micron = 1/25400 of an inch or 1/10000 of a cm

Blood or American system	Spinning count or English system	Micron system
Fine	88s, 80s, 70s	15.0-24.0
Half blood (50%)	62s, 60s	24.9-26.3
Blood (37.5%)	58s, 56s	26.4-28.4
Blood (25%)	50s, 48s	29.3-32.7
Low quarter blood	46s, 45s	34.4-36.0
Common	44s, 42s	36.3-37.0
Braid	40s, 36s	38.1-40.2

7. *Style grading*: This grading system was introduced in Rajasthan which cuts the graders to 32 only. It is based on the recommendation of FAO experts and is followed by wool producing states like Punjab, Haryana, J&K, Gujarat and Karnataka etc. incorporating some appropriate modification in it.

Style	Code No.	Description
Good	1	Wool with good colour, washed, skirted and vegetable matter content of 0- 3 % with reasonable quality and strength.
Good average	2	Wool having yellow colour well skirted with vegetable content of 0- 3% and reasonable in quality and strength.
Average	3	Wool of average washing, well skirted and vegetable content of 3- 6 %
Inferior	4	Wool of poor washed category with vegetable content of above 6%

8. *AGMARK standards:* To maintain the quality control of carpet wool in India, AGMARK devised a grading system to export the wool from India. Wool grading and marketing rules, 1961 defines the quality of various types of wool, permissible the grade specification and lay down the methods of marketing, packaging etc. Agricultural Marketing Advisor to Government of India issues certificate of authorization to the exporters.

Schedule	Wool category
Schedule-I	Indian clipped wool
Schedule-II	Indian pulled wool
Schedule-III	Indian tannery wool (limed) a. Wools other than south India tannery and Aden type b. South India and Aden type wool
Schedule-IV	India mixed wool, clipped -carded, clipped-pulled wool
Schedule-V	Indian Hill wool greasy a. clipped
Schedule-VI	Indian ginned wool

These systems are prevalent in different parts of the country but none of the above grading system is practiced in the country to any significant extent. These grading systems were evaluated by Central Sheep and Wool Research Institute, Avikanagar, Rajasthan (CSWRI). The study revealed that the visual or tactile grading system is highly subjective and does not effectively discriminate among wools of different quality, and there is a marked overlapping of the grades. The Indian wools are highly heterogeneous and maximum variability is among fibers themselves. Grading does not impart any special feature which could improve the performance of graded lots over ungraded lots. So they recommended following provisions:

1. Wool from different agro climatic regions and breeds may be marketed as such.
2. At the time of shearing fleece should be properly skirted.
3. Fleece after skirting may be classed into at the most 2 or 3 grades, like fine, medium and coarse.
4. Bales from individual lots should be sampled, and these samples be subjected to objective quality assessment through laboratory testing for yield, length, average fiber diameter and vegetable matter content.

Properties of wool

True wool is elastic and hygroscopic, non inflammable and non liable to melt. They retain warmth and create heat and forms soft pliable yarn. Wool contains felting property and ordinarily water proof in nature devoid of medulla. The price of wool is basically decided on the basis of fineness, length, elasticity, crimpness, shrinkage, colour and kemp percentage.

Physical properties

1. *Colour*: the normal colour of wool varies from white to near white, brown and black. But demand of pure white raw wool is higher because it can take any of the colour on dyeing.

2. *Tenacity and tensile strength*: the tensile strength of wool fibre is low due to presence of less hydrogen bond. In wet condition when wool fibre absorb moisture then water molecules steadily force sufficient polymers apart to cause a significant number of hydrogen bonds to break. Water molecules also hydrolyse salt linkages in amorphous regions of the strand. Thus swelling of fibre takes place due to explicition of inter-polymer forces of attraction result the loss of strength of wet woollen material. The tensile strength of wool in dry condition is 1.0-1.7 while in wet wool 0.8-1.6. The tensile strength of wool fibre can be improved by using ply yarn and hard twisted two ply yarn and is regarded as assurance for durability. However, tightly twisted single yarn can make the strong fabric. Tenacity is generally expressed in g/tax and can be calculated using the formula:

   Mean breaking load/mean linear density x 100

3. *Elasticity:* elasticity of wool fibre is a process of stretching the fibre through disulphide bonds in amorphous parts of strand or fibre and strand is released the disulphide bonds pull the protein molecules back into their original positions. Sometimes disulphide bonds are fewer (as in case of alkali treatment of fibre) then polypeptide chains slides over one another and induces permanent extension of wool. The natural crimps of fibres help in retaining its natural shape. Pure wool has good elasticity and standard elongation in dry wool is 25-35 percent while in wet wool 25-50 percent. The good elongation and elasticity characteristic of wool fibre protect them from tearing under tension, provides free body movement and helps in better shape retention.

4. *Resiliency:* wool fibre has high degree of resilience and good quality wool is soft and wool fibres wrinkles less while poor quality wool is harsh in feel and wrinkles more.

5. *Hydroscopic nature:* wool is hydroscopic in nature and absorbs moisture. It is due to polarity of peptide group and salt linkages which attracts moisture while amorphous nature of polymer system of fibres absorbs moisture. In dry weather condition wool fibre generates static electricity and water molecules helps in distribution of this energy.

6. *Density and specific gravity:* wool fibre is relatively low density fibre and comparatively light in weight. The specific gravity of wool fibre ranges from 1.30 to 1.32 and the average value of dry non medullated wool is 1.304.

7. *Heat conductivity:* wool fibre is low in heat conductivity thus ideal for use in cold weather. The resilience property of wool makes the fabrics warmth and medulla of wool filled with air enhances the insulating power of fibre. The fibre strand usually grasps moisture in vapour form and protects the body in cold atmosphere.

8. *Dimensional stability:* wool fibres are poor in dimensional stability and shrinks easily. Thus felting or shrinkage is a common phenomenon observed during mechanical action, such as agitation, friction and pressure in presence of heat and moisture. The scales present over wool fibres interlock and prohibit the fibres to return back in its original form.

9. *Refractive index:* refractive index is the ratio of velocity of light in a vacuum to its velocity in a specified medium. It is small in long wool breeds while large in short wool breeds of sheep. The refractive index of wool in general ranges from 1.551 to 1.555. Breeds wise Lincoln has 1.543refractive index while it is 1.547 in Hampshire, Oxford, Dorset, Leicester, and Mongolian, 1.548 in Southdown and 1.551 in Merino and Mouflon.

10. *Lustre*: lustre is the ability of wool to reflect light. Wool with lustre when dyed has brighter appearance than the wool without lustre. Course wool with fewer scales has more lustre than fine wool because of smoothness of fibre.

11. *Crimpness:* natural waviness of wool per cm or inch is called crimpness. The number of crimps per cm or inch area is indicative of wool fineness. More the crimps of wool more are fineness of wool. It varies according to the breed but normally ranges from 2-12 per cm. It can be measured by crimpometer.

12. *Wool fibre diameter:* wool fibre diameter is also indicating the fineness of wool. Wool fibre diameter is directly related to the fineness of wool and to the quality of wool. It is an important criterion to grade the wool in different categories for merchandizing.

13. *Moisture regain:* moisture regain is the capacity of wool to absorb moisture. It is expressed as percent dry weight and varies from 16-18 percent.

14. *Fleece density:* fleece density is the number of fibres grown per unit area. It actually depends on S/P ratio. Fine wool like Merino contains more than 100 million fibres per unit while coarse wool contains fibres in between 10-20 million.

15. *Fineness and medullation:* fineness of wool is basically depending on fibre diameter. Pure fine wool contains no medulla but coarse wool and hair contain medulla. Medulla is a hollow structure in the centre of fibre.

Chemical properties

1. *Heat sensitivity:* wool is slow to burn and on burning produces porous and brittle mass of carbon and produces characteristic sulphur smell. Wool contains plastic quality and helps in moulding it into various shapes at melting temperature (100^{0}C). At temperature between 100-150^{0}C wool losses all moisture and becomes harsh and brittle but on moisture regain again becomes soft, strong and elastic. At 130°C wool keratin readily decomposes into ammonia but on higher temperature wool becomes discoloured and decomposed.

2. *Water sensitivity:* wool is insoluble in both hot and cold water but losses strength on continuous treatment with hot water. However, dyeing affinity enhances on exposure to higher temperature and steam.

3. *Acid resistance:* wool is generally resistant to mineral acids of all strength even at higher temperature. Nitric acid tends to cause wool damage by oxidation and turns to yellow which helps in identification of animal fibre. However, concentrated sulphuric acid completely decompose the wool fibres. The strong acids at higher temperature hydrolysed the peptide chains and dissolve wool fibre completely within few minutes particularly in boiling aqueous solution of 5% NaOH. The decomposition of wool fibre is mainly due to hydrolysis of salt linkages and hydrogen bonds by strong and concentrated acids. The major effects of acids on wool fibre may include absorption of acid with amino group, chemical modification of side chains, hydrolytic degradation of peptide links in keratin etc. Acid damaged wool can be identified by swelling test developed by Krais and Viertel.

4. *Alkali sensitivity:* wool is quiet sensitive to alkali. It completely dissolves on boiling with 5% caustic soda due to break down of amino group. The decomposition of wool fibre with alkalis is mainly due to hydrolysis of disulphide bonds; hydrogen bonds and salt

linkages of wool resulting polymers to separate from each other. Prolonged exposure to alkalis causes hydrolysis of the peptide bonds of wool polymers lead to polymer fragmentation and total destruction of the fibre. However, wool lustre and strength enhances upon treating with concentrated cold caustic soda solution under controlled condition. The alkalis which are considered safe for wool fibre are ammonium carbonate and borax. The wool damaged with alkali can be identified by All Worden reaction or by urea bisulfite test.

5. *Action of salt:* wool should always be washed in soft water because calcium and magnesium salts present in hard water produces yellowing effects upon prolonged boiling. The copper and iron ions produce undesirable metal stains during wool processing.

6. *Bleaching effect:* bleaching of wool with chlorine produces harmful effect on wool and damages the wool fibre. However, bleaching of wool can be done successfully with potassium permanganate and Na_2O_2. Bleached wool can be identified by basic fuchsin test.

7. *Effect of sunlight and weather:* sunlight in particular ultra-violate radiation induces yellow white or dull colour to the wool fabrics. It is due to severance of peptide and disulphide bonds and degradation of wool polymers. Prolong exposure of sunlight weakens the fibre and ultimately damage it badly.

8. *Colourfastness:* to make attractive appearance of wool fibres as well as to enhance the acceptability of fabrics different types of dyes are used. As wool is sensitive to alkalis so most of the time acid dyes are preferred. However, chrome and mordant dyes can also be applied. These dyes exerted their action in the amorphous areas of wool and produces attractive colour.

9. *Resistance to organic solvents:* organic solvents have no adverse effect over wool fibres and can be applied for processing's.

10. *Adverse effect of insects and micro-organisms:* insects and micro-organisms can adversely affect the wool. As wool affected with mildew remains wet for longer period of time. It is noticeable that wool garments contain more number of bacteria than any other textile fibres. However, dry cleaning process reduces 90% of bacteria adhered with wool.

References

1. Basal, G. and Oxenham, W. (2006). Comparison of properties and structures of compact and conventional spun yarns, Textile Research Journal, 76 (7): 567–575.
2. Bergin, W.V. (1968). Physical properties of wool. In: Wool handbook, Vol-1, Inter Service Publishers, London, 168-199.
3. CSIRO, (1979). Proceedings of a Seminar of Staple Length and Strength of Greasy Wool, Division of Textile Physics, Ryde, 7 December 1979
4. Feldtman, H. D., Leeder, J. D. and Rippon, J.A. (1983). The role of fibre structure in wool fibre and fabric performance. *In:* Postle, R., Kawabata, S. and Niwa, M., Objective Evaluation of Apparel Fabrics, Japan, The Textile Machinery Society of Japan, 224–268.
5. Leeder, J. D. (1984). Wool - nature's wonder fibre, Ocean Grove, Vic.: Australasian Textiles Publishers.
6. Moore, G. P., Jackson, N., Isaacs, K., and Brown, G. (1998). Pattern and morphogenesis in skin. J Theor Biol., 191: 87–94.
7. Simpson, W. S. and Crawshaw, G. H. (2002). Wool: Science and Technology, The Textile Institute, Woodhead Publishing, Pp 202-317.
8. Wani,S.A., Malik,A.H., Salahuddin,M., Pal, M.A., Sofi,A.H. and Kirmani,M.A. (2008). Laboratory manual for animal fiber technology, Division of LPT, SKUAST, Srinagar, Pp 1-70.

Chapter **26**

Wool Shearing, Processing and Storage

Shearing is an operation of clipping the wool from sheep body. It is essential to get the wool from animals as well as to provide comfort to the sheep and enhance the economic status of sheep farm. The time of shearing is twice in a year preferably once at beginning of summer (march-April) and second at the start of winter (September - October). However, for veterinary reasons and other requirements of animals, shearing can be performed any time.

Considerable points in shearing

1. Sheep should be washed 10-15 days before shearing and wait for 10-15 days after washing to make the fleece dry and grease retainment to facilitate better shearing.
2. Sheep should not be feed 10 hours before shearing to save fleece from stains of manure.
3. Cleaning of individual sheep is required before shearing which includes the removal of soiled wool, thorns and clipping of urine and dung stained wool.
4. Sheep should be shifted to clean pen and to smooth board platform for shearing and clean wool production.
5. Sheep requires well nourishment for good quality wool and shearing should be done in comfortable weather.
6. Sheep skin should be stretched as well as clipping of sheath; udder and teats should be done before shearing.
7. Shearing blade should be flat at level; strokes should be long, even and regular and fleece should be removed in one piece.
8. Shears should be sharp, clean and well greased and shear cuts must be dressed before release of animal after shearing.

Shearing procedures

Shearing is a skilled operation in which fleece is opened first in all of the methods adopted for shearing. For that purpose sheep setting is done on its rear and between the shearer knees but the direction of sheep should be same as of shearer. It is utmost important to make a line of division in fleece. A skilled person can shear only 15-20 sheep a day with hand shearing while machine shearing can complete shearing of about 100 sheep's in a day.

Generally there are two shearing patterns are in use-*along the sheep pattern* and *around the sheep pattern*. Others are using combination of all these two methods. In *along the sheep* shearing pattern parallel strokes are made from head to tail until back is reached. It is done in one side of sheep first followed by another side of sheep. However, in *around the sheep* pattern of shearing sheep's are allowed to sit on buttock and strokes are made round the sheep's body and fleece is opened at throat, round the neck, shoulder and back etc.

There are two basic methods of shearing the wool -hand shearing and machine shearing. However, chemical method is also adopted in some of the areas but it is uncommon method due to its limitations:

1. *Hand shearing*: hand shearing is an age old practice and induces great stress to the sheep as well as to the shearer. However, it is common method of shearing the wool in India due to its low cost and easy management. In this shearing method, tarpaulin sheet sacks and papers are arranged as per the need of different types of wool. To collect the wool from sheep in a single piece, sheep's should be handled gently and politely. Always avoid making the second cut over fleece, injuries to the sheep, floor contamination to wool etc. Wool should be then spread over the sheets sacks and papers with skin side down and tag bags are used to separate out the tags, facings and arm wool.
2. *Machine shearing*: it is modern method of shearing the wool and adopted all over the world. It produces uniform and smooth wool with high dry yield percentage. In machine shearing of wool little training is required and one time cost involvement. It contains metal comb over which cutter is driven very close to the sheep skin.
3. *Chemical shearing*: though chemical shearing is adopted in some of the sheep farms in USA and other countries but it is very uncommon method in India. In this method cyclophosphamide (CPA) drug is given in feed @24 mg / kg of live weight of sheep. Shedding of wool started in this method on 12th day of drug administration and

wool can be removed within 3 days. However, method is not well adopted due to adverse effect on sheep's body particularly adverse effect of drug on foetus, shedding of wool on patches, residual problem of drug and induction of stress as well as sheep to the adverse environment.

Storage of wool

Shearing of wool decides the quality but its maintenance till further use is also very important. So wool after shearing should be exposed to drying and cleaning and storage of wool should always be done on clean, dry place on wooden floor of sheets. Wool should also be protected from contamination with drugs and droppings, invasion of rodents and moths, molding and staining etc. Wool can be sprinkled with 2.5% malathion or methoxychlorane to protect from moths.

Post shearing operations of wool

Post shearing operations for wool are important steps to refine the wool. So that it can be utilized in manufacturing of fabrics, rugs, blankets and carpets. These operations can further be classified as preliminary processing operations of wool and processing steps.

A. ***Preliminary processing of wool:*** preliminary operations of wool are basically includes the operation which makes the wool ready for various operations. These operations can further enhance the quality by removing the impurities and prolongs the self life of wool. These operations help in enhancement of marketability of wool. Following steps can be categorized in as preliminary steps in wool processing:

   i. *Sorting:* wool sorting is the segregation of wool into various categories depending upon their value. It is different from classing and grading that it makes various sorts from fleece while classing of grading is basically depend on whole fleece. It facilitates the marketing of wool and help in deciding the price of wool. It is a skilled operation and knowledge of wool fibre and quality and impurity are important to sort out the units.

   ii. *Opening and dusting:* wool opening and dusting operations are generally performed by using opener machine. Wool clumps of fibers are opens up into individual staples which help in delivery of uniform wool for scouring. Dusting with opener machine removes the dust and dirt adhered with wool and helps in removal of most wool impurities. The opening and dusting of wool facilitates the proper penetration of scouring liquor into wool fiber and render the scouring thorough and more uniform.

It also reduces cost by saving on soap alkali scouring liquor.

iii. *Scouring:* scouring is the removal of wool impurities by chemical treatment. Generally it is done using aqueous scouring process called detergent method or by solvent degreasing process in which ether or benzene is used. Scouring process is usually accomplished in a series of vats or bowls which may be 3 to 6 in numbers and wool is propelled through these vats by mechanical rakes with intervening squeezers. However, Indian carpet wool is seldom scoured through more than 3 vats. Scoured wool is then subjected to drying through specially constructed dryers.

iv. *Burr picking and carbonizing:* the vegetable matter present in wool is called burr. Its removal from wool is utmost important because it hampers in manufacturing processes, and may damage card clothing and combs. Burr removal is generally accomplished by mechanical or chemical methods. Burr removal by mechanical means includes hand scissoring or burr crushing by crushers. The chemical removal of burr is called carbonizing and achieved by using sulphuric or hydrochloric acid and/or by salts such as aluminium chloride which produces acids on heating.

B. ***Processing of wool:*** The wools are processed on woolen and worsted system and involves following steps:

Woolen yarn	Worsted yarn
Intermingled fibres with bulky or lofty threads which appears rough and fuzzy.	Fine, smooth and compact fibres.
Mixed fibres with different length. Usually short fibres (0.25 to 2-3 inches).	Parallel to the length of yarn. Longer fibres (>2.5 inches)
Used to manufacture soft, rough and fuzzy fabrics.	Used for smooth suiting and shirting cloths and knitting yarns.
Yarns with greater bulk density and filled with trapped air.	Usually carded and undyed. Spin into worsted yarn.
Good in insulating property and fabrics keeps body warm.	Less warmer, used for short spinning (1.5 inches) into knitting goods with soft handles.
Used in manufacturing of tweeds and blankets like fabrics.	Only virgin wool is used.
It is made up of one type of top.	Rarely made up of one type of top.
Less regular, uniform and not in good strength.	More regular, uniform and good in strength.

Processing steps for woolen and worsted yarns

Woolen system	**Worsted system**
Raw wool	Raw wool
↓	↓
Scouring	Scouring
↓	↓
Loose/scoured/recovered wool	Oiling
↓	↓
Oiling	Carding
↓	↓
Willowing	Back washing
↓	↓
Carding	Gilling
↓	↓
Mule spinning	Combing
↓	↓
Yarn scouring/ weaving	Slubbing Dyeing/ Gilling and/ or recombing
↓	↓
Yarn dyeing/ Piece scouring	Drawing
↓	↓
Carpet yarn/ Milling	Spinning
↓	↓
Piece dyeing	Yarn scouring/Weaving or knitting
↓	↓
Finishing	Yarn dyeing/ Piece scouring
	↓
	Piece dyeing
	↓
	Finishing

Steps in processing of wool

i. *Oiling*: the basic purpose of oiling the wool is to provide lubrication, minimize breakage, reduces fly waste, static electricity and enhancement of cohesion of fibers in loose slivers during carding, drafting and spinning. Mineral oils emulsified with ionic detergents are generally used @3-5% of wool weight. In Indian carpet industry, Mahua oil emulsified with crude soap is generally used.

ii. *Willowing*: willowing is a combined operation of oiling and opening. It is usually applicable in worsted yarn processing and 0.5% per cent or even less oil emulsion is applied.

iii. *Carding:* Carding is a method of separating wool fibers clinging together. It is processes in yarn manufacture in which the fibres are brushed up, made more or less parallel, have considerable portion of foreign matter removed and are put in to a manageable form known as sliver. The purpose of woollen carding is to further open the wool, disentangle locks, straighten the individual fibers, removal of natural impurities, stock mixing and its convenient delivery to spinning frame. Woollen carding is accomplished by a 2 -3 or 4 card systems. However, worsted yarn carding includes placement of wool fibres parallel to each other and arranged into continuous sliver of definite weight and thickness. It also facilitate removal of impurities. In general short fibre wool (<2.5 inches) is used in carding while longer wool is purified by combing. In final step of carding fibre web is divided into small strips called pencil rovings. These are collected on large spools on the end of the card and placed on the spinning frame to make yarn.

iv. *Spinning:* carded yarn is straight without any twist and held together by oil and natural hooks existed on the surface of wool fibers. The actual twisting of roving takes place on spinning frame and turns into yarn which is collected on wooden bobbins. The spinning frame can spin up to 90 threads at one time. It is sufficient to spin one ply yarn having single stranded yarn but for handling two or more ply yarn and to make it twisted together, plyer with several cones onto fewer spools is used. *Flayer spinning* is used for coarse yarn, *cap spinning* for finest yarn, *ring spinning* is preferred for medium thickness yarn while mule spinning is done for woollen yarn. For mule spinning ambler super drafter machine is used in which movement of fibre can easily control and raper auto leveller helps in drawing of yarn. Spinning of worsted yarn is generally performed by cap or ring spinning. Irrespective of method employed basic aim of spinning remains in drafting, drying, twisting and winding on package.

v. *Gilling:* gilling is a process of forceful arrangement of fibers through drafting, attenuating or drying through pins. It is necessary to make the homogenous mixture of fibers and distribution of fiber with uniform weight sliver. Generally carded sliver are subjected to gilling on auto leveler to make them parallel for combing operation.

vi. *Combing:* combing is a process of separation of short fibers, vegetable material, slubs and neps. It also makes the fibers parallel to each other. So they can make ready for weaving and further processing. The fibers obtained after combing is generally termed as top. Basically two combing systems are generally adopted -French combing system and Brad ford combing system. Indian wool is generally course and medium type. French system is mainly preferred for medium wool type and can easily be adopted in Indian conditions.

vii. *Top finishing:* the combed wool is generally subjected to top finishing for making the sliver regular and of desired weight, maintenance of parallel state of fibers and proper packaging.

viii. *Weaving and knitting:* weaving is a process by which yarn is turned into fabric garments. In this process warp and filling threads are interlaced in loom. But weaving actually involves number of preliminary processes like cone binding, warp preparation and sizing, pirn binding of welt yarn, tying and drying of warp etc. In weaving process looms have two types of motions such as primary motion or basic motion and secondary motion. Basic motion includes shedding, picking and beating while in secondary motion let off and take up process is completed. In weaving process generally two types of weaves are achieved- plain weave (rib weave and basket weave) and floating weave (twill weave, satin weave or sateen weave)depending on the type of cloth preparations. In plain weave process interlacing is done by passing the filling threads alternatively over and under the warp threads while in floating weave fillings threads are passed one over and 2 under or more warp threads as in twill fabrics.

Generally weaving and knitting terms are used in similar sense but technically weaving is a process of interlacing two sets of yarn at right angles by hand or a power loom while in knitting process one set of yarns form loops and one loop caught into another and one row of loops hanging on the one below and performed by knitting machines.

ix. *Dyeing*: dyeing is done to provide various colours to wool. Wool is the most reactive of all textile fibers towards different types of dyes like acid dyes, metal-complex dyes, chrome dyes, vat dyes, reactive dyes and direct dyes. Among different types of dyes used for wool colouration, acid dyes are most suitable which can be used in different variants such as chrome dyes and vat dyes. The acid dyes containing sodium cations and dye anions are responsible for colour development in wool. In colour development process dye anions interact with fiber and displace already adsorbed ions, such as chloride ions, by a process of ion exchange. Colour development is also dependant on the affinity of substrate to hydrostatic attraction through hydrogen bonds. There are two regions are generally found in wool such as amorphus and crystalline region. In which amorphus region provides well penetration of dyes and took dyes well.

Type of dye	Affinity to wool
Basic dyes	Basic dyes generally stained convex outer portion of crimp curvature such as orthocortex while paracortex is less accessible to basic dyes and contains higher sulphur. These dyes give bright shades to wool parts.
Acid dyes	Preferentially stained concave inner side of crimp curvature such as para cortex. These are most important dyes for proteinous fibers and suited for wool industries followed by metal complex and basic dyes in order of preference. The examples of acid dyes generally used for the purpose are sandoz yellow 4GL, turquoise AS, sand navy 5 RL, sand blue BR, sand red RS, sand red 3 BN, luganil orange FBRL, luganil grey FBSBL , navidol black MSRL, sand brown G etc.
Chrome dyes	Wool tip contains reducing groups such as aldehyde (-CHO) and sulfhydryl or mercaptan (-SH) which prevent full development of shade for many chrome dyes.
Metal complex dyes	1: 1 and 1:2 metal complex dyes can be used for wool dyeing.
Reactive dyes	Best suited for cellulose fiber but can be utilized for protein fibers. There are two types of dyes are generally used cold brand dyes (suitable at room temperature) and hot brand dyes (used at 60°C to 70°C and even at 80°C).
Azoic dyes	Most suitable for cellulose dyeing but can be used for wool dyeing and examples are Brimthol and Napthol.
Vat dyes	Vat dyes as such are suitable for wool fiber but modified vat dyes or solubilized vat dyes can be used for wool fiber dyeing.

The effective dyeing of wool requires certain stabilizers and dyeing agents. Important dyeing agents used for the purpose are silicate, camaqua and scourex 400. Certain dyeing agents such as exhausting agent (Common salt, Glover salt, Sulphur), pH exhausting agent (acid), leveling agents (Lyogen, SMK, Ammolan FBSK Livocod LA), hard water softening agents

(Soda Hexa Meta Phosphate) and defoaming agent or anti foaming agents are of great value.

x. *Finishing*: finishing is a process of making the wool fiber more attractive and acceptable. The basic aim of finishing is to remove impurities such as oil and lubricant, size and dirt, present in grey fabrics. Finishing is actually completed in two steps -preliminary processes and actual finishing. Preliminary processes includes numbering, weighing, perching, picking, knotting and mending while actual finishing of woolen fabrics includes washing in rope washer or openening with scouring machines using synthetic detergents, alkalies, emulsifiers etc. However, final finishing is decided by type, raw wool used as well as design and structure of fabric produced.

xi. *Milling*: milling is a process of shrink the fabrics in desired degree and thickness to make it acceptable. In this process wool fabrics are makes good in appearance with lustre; wrinkle free by beaming and wet decatising with combined application of moisture and tension. Milling can automatically be done by stock or rotary machines but rotary machines are widely used for milling of fabrics.

xii. *Raising:* raising is a process of making the fabric more attractive and even. To achieve the evenness in wool fabrics, fibers are entangled or lifted out the body of fabrics with sharp pointed wire rollers.

xiii. *Shearing:* brushing generally raises the protrusions which make the fabric uneven and disturb the fiber pile. So to make the fabric even and good looking shearing is done to separate out the protruding fibers from fabrics. It is generally followed by pressing and cooling to achieve the fabric with high lustre, permanent setting and good in appearance.

Wool fabrics for better heat stability and suitability as textile fabrics can be achieved by following the processes as discussed earlier. But better quality and stable fabrics can be achieved by following certain additional processing steps such as stretching, use of water repellents, stain resistant's, moth proofing and shrink proofing agents etc. Thus a fantastic quality fabric can protect the human body in better way.

References

1. Basal, G. and Oxenham, W. (2006). Comparison of properties and structures of compact and conventional spun yarns, Textile Research Journal, 76 (7): 567–575.

2. Bergin, W.V. (1968). Processing of wool. *In:* Wool handbook, Vol-1, Inter Service Publishers, London, 211-247.

3. CSIRO, (1979). Proceedings of a Seminar of Staple Length and Strength of Greasy Wool, Division of Textile Physics, Ryde, 7 December 1979

4. Feldtman, H. D., Leeder, J. D. and Rippon, J.A. (1983). The role of fibre structure in wool fibre and fabric performance. *In:* Postle, R., Kawabata, S. and Niwa, M., Objective Evaluation of Apparel Fabrics, Japan, The Textile Machinery Society of Japan, 224–268.

5. Leeder, J. D. (1984). Wool - Nature's wonder fibre, Ocean Grove, Vic.: Australasian Textiles Publishers.

6. Moore, G. P., Jackson, N., Isaacs, K., and Brown, G. (1998). Pattern and morphogenesis in skin. J Theor Biol., 191: 87–94.

7. Simpson, W. S. and Crawshaw, G. H. (2002). Wool: Science and Technology, The Textile Institute, Woodhead Publishing, Pp 202-317.

8. Wani,S.A., Malik, A.H., Salahuddin, M., Pal, M.A., Sofi, A.H. and Kirmani,M.A. (2008). Laboratory manual for animal fiber technology, Division of LPT, SKUAST, Srinagar,Pp 1-70.

❑❑❑

Chapter 27

Physical, Mechanical and Chemical Testing of Wool

Wool is a natural fiber and considered as renewable, sustainable and environmental friendly. It is capable to keep the body warm and can be utilized as casual bears and also in formal bears and provide comfort to the human body in both of the active and passive situations. So to maintain a standard quality of wool for fabric development it is utmost important to test the wool fiber for certain qualities. Testing of wool fiber is also important to retain the unique physical and chemical properties of wool which makes this fiber versatile. Fiber quality is in real sense is a set of characteristics and defects in the fleece; both inherited and acquired, which influence its end use. The term quality testing includes a process of critical examination of material to draw the information's related to qualitative or quantitative aspects of wool fibers. There are number of standard test procedures are in prevalence but most commonly followed test procedures for wool are American Society for Testing Materials (ASTM), British standards, Indian Standard Institution (ISI) or International Wool Textile Organization (IWTO) etc.

Wool Sampling

The basic principle of sampling is to draw a portion of material which is true representative of a lot or mass. Though wool is a non-uniform material thus requires careful drawing of sample specimens for representation of bulk with predictable degree of error. Sampling should always be done by keeping in mind that every fibre of wool has equal chances to be selected. The sampling of raw wool is more difficult than sampling of top or yarn. Raw wool samples are generally drawn by coring or zoning methods. Coring gives more accurate results for the assessment of fiber diameter, grease or oil content and vegetable matter than hand sampling. If fiber length is not a criterion of examination then sample can be drawn using a hole placed in table or sample board. The wool material is laid over the table or sample board and sample specimen is drawn by pinching are and small sliver is obtained by hands. Sample size depends on the test is to be performed such as physical testing for fibre length, stable length, crimp, fibre diameter etc requires 10-20 g of sample while chemical tests like scouring yield, contents of grease, suint, burr etc. are carried out with 40-100 g of wool sample. Some of the important sampling procedures followed for wool testing can be described as:

1. *Hand sampling technique*: In the hand sampling technique sample is drawn by using human hands. The examples of hand techniques are zoning and halving, board sampling, in process sampling and top sampling.

   i. *Zoning and Halving:* zoning and halving sampling technique is opted when wool is not tied in bales or in open form and core sampling is impossible. In this technique hand drawn is performed randomly but amount remains same in each draw. Then half of the drawn is discarded each time till half of the lot is separated.

   ii. *Board sampling*: in board or table sampling technique wool is laid on table or boards and sample is drawn through randomly placed holes by pinching. But the sample drawn by this technique is not suitable for estimation of fiber length because long and short fiber segments are placed together.

   iii. *In process sampling*: in this sampling technique wool sample is drawn during processing. But care should be taken that sample should be drawn from all parts of machine or from card across the apron or yarn from many spindles by hand.

   iv. *Top sampling*: top sampling is generally used for collecting the wool specimens from top, roving or other parallelized fibers. But care should be taken that sample should always be unbiased by the presence of excessive ends of long fibres. So squeezing off one end and drawing off one side length of fibres is always done before collection of samples.

2. *Grab sampling technique*: Grab sampling technique for wool was developed by Commonwealth Scientific and Industrial Research Organization (CSIRO) in 1970's in Australia. Grab sampling of wool is generally carried out by mechanical grab apparatus. This machine may be automated or manually operated and may have 1-9 grab arms. The Mechanical Tuft Sampling Machine can also be used for grab sampling. Grab samples are generally collected from each bale in a lot. The beauty of grab system is that every portion of wool in a lot has an equal chance of being selected and each bale within a lot

is equally represented in a sample. It is suitable sampling technique for the determination of staple length and staple strength.

3. *Core sampling technique*: Core samples collected from a lot may have one or more bales. Generally core sampling is done by manual hand core device consisting of long tube with a slit along the length of tube and a replaceable cutting tip. It can also be collected by mechanical machine developed by CSIRO in Newzealand in 1960's. Core sampling technique is generally preferred for measurement of fiber diameter, grease, suint contents and vegetable matter.

Wool Yield

In general term wool yield is defined as the weight of washing wool or scoured wool in which wool is scoured to remove impurities like dirt, wax, suint and grease following subsequent drying. The obtained weight of wool is then expressed as wool yield. In 1960s IWTO developed a technique for wool yield estimation by the name of IWTO-19. In IWTO-19 technique wool samples are initially blended mechanically for uniform mixing of cores of bales. Then about 150 g sub-samples is drawn from the mixed sample and scoured using laboratory scouring machine or by modern laboratory scouring line. The samples are then subjected to drying under hot air oven at 105^{0}C or through multi-head driers. The residual content of wool like *grease, suint* and *wax* is estimated by solvent extraction with alcohol using 10 g specimen sample or by non destructive method like NIRs. The *residual dirt or mineral matter* is measured by burning 10 g specimen at 800^{0}C and measuring the ash value. The *vegetable matter* estimation can be done by immersing 10g scoured wool sample in hot 10% solution of sodium hydroxide. The remaining weight of scoured wool is then considered as percent wool yield. The *scouring yield* and *clean wool yield* can be calculated using the following formulas:

Clean wool yield= Scoured yield – Vegetable content

$$\text{Percent scouring yield} = \frac{\text{Weight of scouring}}{\text{Weight of raw or grease wool}} \times 100$$

X-ray scanning technique which is generally used in security at airport can also be utilized for rapid determination of wool yield.

Shrinkage test

Shrinkage in raw wool can be tested by core test. In which core sampling is performed along with analysis. It is a reference method of United States Department of Agriculture (USDA). It is simply the indication of impurities present in wool and indicates the reciprocal clean fleece weight or yield. The most commonly used instrument for shrinkage estimation is Squeeze Box. It is an invention of P.E. Neale of Mexico.

$$\text{Percent shrinkage} = \frac{\text{Weight of raw wool - Weight of scoured wool}}{\text{Weight of raw or grease wool}} \times 100$$

Measurement of vegetable matter

Vegetable matter present in wool is generally termed as burr. It can be determined by various methods like hand picking method, carbonizing method, comparison method and caustic soda method. In *hand picking method* vegetable matter is separated by hand. It is accurate method but takes lot of time. So it cannot be used for commercial purpose. Chemical method of removing burr is called *carbonizing*. In this method certain acids like sulphuric, hydrochloric and salts of aluminium chloride, magnesium chloride and sodium bisulphite is commonly used which produced acids on heating. Among these carbonizing compounds sulphuric acids works better at 100 to 170^0 C, hydrochloric acid and sodium bisulphite at 125 to 130^0 C as well as aluminum chloride and magnesium chloride at 125 to 150^0 C. Among all most commonly used carbonizing agent is dilute sulphuric acid. The *comparison method* of determination of vegetable matter in wool was developed by Wollner, Tanner and Michelson. In this procedure soured wool sample is immersed in a mixture of monochloronaphthalene and petroleum distillate having same refractive index (1.555) as wool. The illumination can be observed with the help of a special instrument called Transparizer and matching is done with standard photographic transparencies. But quantitative evaluation of vegetable matter in wool is a difficult task to be achieved by this method. The *caustic soda method* for estimation of vegetable matter in wool is common and rapid test. In which 40 g of wool is dissolved in two liters of boiling 3% sodium hydroxide solution for about 1-2 minutes. The sodium hydroxide solution dissolves the lignin and other components of vegetable matter and rest of the residues can be weighed and result can be interpreted accordingly.

Assessment of wool purity by Benzene test

The purity of wool fiber can be assessed by using Benzene test. The test is basically based on visual judgment. In this test when pure wool fibers are immersed in benzene solution then they becomes invisible. Contrary to this course fibers or fibers with gas, air or medulla appears like a white streak in benzene solution. The heterotype wool fibers show same patterns but some fibers disappear and some appears as streak.

Determination of wool pH

The pH of wool is determined by colorimetrically method using commercially available indicator solutions or papers or by electronic pH meter. Generally accurate pH determination can be achieved by electronic pH meter and making a solution of wool in which both wool and water reaches to equilibrium. This state can be achieved by taking 10g of wool and making the wool pieces in the size of ¼ inch length. These wool pieces are then immersed in 200 ml of freshly boiled distilled water in a closed clean flask. These wool pieces are soaked at room temperature for at least 2 hrs and sometimes up to 24 hrs with constant gentle agitation. Alternatively, wool pieces can be soaked in boiling water of same amount as discussed earlier followed by cooling for 30 minutes in Soxhlet apparatus. The pH reading can be noted down using electrode and monitor of electronic pH meter.

Estimation of moisture

Moisture in wool can be determined by drying the sample in hot air oven at 100^0C till the constant weight is reached. In this method 10 g of wool sample is subjected to drying in hot air oven till constant weight. Specific type of ovens like Emersion oven (handles two samples of half pond size) and Braebender oven (for 10 samples of 10 g each) can also be used for the purpose. The moisture content in wool and moisture regain by wool can be estimated by the following formulas:

$$\text{Percent moisture} = \frac{\text{Air dried weight of sample - Oven dried weight of sample}}{\text{Air dried weight of sample}} \times 100$$

$$\text{Percent moisture regain} = \frac{\text{Air dried weight of sample - Oven dried weight of sample}}{\text{Oven dried weight of sample}} \times 100$$

In recent days Forte electronic moisture content analyzer is used for accurate results. It is considered as non destructive method of moisture measurement in textile industry. Some other techniques such as electrical capacitance near infrared reflectance spectroscopy (NIRs) and microwave radiation can also be used for online estimation of moisture. However, these techniques are not sufficiently recognized by International Wool Textile Organization (IWTO) certification.

Estimation of wool ash

Wool ash is determined by ASTM-D method. Samples are generally drawn for ash estimation by core method rather than hand sampling. For test 5 g of scoured or clean wool is burned over the Bunsen burner under crucible till volatiles are driven off. Then the burned sample is ignited in muffle furnace at 700^{0}C until all the carbon has been burned off. The weight of finally ignited sample is drawn and calculates the ash content in respect to the initial weight of sample used for test. The ash content is usually expressed in percentage.

$$\text{Percent ash} = \frac{\text{Weight of ignited sample}}{\text{Weight of scoured wool}} \times 100$$

Colour identification test

The wool colour is an important parameter to grade the wool and visual examination is still a prevalent method for colour differentiation. But differentiation in shades of white can be achieved only by certain instruments. Indian wool is variably yellowish in colour but Merino wool in growing stage may be very white and bright. The wool colour can be initially measured using balanced illumination method developed by CSIRO. In this method 0.25-0.50 g of washed and carded core sample are spread thinly between glass plates and illuminated with dual source of light from below and above. The specimens are examined under 2 x magnifications. The wool colours after dyeing can be differentiated by colour illuminators and anthraquinone blue SWF dye test. The addition of chlorophyll in wool can be measured by digestion of chlorophyll by hot alcohol. Chlorophyll presence in wool can also be identified by colorimetric tests using Lumetron or colour assessing instruments.

Optical tests

A. Fiber identification test

The identification of natural fibers and manmade fibers is of utmost important criteria to accept the fibers for various industrial uses. These fibers can be identified by using microscopic, chemical and physical tests.

1. *Microscopic methods of fiber identifications*

Fiber type	Salient features in longitudinal section	Salient features in cross sections
Wool	Flat scales on surface and free end are always pointed towards fiber tip.	Fibers appear oval or round.
Cotton	Fibers have smooth surface, almost cylindrical but sometimes irregular twist convolution are observed.	Round to oval with centrally located lumen in mercerized cotton while bean shaped in pure cotton.

Silk	*Cultivated or Mulberry silk* is with smooth surface and uneven in width and contains fold on surface. *Wild silk or Tussar silk* shows pronounced striations and fibers lies parallel to long axis.	*Mulberry silk fibers* are triangular in shape and sometimes elliptical shape with two triangular fibers. *Tussar silk fibers* are oblong to wedge shaped.
Rayon	*Viscose rayon fibers* are striated and run parallel to long axis. *Acetate rayon fibers* are with few striations (2-3). *Cuprammonium rayon fibers* are uniform with no marking on surface.	*Viscose rayon fibers* show circular and oval to ribbon shaped serrations on periphery. *Acetate rayon fibers* are round to smooth but usually clover leaf shaped with 2 to 4 individual lobes but usually 3 in number. *Cuprammonium rayon fibers* are round to oval.
Nylon or polyamide fibers	Fibers are cylindrical with smooth surface without any marking.	Round and uniform in diameter.
Dacron	Highly transparent, smooth and uniform in diameter.	Round fibers.
Orlon	Transparent but irregular striation on surface with apparent lumen.	Fibers are dumb-bell shaped or dog bone shaped

2. *Staining methods for textile differentiation:* Staining test is used to differentiate various types of fibers. It is based on the principle of fiber colour behaviors against dyes. The numbers of stains are used for this purpose but major ones are Shirlastan-A and zinc chlorideiodine. Shirlastan-A gives pinkish violet colour (lilac) to scoured wool, violet blue to bleached cotton, purple to mercerized cotton, bright pink to viscose rayon and bright blue to cuprammonium rayon while zinc chlorideiodine give no colour to scoured and bleached cotton and blue colour to rest of the fibers mentioned above.

3. *Solubility and swelling test*: The solubility and swelling characteristics of different fibers are somewhat different. So on the basis of swelling and solubility of various fibers in different solutions can be differentiated. For example wool can be completely dissolved in 5% sodium hydroxide but it does not dissolve in concentrated hydrochloric acid for 15 minutes. However, silk fibers easily dissolve

in this solution. Similarly textile fibers like secondary acetate is soluble in acetone and cold glacial acetic acid, triacetate fibers in chloroform, polyester in hot metacresol and Dacron or polyacrylonitrile in dimethyle formalin solution. Nylon fibers are quite soluble in 85% formic acid and 90% phenol but insoluble in cold glacial acetic acid. Swelling with acids damaged wool can be identified by caustic soda and concentrated ammonia solution.

B. Fiber testing

1. Fiber diameter
2. Fineness or crimpness of wool
3. Staple length
4. Staple strength
5. Fiber length
6. Tensile strength

1. *Fiber diameter measurement*: Wool fiber diameter can be measured by airflow instrument or projection microscope. In airflow measurement technique porosity of a compressed plug of fiber of a fixed mass is adjusted to a constant moisture value. Then instrument is adjusted to a constant air flow and variation in pressure is correlated with diameter. Sonic air flow meter can also be used for the purpose. Another method developed by IWTO for fiber diameter measurement is known as IWTO-28. Australian Wool Testing Authority (AWTA) in 1982 invented another method of wool fiber diameter estimation in which video camera and frame grabber is used to capture the digital image of fiber snippets distributed on a microscope slide. Later the instrument was replaced by Sirolan Laserscan and OFDA-100 techniques for fiber diameter measurement. Now these instruments and techniques can measure the wool fiber diameter in online system and record can be maintained for longer period of time.

2. *Fiber fineness or crimpness measurement:* Crimpness in wool is the indication of fineness of wool fiber and more crimps is related to more fine wool. Crimpness in wool can be measure by using *crimpometer* and expressed in terms of crimp per inch or centimeters. For fineness of wool measurement *Ermascope* (a type of microscope) is of great importance. It is based on projection of highly magnified (about 500 times) images of short fiber segments on screen and measuring and calculating the average fiber fineness of wool. Wool

fineness can also be measured using *air flow apparatus.* In which air flow is measured by manometer with respect to average fiber diameter. In 1976 CSIRO developed *Fiber Fineness Distribution Analyzer* (FFDA) in which reduction in intensity of light transmitted by laser and subsequently detected in photo-detection during its transaction of fiber in a transport fluid through a cell. The magnitude of drop in intensity of light during transaction of fiber is directly related to the wool fiber fineness. The recent techniques such as *WIRA fineness meter* and *Palmer wool fineness meter* are also of great importance in wool fineness measurement. The frequency of crimp in staple can be measured using ATLAS instrument.

3. *Staple length measurement:* In general method staple length is measured using a ruler. In this method wool staples are carefully laid on a velvet board and measured by ruler. Then average staple length is obtained by calculations. A technique developed by CSIRO in the name of ATLAS can be used for staple length measurement. In this system staple length is measured by passing a fixed speed light beam over the staple. The time taken by light beam to pass the staple is considered as staple length.

4. *Staple strength measurement:* Initially staple strength was measured gripping the fiber in hand and applying the force by flicking the staple with middle finger and staple length was measured using ruler. The staple strength can be measured by using the peak force applied to break the staple into two different pieces. Staple strength can be measured using strength tester and Instron strength measurer instruments. Wool strength is important in assessing how well the wool will perform during processing. The major factors responsible for staple strength are variation in fibers diameter along fibers, variation in fibers diameter between fibers, follicle shutdown, intrinsic fibers strength etc.

5. *Fiber length measurement*: Fiber length in wool sliver is an important parameter to assess the quality of wool during processing because it has direct bearing on the spinning performance. Almeter instrument can be utilized to capacitance to estimate fiber length. AL-2000 instrument and IWTO-17 method can also be applied for measurement of fiber length. A new instrument OFDA-4000 is capable to find out the relations between fiber length and diameter. An instrument called *WIRA fiber diagram machine* can also determine the average fiber length.

Colorimetric tests

The wool fibers are basically damaged during processing. These damages can easily identified by colorimetric tests. These tests are quite effective in identification of fibers damaged with acid, alkali, oxidation, microorganisms and insects. Colorimetric tests are basically based on the chemical state of keratin and can be identified by the changes takes place in sulfur, cystine, and nitrogen contents. But colorimetric test are not applicable in dyed fibers and fibers damaged through chemicals and mechanical means. So identification of mechanically damaged fibers requires certain microscopic tests as discussed earlier in this text. Some of the common colorimetric tests can be listed as:

Test	Principle	Procedure	Findings
Methylene blue absorption test	Stain retention by keratins.	One litre of methylene blue absorption solution is prepared using 1.279 g stain, 6.81 g of potassium dihydrogen phosphate, 29.63 ml of 1N caustic soda solution. One gram of sample initially soaked in O.1N hydrochloric acid for 1 hour and rinse 10 to 20 times by immersing in 200 ml stain solution at room temperature. After 24 hrs samples are rinsed in running water for 20 minutes.	Undamaged fibers stain light blue and damaged fibers dark blue
Pauly or Diazo Reaction test	The amino acid, tyrosine, present in the keratin of fibrous layer yields azo colour reaction.	Fibers are immersed in diazobenzene sulfonic acid solution.	Injured wools are coloured orange – yellow to a full red in soda alkaline diazo – solution.
Benzopurpurin test	Stain retention by keratins.	One gram of neutral wool is placed in 100cc of benzopurpurin 4B solution (0.1g/litre) Boiling for one minute. Wool washing in hot water until all the excess dye is removed followed by drying.	Undamaged wool shows only a slight pink colour while damaged wool takes pink to a dark red colour.
Rimington Pauly test	More scales breakage indicates intense colour.	Mixing of 2 cc of conc. hydrochloric acid to a mixture of 10cc of 10% sodium sulpfanilate and 5 cc of 8% sodium ni trate and keep undisturbed for 1 minute. Addition of 15 cc of 9 % sodium carbonate solution contains 0.1g sample and keep undisturbed for 10 minutes. Remove sample and wash sintered glass crucible with 300cc of distilled water. Drying of sample in watch glass in a dark room. Properly dried sample is added with 50 cc of 2 N sodium hydroxide and allow to stand for 18 hrs.	Rimington defined 100 units of damage to be such that a 0.1 g sample after treatment yield 25 cc of solution with exactly same colour intensity as the 0.1 % new acid brown S.

		Shake well and compare with 0.1% new acid brown S solution using colorimeter and artificial light.	
Kiton Red test	Higher intensity of colour indicates more damage to elasticum.	All reactions should be performed under a constant temperature of 70 ± 1o F with freshly prepared solutions. One litre staining solution is prepared by adding unhydrous Kiton Red G (0.307g in 250 ml distilled water) in 50 ml of 0.1 N hydrochloric acid. About 1 gram of wool sample wetted thoroughly and immersed for 10 minutes in 50 ml of 2 % borax solution. Rinsing with 10 ml of stain solution in stopper bottle. Shaking for one hour and again rinsing.	Undamaged wool does not absorb the stain but partially damaged wool turns pink and heavily damaged wool turn red. Microscopic examination revealed quantitative values based on particular stain.
Basic Fuchsin test	Simple and quick stain test and capable to distinguish oxidative bleached wool with cashmere.	Stain is prepared using 0.1g of basic fuchsin in 70 ml of isopropyl alcohol and 30 ml of distilled water. The fibers are then immersed in solution and results are interpreted.	Damaged fibers stain dark red; undamaged light pink. Quantification can be done by microscopic test.
Lead Acetate test	Action of oxidation on wool induces free sulfur compounds and reacts with heavy metals such as tin and lead and develops brown to black metal sulfides.	Test is performed by using 0.5 % solution of lead acetate prepared with 200 cc of 2.5 % lead acetate, 68 cc N acetic acid and 712 cc of distilled water buffered to pH 5. One gram wool sample is boiled for ¾ hour in lead acetate solution followed by drying at room temperature.	The unbleached wool appears dark brown or black while peroxide bleached wool remains unchanged.

Identification tests for acid, alkali, oxidation and microbial damage

The textile fiber damaged by acid, alkali, oxidation and microbes can easily be identified by using certain tests specifically designed for the purpose. They may be classified as:

Test	Principle	Procedure	Findings
Alkali damage test (Allworden reaction)	Best known test for confirmation of alkali damage. Test is based on fact that epicuticle of wool fiber is readily dissolved by alkalis but not by acids or most other degradative factors.	Degreased wool fibers with alcohol are mounted on microscopic slide in a solution prepared with equal volume of distilled water and freshly prepared chlorine or bromine. The process alters the osmotic pressure by chlorokeratin compounds under the epicuticle and increases its extensibility and expandability.	Characteristics bubble formation in epicuticle along the fiber surface in undamaged fiber while no bubble appearance in damaged epicuticle or fiber by alkali. Presence of alkali in wool can be detected by boric acid test.
Alkali damage test (Urea bisulfite test)	Alkali treated wool decreases solubility while acid treated wool increases solubility.	Wool is immersed in urea bisulfite solution and observed the degree of wool solubility.	Alkali treated wool decreases its solubility in urea-bisulfite solution while solubility increases in acid treated wool.
Acid damage tests	It is combined chemical and optical test but requires microscope.	A swelling solution is prepared by using 20 g caustic soda in 50 cc concentrated ammonia after proper cooling. Few drops of swelling solution are poured near cover slip mounted with wool fiber. Fiber shows accumulation of caustic soda and observes the swelling reaction.	Acid damaged wool shows swelling within 1-2 minutes while undamaged wool does not show swelling in less than 8 to 10 min.
Oxidation damage test (Alkali solubility test)	Action of oxidation on wool induces free sulfur compounds and reacts with heavy metals such as tin and lead and develops brown to black metal sulfides.	Normally oxidizing agents treated wool swells 11-14 % in 0.1 N sodium hydroxide solution and increases degree of chemical degradation. But solubility above 20% in NaOH solution indicates severe wool damage by oxidation agents.	Oxidizing agents such as hydrogen peroxide, chlorine and bromine and exposure to light shows increased solubility in alkali treated wool. It is best test for chorine damage wool.
Microbial damage test	Bacteria and fungi shows specific pattern in a particular stain.	Microscopic test using gram's stain for bacteria, lactophenol and cotton blue for fungi.	Identified on the basis of specific pattern of micro-organism.

There are number of other tests can also be helpful in assessment of wool quality. Yarn quality can be identified by using spinning count, strength, evenness and twist capacity while fabrics should be tested for strength, elongation, breaking test, thickness, compression and resilience, thermal properties, pilling, abrasion resistance, crease recovery and relaxation shrinkage. Spinning count or yarn number defines the linear density of textile strand. Spinning count is actually the number of bundles per pound. Wool evenness is measured by evenness tester, strength by strength tester or Instron tester. Breaking tests of fabric can be determined by Grab and Ravel strip tests.

References

1. Basal, G. and Oxenham, W. (2006). Comparison of properties and structures of compact and conventional spun yarns, Textile Research Journal, 76 (7): 567–575.
2. Bergin, W.V. (1968). Physical properties of wool. *In:* Wool handbook, Vol-1, Inter Service Publishers, London, 168-199.
3. CSIRO, (1979). Proceedings of a Seminar of Staple Length and Strength of Greasy Wool, Division of Textile Physics, Ryde, 7 December 1979
4. Feldtman, H.D., Leeder, J.D. and Rippon, J.A. (1983). The role of fibre structure in wool fibre and fabric performance. *In:* Postle, R., Kawabata, S. and Niwa, M., Objective Evaluation of Apparel Fabrics, Japan, The Textile Machinery Society of Japan, 224–268.
5. Leeder, J.D. (1984). Wool -Nature's wonder fibre, Ocean Grove, Vic.: Australasian Textiles Publishers,
6. Mizzel, L.R. and Harris, M. (1943). Nature of the reaction of wool with alkali. J. Res. National Bureau of Standards, 30: 47–53.
7. Simpson, W.S. and Crawshaw, G.H. (2002). Wool: Science and Technology, The Textile Institute, Woodhead Publishing, Pp 202-317.
8. Wani,S.A., Malik, A.H., Salahuddin,M., Pal, M.A., Sofi,A.H. and Kirmani, M.A. (2008). Laboratory manual for animal fiber technology, Division of LPT, SKUAST, Srinagar,Pp 1-70.
9. Wood, E. (2002), 'The basics of wool colour measurement', Wool Tech Sheep Breed, 50: 121–132.

Index

C

T

FSC
www.fsc.org
MIX
Papier | Fördert gute Waldnutzung
FSC® C083411

Zeitfracht Medien GmbH
Ferdinand-Jühlke-Straße 7
99095 Erfurt, Deutschland
produktsicherheit@kolibri360.de